MONUMENTAL CURES

Dr. Micozzi's Definitive Guide to Surviving Mainstream Medicine

D0187744

Marc S. Micozzi, M.D., Ph.D.

OV2B000486

Table of Contents

Part 3: Brain-Healers from Behind the Curtain

Part 4: Master Your Heart Health—Naturally

Part 5: Conquering Everyday Health Problems

Part 6: 9 Secrets to Stop Aging in its Tracks

Part 7: A Drug-Free Guide to Defeating Your Depression

Part 8: Natural Answers for an Ironclad Immune System

Part 9: Natural Ways to Nurture Your Health

Introduction

Humans possess an innate self-healing potential, an "inner wisdom of the body." Accessing this self-healing system is the primary goal of the healing arts. And addressing the cause of any illness is the first step towards accessing the body's own healing potential. However, modern medicine's primary focus is on suppressing symptoms instead. The problem is, suppressing symptoms with pharmaceutical drugs can compromise and diminish the body's natural ability to heal itself. Which is why natural, nonpharmaceutical measures should generally be the first approach—not the last resort. Unfortunately, far too many promising natural therapies—and cures—have been derailed for the sake of profit and political gain. But in the following chapters, I'll tell you how you can find these effective treatments—and put them to use for you and your loved ones starting today.

Always on the side of science,

Marc S. Micozzi, M.D., Ph.D.

PART 1

CANCER ANSWERS FROM A TRUE INSIDER

Chapter 1

The "ONE WORD" battle plan
to crushing cancer

Until this very moment in medical history, the common notion in the mainstream crusade against cancer is: *Chemo is as good as it gets.*

Of course, I've always known this was untrue. And if you've been curious enough to poke your head up from the sea of cancer misinformation we're drowning in, maybe you've glimpsed the truth for yourself.

Chemotherapy is a desperate grasping at straws in an effort to "kill the cancer before we kill the patient." But it also blatantly ignores the mountains of complementary medical research proving that cancer can be prevented and treated without this.

But in the last few years, even some of the most die-hard mainstreamers have taken notice of a new form of cancer treatment called anti-angiogenesis. It's radically different from the "poison and pray" chemo approach to treatment. An approach many of us have had to watch loved ones suffer through. But as you'll see, the difference in methodology is only the first of many reasons to have hope.

The "AH-HA!" moment
modern medicine was praying for

In 1998, *The New York Times* created a media frenzy…they reported a scientist by the name of Dr. Judah Folkman had discovered a way to eradicate tumors in mice. The frenzy swelled to such heights that Nobel laureate, Dr. James Watson was quoted as saying, "Judah is going to cure cancer in two years." And, in effect, he did. So why haven't you heard about it over the past decade?

Indeed, Dr. Folkman was a special kind of scientist. I admired his natural instincts in following the science so much, in fact, that even before the media frenzy in 1998, I personally invited him to speak in

Philadelphia to a standing-room only crowd of distinguished physicians and scientists. (This was when I was director of The College of Physicians of Philadelphia, and I was honored to have him come and enlighten my guests).

At that point, Dr. Folkman had already been following this particular scientific revelation for over 30 years.

It all started with the question…how can tumors grow so fast and so aggressively?

During his time at the National Naval Medical Center in Bethesda, MD, he had noticed cancer cells were unable to organize into tumors bigger than a few millimeters *in vitro* (meaning in test tubes, outside of the body). So somehow tumors were dependent upon the human body for growth.

And then he saw it.

Your body is being hijacked

Dr. Folkman was already considered to be the founder of angiogenesis research, so he knew what to look for. But what exactly is angiogenesis?

It's your ability to grow new capillary blood vessels in the body. It's a special process. And in balance, it shouldn't happen too often (mostly during menstruation for women, wound healing, and of course, while a fetus is still within the womb).

But when the body needs to divert more blood and nutrients to a specific area, it activates endothelial cells in the lining of blood vessels to release enzymes called proteases. These allow endothelial cells to "bust out" of the current capillary they're in and form new capillaries. This ability to form new blood vessels obviously helps with the healing process, human growth, and supplying much-needed nutrition throughout your body.

But it can turn deadly…

The big break came when Dr. Folkman applied his knowledge of angiogenesis to cancer research. For decades, researchers had marveled at a tumor's ability to grow exponentially larger in such a short amount of time. But what if these cancerous tumors were *using* your body to feed themselves and even spread elsewhere?

It wasn't long after that Dr. Folkman proved tumors secrete angiogenesis-inducing factors (mitogens) which cause neighboring normal capillaries to extend and supply blood to the tumor.

It was an incredible step—one that could eventually lead us away from the "poison and pray" treatment of chemotherapy, which oncologists appear so eager to administer these days.

This single hypothesis spawned nearly uninterrupted breakthroughs for almost 40 years. It's the kind of watershed moment about which every scientist dreams. Two of the biggest breakthroughs came in identifying a whole family of angiogenic peptides and in showing that once you shut them down, you can choke tumors out of existence.

What does that mean for you and your family?

"Angiogenesis research will probably change the face of medicine in the next decades, with more than 500 million people worldwide predicted to benefit from pro- or anti-angiogenesis treatments"

That is a quote from the January 2006 issue of *Nature*—and they're right.

Anti-angiogenesis therapy is already turning heads in research facilities and hospitals all over the world. That's why over $4 billion has recently been spent researching anti-angiogenesis, making it one of the biggest medical research initiatives in history.

In fact, there are already 374 clinical trials in the works and vested interests are practically drooling over the profit potential.

Sadly, Dr. Judah Folkman passed away recently at the age of 75, but the research he started is now finally thriving. New angiogenesis inhibitors are being discovered all the time. Doctors are now witnessing tumors shrink and in some cases wither away completely. In fact, this therapy should be able to make chemotherapy extinct someday.

But the best news is that you don't have to wait another minute to start putting this revolutionary technique to work for yourself. As usual…

Nature is already seventy steps ahead of us

…And counting. The great news for all of us is that these angiogenesis revelations have shone light on an entire world of <u>natural</u> anti-angiogenesis compounds.

Much in the same way you might support your immune system with vitamin C, or your joints with Boswellia or your prostate health with saw palmetto…there are safe and natural ways to support your body's angiogenesis balance.

I'll reveal some of nature's most powerful—and readily available—anti-angiogenesis treatments in chapter 3. But first, a closer look at one of the most powerful cancer cures ever discovered—and the insidious story of how it was derailed by the very people in charge of "protecting" our health.

Chapter 2

The natural cancer secret: The C6 Protocol

The proven cancer revelation— pushed aside for profits!

In 1984, a senior staff scientist for the National Cancer Institute (NCI) and a personal friend of mine was on the verge of a medical epiphany. She had gathered towering piles of PROVEN research regarding a downright *ordinary* substance. Vitamin C.

She was a part of the "crash program" to uncover as much as we could on the relationship between diet, nutrients, and cancer. And had taken it upon herself to gather and review a decade's worth of small, very sound studies on vitamin C. And what she found was staggering.

In fact, this tireless researcher reviewed over 46 separate epidemiological studies. She found that 33 of them revealed vitamin C offered **significant protection against cancer…particularly for esophageal, pancreatic, stomach, lung, and breast cancers**.

Thirty-three out of 46. That's a 71% rate of positive results!

And in subsequent studies, vitamin C continues to produce jaw-dropping results…

- One study in mice showed vitamin C could rob a tumor of its power source—literally halting any new growth.

- In the prominent medical journal *Prostate*, it was reported to be a "potent anticancer agent for prostate cancer cells."

- It was shown to be a CRITICAL element in your body's ability to resist neoplasia—the formation of abnormal cells.

Research had even been performed by two-time Nobel laureate, Linus Pauling leading him to controversially proclaim, "This substance can prevent cancer."

Imagine. A real cancer breakthrough sitting right under the nose of the NCI the whole time. And all they had to do was look beyond the cutting, burning, and poisoning. To consider safer, natural approaches. And they didn't even have to look far. This secret weapon was found just starting with the basics! Of all things, vitamin C.

And yet, tragically, chances are you still haven't heard the potential of vitamin C for the prevention and treatment of cancer.

There was one BIG PROBLEM…

When this dedicated researcher finished her work, she went proudly before our political bosses to deliver the revolutionary news. Was she congratulated? Was she asked to present her findings to an expanded panel of her superiors? *Was she even listened to?*

No. The National Institutes of Health (NIH), the guardian of this nation's health and wellbeing, wasn't interested in her findings. They weren't interested in the success rates, shrinking tumors, or how amazingly simple, affordable, and effective her discovery was.

I know it sounds unbelievable. We're talking about a senior scientist, with a stack of credible research in hand. The sheer weight and height of which she actually carried into her superior's office to try to convey the potential in person.

But the sad truth is…the NIH already *had* a "natural cancer plan." And vitamin C didn't fall in line. The "science bureaucrats" ignored a hard-working, dedicated scientist with more-than-promising results in hand. All because they had already invested themselves in a plan that would just be too hard to stop.

What was so good that they could afford to ignore this colleagues' staggering scientific findings?

Beta-carotene. Those two words (and tens of millions of dollars) single-handedly derailed this nation's entire medical establishment—for decades—from finding a PROVEN cure for cancer. Because in 1984, a monumental initiative was mandated. The goal was to make beta-carotene the *cancer treatment darling* for the upcoming century.

One study is all it took to get the NIH frothing at the possibilities. Just one study, compared to the stack of research my colleague uncovered on vitamin C.

You see, beta-carotene is a plant-derived form of vitamin A. And in 1981, an influential English scientist (who had studied in Nazi Germany during their earlier war on cancer) in an influential English scientific journal, simply asked a simple question based on a study showing the higher one's vitamin A levels; the less likely they were to develop lung cancer.

Beta-carotene was of interest because it's a water-soluble, plant form, that can be converted in humans to Vitamin A, which is fat-soluble (and therefore potentially toxic). So, NCI was really looking for Vitamin A activity thru giving "safe" beta-carotene. Of course, we now know that even that thinking was faulty. Many people do not convert beta-carotene to Vitamin A at all, or only a little, or only under certain conditions.

So, beta-carotene can not be considered a reliable source of Vitamin A from plants. So, the NCI immediately jumped to all the wrong conclusions.

And conveniently for the NIH, there was a synthetic form of beta-carotene already on the market. Readily available for testing. So they jumped right in. (Though it's likely that's not the only reason, which I'll explain in just a minute.)

Flash forward two years and the NIH had issued a large-scale clinical trial. (The cost of which soared into the tens of millions.) And word had spread to the press that "beta-carotene would save us all from cancer!"

All the while, several colleagues from the USDA Human Nutrition Research Center and I were uncovering evidence of the exact opposite.

We actually looked to the past and reviewed a dozen smaller studies on beta-carotene. And we found no correlation between blood levels of beta-carotene and cancer.

We also looked at over 30 studies following the results of the British Empire Cancer Campaign. We looked at the foods that consistently showed protective effects against cancer. Then we used the latest, state-of-the-art technology to identify the carotenoid content of each of these foods. And they were *not* high in beta-carotene. But they *were* high in vitamin C and other nutrients.

There was essentially no reason for the NCI to "bet" on beta-carotene. No reason to proceed with multi-million dollar, taxpayer-funded clinical trials that gave synthetic beta-carotene to people already at increased risk for cancer.

But it was too late. The NIH had already let word leak out to the media about their new "darling." And seemingly overnight, thousands of everyday citizens were taking beta-carotene for cancer. All before a full-scale clinical trial had even started!

In fact, once the clinical trial got underway, it was hard to organize the control group of patients *because so many people were already taking beta-carotene*. In the medical science world—that's counting your eggs long before you even have the chicken…

But why, oh why was the NIH throwing caution (and a proven cure!) to the wind?

Because the reward was just too great. And unfortunately, I'm not talking about saving lives. When it comes to questionable judgments taking place in our more *"infallible"* institutions—always look at the advisory board.

In this particular case—a member of one of the *National Cancer Institute's* advisory boards happened to be a senior science officer at the manufacturer of a leading synthetic beta-carotene available at the time. And there it is. The shameful dots should be easy enough to connect. If beta-carotene became the "chosen one" amongst the NIH, record profits were *guaranteed. Even before results were ever gathered, and regardless of what the results showed.*

All the while, sealing the fate of a TRUE CANCER ANSWER to sit on the shelf, collect dust, and be kept from you.

One day I asked another scientist how the NCI could continue to ignore all the evidence about vitamin C. He explained that two-time Nobel Prize winner Linus Pauling had given vitamin C a "bad name." In the government's eyes, he was too vocal about its benefits. And the NCI couldn't afford to be seen as "kooky" or "fringy." Better to be just plain wrong. Meanwhile, Linus Pauling single-handedly held as many Nobel Prizes as the entire scientific bureaucracy of NIH put together. But the NCI prefers to be "often wrong, but never in doubt."

In fact…

We discovered many things when we began to do research with the USDA. First, we found that the nutritional quality of foods had declined drastically each decade during the 20th century right through the 1980's.

Second, almost all the healthy foods that are known to prevent cancer in fact are not high in beta-carotene. But we did find that these foods *are* high in vitamin C and a lot of other carotenoids that no one had heard of before, including **lutein, lycopene**, and **beta-cryptoxanthine**. All powerful nutrients that you can easily stock up on through the green, leafy vegetables you get at the grocery store.

And all the NCI managed to prove, tens of millions of dollars later, was that beta-carotene did *not* prevent cancer. And that, in fact, **cancer could actually increase by over 25% in some when using the synthetic, isolated beta-carotene of our friendly drug company**.

And all along, this flawed approach of the NCI—using the wrong doses, forms, and isolated synthetic nutrients—led to mixed results. Which of course opened the door to criticism by pharmaceutical-led mainstream medical science and oncology. Who continue to argue that nutrition won't work against cancer.

I even went so far as to formally predict the failure of this flawed approach. I knew it wouldn't work thanks to my work with the USDA, who actually knew something about nutrition. So I wrote up a scientific paper using the flawed and ill-fated example of beta-carotene. But my paper got caught up by my "political" bosses at the NCI…protecting their cancer empire, covering up their ignorance of human nutrition, and their waste of time and tax dollars.

Finally, once I left the NCI to work at Walter Reed Army Medical Center, and away from my "political" bosses…my paper was published in the *Journal of the National Cancer Institute* itself. Fortunately, the journal is reviewed by non-government scientists independent of the NCI itself. And I was awarded the Young Research Investigator prize for this work at Walter Reed.

It wasn't until 2002 that there was finally general recognition among physicians that using RDA guidelines to treat diseases was not adequate. Thanks to the publication of a pair of papers by Fairfield and Fletcher in the *Journal of the American Medical Association.*

The stage was finally set for accepting that nutrients should be taken in adequate doses and in natural combinations in order to prevent and cure diseases such as cancer. Three-quarters of a century after the British initiated their first efforts in the war on cancer.

Vitamin C breakthrough for cancer targets tumors at the source

Despite the best efforts of the Medical Mandarins at the National Institutes of Health, research on vitamin C and cancer HAS continued… And the results of several new studies have allowed me to bring a lot of thinking and observations from the past 35 years together. Into a rare—but very real—honest-to-goodness cancer breakthrough.

There has been a lot of interest in the ability of vitamins and minerals to lower the risk of cancer for many decades. But the way a lot of the research is done just doesn't get it right. They use the wrong nutrients, the wrong forms of administration, the wrong doses, for the wrong reasons. Then, if they don't find a positive result, the "experts" have been all too quick to say, "See, it doesn't work!"

Vitamin C has endured more than its share of this shoddy research and scientific bias. Especially when it comes to this nutrient's anti-cancer potential.

And thanks in large part to this inept research, many "experts" have been warning cancer patients against vitamin C for years.

When we began offering high-dose, intravenous vitamin C to cancer patients at Thomas Jefferson University Hospital 10 years ago, we first had to prove to a number of hospital review committees that it would be safe. (It was.) And that it wouldn't interfere with other treatments (chemotherapy and radiation). (It didn't.)

And now, a new toxicology study has been performed on intravenous vitamin C. And the results are very revealing. The dose administered was 1 gram (1,000 mg) <u>per minute</u> over 4 consecutive days each week for a total of 4 weeks.

That dose—1,000 mg—is more than the government's recommended <u>daily</u> allowance of vitamin C. And the subjects in this study got 1,000 mg every *minute*.

Researchers then determined how quickly vitamin C is eliminated from the body. They did this by finding the nutrient's "half-life." (Half-life means the time it takes for the concentration in the blood to be reduced by half. The radiation oncologists who burn out cancers are familiar with radioactive half-life.)

The half-life of vitamin C was measured as 2.0 hours (plus or minus, 36 minutes). In this sense you would think of vitamin C as "short-acting" if it were a drug. But the clearance time for all vitamin C to be eliminated from the body was 21 days, plus or minus 5 days.

I think a possible reason for this difference is that the body (particularly the muscles) acts as a reservoir for vitamin C—and can take up and store a large amount .

But it's important to note that <u>none of the study participants suffered any ill effects from this high-dose intravenous administration of vitamin C.</u>

This basic toxicology information is very important. (I wish my colleagues and I had been authorized to study vitamin C like this back in the 1980s instead of just looking at carotenoids. Although at least we were able to discover the importance of lutein and lycopene at the same time I was exposing the lack of any real evidence for beta-carotene. But I digress…)

The new study also tells us that it is probably impossible to achieve blood levels of vitamin C high enough to <u>treat</u> cancer by taking oral supplements.

IV vitamin C enhances chemo

So that answers the safety question about vitamin C for cancer patients. But what about the concerns regarding vitamin C's impact on other cancer treatments?

Well, new lab studies show that IV vitamin C actually *enhances* chemotherapy drugs like gemcitabine and erlotinib against pancreatic cancer cells (notoriously difficult to treat). Researchers observed this effect even in cancer cells that are otherwise resistant to gemcitabine treatment.

This means doctors may be able to lower the doses of toxic chemotherapy drugs they give their patients if they also administer them with safe IV vitamin C.

So this new (and long overdue) research finally allows us to set aside old myths and misconceptions about administering vitamin C to cancer patients.

Of course, even after all of this has been settled, there will undoubtedly be the hardened skeptics who will refuse to believe it until someone answers the age-old question "but <u>how</u> does it work?"

Well, new scientific research now has that aspect covered too…

Not just an anti-oxidant

Early theories about the role of vitamin C (ascorbic acid) in preventing cancer focused on its role as an "anti-oxidant."

But oxidation and anti-oxidants are more complicated than it seems. It all goes back to Chemistry 101: Chemically, any oxidant can become an anti-oxidant, and any anti-oxidant can become an oxidizing agent, depending upon the surrounding molecular environment, acid-base balance, and other factors.

And this probably explains why test tube laboratory studies showed that high enough levels of vitamin C actually cause direct cancer cell death. When ascorbic acid gets so high, it may reverse action and become an oxidant, or may simply just act as an acid. Which poisons cells.

However, in lab studies, vitamin C was also effective against experimental tumors even at lower doses that could not kill cancer cells directly.

So, how does it work? Well, it turns out you don't have to kill cancer cells outright (and risk poisoning yourself).

Starve cancer cells to death

There is a two-stage model of cancer. (This model was key to my own PhD dissertation research, which recognized the importance of early childhood nutrition in the long-term risk of cancer.) The first stage involves some chemical damage that alters the DNA in normal cells, "mutating" them into individual cancer cells. This is called cancer initiation.

Then the cells have to grow into actual tumors. This stage is called cancer promotion. The ability of cancer tumors to grow (promotion) is based upon them hijacking the body's blood supply—which you know now as angiogenesis

And it now appears anti-angiogenesis is an important mechanism by which an agent can prevent cancer without having to actually kill the cells (which is the toxic property of today's cancer drugs). If you can prevent the cancer from getting blood supply, the cells will starve to death, without having to actually poison them.

And a convincing new study shows the anti-angiogenic properties of vitamin C. In fact, three of them.

A triple play against tumor growth

In lab models, researchers used an intravenous vitamin C dose of 25 to 60 grams. (A dose you could safely get in 25 minutes to one hour with the "1-gram-per-minute" approach used in the human toxicity study reported above.)

First, the vitamin C inhibited endothelial (blood vessel) cells from multiplying—without harming normal, healthy endothelial cells. (Remember, chemotherapy drugs prevent cells from multiplying by poisoning normal cellular metabolism.).

Second, the vitamin C also decreased the migration of endothelial cells. This prevented new blood vessel cells from going to the cancer.

And, finally, the vitamin C prevented the endothelial cells from organizing into new blood vessel structures.

That's a triple play against cancer tumor growth.

Oral vitamin C supplements aren't enough to treat cancer

So, vitamin C turns out to be an "anti-angiogenic" powerhouse at doses that are very high, yet well-tolerated by humans. But it has to be administered intravenously to reach the doses that are safe and effective against cancer growth.

Now it's true there is a lot of evidence that lower oral doses of vitamin C (but still higher than the RDA) will *prevent* development of cancer in the first place. But you have to give vitamin C intravenously—directly into the bloodstream—to get high enough levels, long enough, to stop cancer once it is growing in the body. (So any "negative" studies using only oral doses to try to treat cancer don't really mean anything.)

This may sound extreme. But all cancer patients receive various intravenous therapies anyway. In fact, chemotherapy drugs are so toxic they have to be administered intravenously. If you swallowed them, they would poison and destroy the gastro-intestinal tract. Of course IV chemotherapy drugs cause enough physical devastation as it is (nausea, hair loss, fatigue, weakened immunity, another cancer—the list goes on). Intravenous vitamin C can be just as effective against cancer—if not more so. And it doesn't cause ANY of these toxic effects.

So you only have to ask yourself one question: which would you rather get?

Getting an IV vitamin C infusion is similar to having kidney dialysis— but much less invasive. You have to sit for awhile in the doctor's office while the nurse is monitoring and administering the infusion. At Thomas Jefferson University Hospital I set things up so that patients could also listen to mindfulness meditation oral exercises, visualization, and other mind-body approaches to make the time pass more pleasantly and productively.

The Clinical Laboratory Inspection Act governs the laboratories which formulate vitamin C intravenous infusions to ensure they are accurate, potent, and fresh. So look for a licensed physician that offers intravenous vitamin C infusion with an on-site certified laboratory.

Chapter 3

Natural treatments beyond vitamin C: An anti-angiogenesis arsenal

Vitamin E (alpha tocopherol)

It's important to note that natural vitamin E consists of four tocopherols and four tocotrienols. The reason for the mixed media on vitamin E is that the current cancer establishment insists on testing d-alpha tocopherol or dl-alpha tocopherol, both of which will not yield anti-cancer effects.

However, alpha tocopherol can neutralize the effects of certain cancer-causing compounds (such as N-nitrosamines). It may also stimulate the release of antitumor factors from the immune system. Animal studies suggest it can prevent some chemically induced cancers and it may reduce the size of tumors. One study, in humans, suggested a beneficial effect associated with the use of vitamin E in patients with superficial premalignant lesions in the mouth.

And it can be used in conjunction with some of today's more popular cancer treatments. It has been reported that a supplement of 800 mg per day of alpha-tocopherol, taken during radiation therapy for breast cancer, reduced side effects and improved general well-being.

One of the best ways to work vitamin E into your diet is by enjoying a favorite fruit of mine. It's known around the everglades as "the alligator pear." You'll know it as the avocado. This fruit is jam-packed with vitamin E as well as 20 essential nutrients like fiber, potassium, B-vitamins, and folic acid. And healthy essential fatty acids.

If you're going to supplement, I would recommend 100 IU of vitamin E per day.

The "Sun-Maid" Secret—Resveratrol

You may recognize the name of this plant compound for the "anti-aging" claims that are made. That may all be well and good, but there's a much more intriguing potential to resveratrol you may not hear elsewhere—it's potential to act against angiogenesis. This phytochemical compound is found in grape skins and grape seeds—and so in wine. In laboratory studies, it has shown anti-cancer effects by inhibiting the growth of over 12 different types of cancer cells, including prostate, breast, colon, pancreas, and ovarian carcinomas.

Recently, resveratrol has been reported to be an angiogenesis inhibitor that is sufficiently potent in suppressing FGF-2 and VEGF-induced neovascularization *in vivo*. Resveratrol has been shown to directly inhibit bovine endothelial cell proliferation, migration, and tube formation *in vitro*.

In fact, resveratrol has the unique, balanced ability to provide either pro- or anti-angiogenesis effects depending upon the circumstances. In cancer, resveratrol has been shown to inhibit angiogenesis in tumors.

The skin cancer savior—Genistein

This is a naturally occurring isoflavonoid found in soy products and certain other legumes like fava beans. It has been found to have anticancer activity in multiple tumor-cell types. In one study, genistein was found to inhibit angiogenesis in melanoma cells both in vivo and in vitro. It has also been found to play a potential role in cervical cancer and prostate cancer. Epidemiological studies have shown there is an inverse relationship between dietary intake of genistein and cancer incidents, including breast, colon, and prostate cancer.

A generally recommended dose is 50 mg per day. I recommend a brand called Bonistein™ Genistein.

Curcumin

This powerful spice from India has been associated with dozens of health benefits by this point, as is usually the case with these natural wonders, but its anti-angiogenic properties are all but unsung.

More commonly known as turmeric, this spice has been used in

Ayurvedic medicine for centuries and can serve as an antioxidant, analgesic, anti-inflammatory and antiseptic. Curcumin affects a variety of growth factor receptors and cell adhesion molecules involved in tumor growth, angiogenesis, and metastasis. In fact, curcumin is currently being examined specifically for effects on head and neck cancers, the sixth most common cancer worldwide.

While the research still hasn't pinpointed an ideal dosage for fighting cancer, studies have used anywhere from 3,000 to 10,000 mg per day. A safe average dosage is 3,000 to 4,000 mg per day of a standardized supplement. Or, some recommend eating 1 teaspoon of turmeric per meal, more like a food quantity as a spice.

Fisetin

This naturally occurring pigment is found in many fruits, including strawberries, grapes, mangoes, and others as well as green tea. Recently, Indian researchers set out to determine if fisetin inhibits angiogenesis. The researchers first exposed endothelial cells to fisetin and found that it strongly inhibited the grown of endothelial cells and the ability of these cells to organize into new capillaries.

Even better, fisetin strongly suppressed production of two key regulators of angiogenesis: vascular endothelial growth factor and endothelial nitric oxide synthase.

All of this combined shows that fisetin inhibits angiogenesis both in vitro and in vivo and helps to squash many of the pro-angiogenic factors produced by cancer.

Piperine

Piperine (*Piper nigrum*) is the compound in black pepper that gives it its kick. It has a long history of use in Ayurvedic and Southeast Asian medicine—used as a general restorative tonic. Piperine has been shown to substantially increase the body's ability to absorb the nutrients in foods and supplements. It has been shown to work a few different ways: by interfering with the body's ability to metabolize (or use up) substances, stimulating absorption of nutrients through the intestinal lining, and actually slowing down the action of the intestines in order to give the body more time to absorb the nutrients there. Similar to super-antioxidants that support other antioxidants, piperine can increase the effectiveness of other beneficial nutrients, including antioxidants enzymes.

Research has shown it can boost the bioavailability of cancer-fighter curcumin substantially. This is important, since curcumin is not easily absorbed by the body. In addition to these complementary effects, piperine has been shown to have direct antioxidant, anti-tumor, and anti-inflammatory properties. A recent in vitro study showed piperine is able to directly stimulate immune cells. And in recent tests on mice, piperine was shown to inhibit the spread of breast cancer cells in vitro and in vivo.

A generally recommended dose is 20 mg per day of a brand called Bioperine® Piperine, which is a 50:1 standardized extract of Piper *nigrum* fruit.

And the list goes on…

These are just a few of the anti-angiogenic compounds we know about today. It's quite remarkable just how many researchers are finding— and with the growing list, it's becoming quite easy to integrate these compounds into your daily diet. Below is a list of some of the most readily accessible natural, anti-angiogenic compounds from foods and spices.

If you're concerned about cancer, one of the most important steps you can take is to load your plate, meal after meal, with a large variety of these anti-angiogenic foods. And be sure to experiment with the use of fresh herbs, to add even more protective benefits to each meal. And of course, keep them organic and pesticide-free if you can.

Fruits:
Apples, blackberries, blueberries, cherries, clementine tangerines, cranberries, grapefruit, lemons, nectarines, oranges, peaches, pomegranates, raspberries, red grapes, strawberries, and tomatoes.

Herbs & Spices:
Basil, black pepper, cilantro, cinnamon, cloves, cocoa powder, flaxseed, garlic, ginger, ginseng, lavender, licorice root, nutmeg, oregano, parsley, rosemary, tarragon, thistle, thyme, and turmeric.

Vegetables:
Artichokes, beets, bok choy (Chinese cabbage), broccoli, Brussels sprouts, red cabbage, carrots, cauliflower, chard, collard greens, endives, fennel, garlic, kale, mustard greens, olives, onions, peas, parsnips, peppers, pumpkins, radishes, salsify, scallions, shallots, soybean sprouts, spinach, string beans, sweet potatoes, tomatoes, turnips, watercress, and winter squash.

Mushrooms:
Enoki mushrooms, king oyster, maitake, matsutake, oyster mushrooms, reishi mushrooms, and shiitake.

Seafood:
Cuttlefish, flounder, haddock, halibut, herring, mackerel, oysters, salmon, sardines, sea cucumbers, seaweed, shrimp, sole, squid, squid ink, and tuna.

Legumes:
Almonds, cashews, chestnut, edamame, fava beans, lentils, lima beans, pine nuts, tofu, natto, and walnuts.

Beverages:
Apple cider, cocoa powder, coffee, green tea, miso, red wine, soy milk, and white wine.

You'll recognize many of these foods from the list of cancer preventive foods compiled by the British Empire Cancer Campaign of the 1920's and promoted as part of the Nazi War on Cancer during the 1930's. Decades later, the U.S. National Cancer Institute seized on their misunderstanding about beta-carotene as the "magic bullet" ingredient that explained the anti-cancer activity of these foods. But they missed the boat when it comes to the vitamins that are really important, and now we have the new evidence about the role of anti-angiogenesis factors in these foods.

The Tane Secret that could finally put Cancer in the Crosshairs

The story of what I call the *Tane Secret* (pronounced Tah-Neigh) is one of the most fascinating in all of natural medicine—and highlights a very important point about the true nature of scientific research.

As I've always said, for the truest advancements in medicine, *follow the science no matter where it leads.*

But what many researchers, doctors and certainly pharmaceutical shills often fail to see is that science will usually point to the past for some of the breakthroughs that will change our future.

A better name for a new revelation

So why *Tane*? Tane is the Polynesian god of nature and in an even broader sense, the god of good.

I feel it's a fitting name because as you'll see…this natural wonder that has been helping the peoples of the South Pacific for centuries, and is now astonishing scientists in the world's most modern laboratories. And yet, it *still* had its traditional name dragged through the mud for nearly a decade.

I'd like to do my small part in righting a huge medical wrong.

The Tane Secret revealed: Kava

Kava root extract is the medical secret that could revolutionize modern medicine. Its specific origin within the South Pacific is highly debated, but most recent work places the origin and domestication of kava (*piper methysticum*) on a tiny cluster of islands known as Vanuatu.

Widely recognized as one of the premier unspoiled scuba diving destinations on the planet, and known traditionally for the daring "tower jumpers" who leap from great heights held back only by tree vines that let them fall within inches of the ground far below, Vanuatu may someday be better known as the birthplace of a true cancer prevention breakthrough.

Religion within the Polynesian culture is intertwined with many aspects of everyday life. Of course, when one thinks of far away South Pacific islands, the mind immediately recalls the famous heads first discovered on Easter Island by the Dutch in 1722.

These statues likely represent supreme chiefs, vital to the history and growth of this ancient civilization. Over 800 of them still stand on likely burial grounds and help exemplify the passed-down dedication to religion throughout the South Pacific.

Today, as a result of thousands of missionaries from Europe at the end of the 19th century, Christianity is the prevailing religion. However, whether it is the polytheism of sun gods and ocean gods or the monotheism of Christianity, kava has always persisted within the culture of the South Pacific.

What looks like an ordinary shrub, this hardy plant is fast-growing with multiple light to dark green stems. But the root system is its most-sought asset.

These roots (fresh or dried) are pulverized and brewed into a tea, traditionally used as a stress reliever, with many drinking it at the end of nearly every day. Forget about those fake "Polynesian" cocktails with the paper umbrellas—this is the real "Polynesian Cocktail Hour."

On the other side of the Pacific, the citizens of Vanuatu take their cultivation of kava very seriously. In fact, exportation is strictly regulated only to strains deemed as "noble" varieties. Their laws also mandate that exported kava must be cultivated at least five years and farmed organically.

I am up-to-date with the latest observations on traditional use of kava from my research associate who just came back from doing field work in the South Pacific.

New research in the 1980's changed everything

In 1985, *The Hawaii Medical Journal* baffled scientists by publishing a paper, the likes of which few scientists had ever seen before.

Just a few years prior, The South Pacific Commission Cancer Registry was formed. Its mission was to survey and monitor cancer rates for men and women throughout the Pacific Island nations. The researchers used Los Angeles Caucasians as a point of reference.

What it found absolutely confounded the commission.

Following are the cancer incidence rates per 100,000 males in the areas surveyed…

Los Angeles—307.2
Western Samoa—90.2
Fiji—75.0
Vanuatu—70.9

For nearly a decade following the initial survey, medical professionals tried to figure out what could possibly be making such an impact on the citizens of these island nations. Their diets were analyzed, smoking rates were analyzed, even the kind of tobacco commonly used was analyzed. And yet…researchers could not explain these incredibly low cancer rates.

Having done my own scientific field work in the South Pacific during the late 1970s, I had worked with many of these same researchers on other studies regarding diet and health in the Pacific during the 1980's and early 1990's.

The kava connection unfolds

As it turned out, just as the South Pacific Commission was completing their survey, statistics were being gathered for a growing industry within the South Pacific—the kava industry.

And when these two surveys were looked at side-by-side—cancer rates and kava consumption—a breakthrough correlation began to form.

In every country where both these figures were studied, the more kava consumed, the lower the cancer incidence.

This inverse relation was measured in kilograms of kava consumed per year versus cancer incidence per 100,000 males.

So let's recap—the lung cancer rates in Fiji during the 1980's were 76 percent lower than those in Los Angeles at the time. In Vanuatu it was even lower—Seventy seven percent less.

And it appears one of the primary reasons may very well be this time-tested, culturally-renowned herbal tea.

So what happened? Why hasn't so much more already been accomplished on researching this time-tested, natural cancer breakthrough?

A tempest in a teapot...

Supplement sales for all kinds of herbs and vitamins began to really boom in the 1980's, and kava was no exception.

But before too long the brakes were slammed on operations amid a controversy which some still hotly debate to this day...

And new emerging science continuously calls the origin of this controversy into question.

Liver toxicity reports caused the United Kingdom's FDA counterpart to ban kava sales in the 1990's. Suddenly, the kava industry shrank by 50% and all of the promise behind kava and its active compound, *kavalactones* seemed to vanish from the mainstream.

Luckily, botanical researchers kept its potential alive with bold new studies. The kava industry fought hard to clear its name, refuting the earlier studies that were using unproven and unverified forms of kava. And citing centuries of traditional use with no adverse reports.

In 2003, I asked leading European researchers to prepare a review of scientific studies showing the lack of toxicity of kava and published it in the premier volume of my scientific review journal, *Reviews in Integrative Medicine*, published by the same medical publisher as my leading textbook. That review found that observations on kava were confounded by patients taking prescription drugs that are toxic to the liver. It wasn't the herb that was at fault, it was the drugs!

But perhaps the strongest case for kava comes from the current crop of studies using verified kava, which show no adverse effects regarding liver toxicity.

And these studies are finally revealing kava's true potential…

20 years later—science finally prevails

The floodgates are now open and kava is finally prepared to take its place in the medical limelight. We could begin almost anywhere with this torrent of medical research. To date, over seven forms of cancer have been tested in preliminary studies, all with positive results.

Bladder cancer: Studies using mouse models performed at UC Irvine in 2002 and funded in part by the National Cancer Institute revealed an active component within kava, flavokawain A. Researchers found that flavokawain A encourages cell death in pre-cancerous cells by overcoming the effects of mutated proteins. This property is similar to a chemopreventative effect. All three bladder cancer mouse models responded well…and unsurprisingly, there was no evidence of toxicity from the falvokawain A.

Bone cancer: Likewise, a report published in 2013 highlights another active component of kava, flavokawain B. This compound was shown to halt osteosarcoma cell lines and promote cell death. This was shown to be a chemotherapeutic and chemopreventive compound. In other words, it may help prevent *and* treat cancer.

Colon cancer: An animal model designed to determine whether kava consumption reduces markers of colon cancer opened eyes even further in 2012. This 14-week trial revealed that kava-consuming groups had significantly fewer precancerous lesions compared to the control group. The results support that kava may help reduce colon cancer risk and that kava is safe to consume.

Lung cancer: Another mouse-model study was conducted at the University of Minnesota. Researchers used a mouse model that is routinely used to predict lung cancer behavior in humans. The results were astounding. Researchers identified naturally occurring components of kava that appear to prevent the formation of up to 99% of cancer cell lines.

One of the leading researchers called this research **"truly unprecedented in its potential impact."**

And all of this research is just the beginning…

What YOU can do now

It is great news that while medical research on kava went into a near 20-year hibernation period, the production of kava never did.

Traditionally, people in Fiji drink quite a bit of kava tea every day. It can add up to anywhere from 1 to 4 kg of kava per year. That comes out to a whopping 11,000 mg per day—essentially a small bucket-full of kava tea.

So a more practical approach, if you aren't able to incorporate so much of any tea into your daily life…would be to take a kava supplement along with drinking the tea. You can buy raw kava root and make your own tea at home. It's simple to do, but most American palettes might not find the flavor to their liking. For recipes, visit, www. gokava.com and visit their recipe page for teas, smoothies and even a French press recipe.

For use as an everyday supplement, I recommend at least 400 mg a day and always an organic, preferably grown in the South Pacific. To find a form that meets all of these requirements, visit www.herbal-island. com and look for their Kava Kava root extract.

Chapter 4

Antioxidants for prevention of cancer cell formation

Vitamin C is probably the most well-known antioxidant, along with vitamins A, D, and E, and selenium. All of these are readily available and the research is extensive. However, the following are a few antioxidants you may not have heard of for fighting cancer.

The accumulation of free-radical ions at the cellular level is thought to trigger the process of carcinogenesis—the development of cancer cells. These free radicals are in the atmosphere and are formed by the ionizing effects of the sun. They can also come from external toxins, such as pesticides and other chemicals in our food. But they're also formed naturally as a byproduct of certain processes in the body.

Substances called antioxidants help keep free radicals in check, thus helping to prevent the formation of cancer cells. The body produces some antioxidants on its own. But you also get them from the foods you eat. Plants in the natural environment include a wide variety of potent antioxidants. Plants, like people, must protect themselves from the oxidative effect of free radicals in the atmosphere and from solar and other radiation.

Many plant compounds have been developed and tested for the ability to serve as antioxidants. In addition, various basic nutrients, such as vitamins, minerals, and amino acids have been found to have antioxidant properties. And when combined, antioxidant ingredients have been shown to work together to multiply their effects as a whole.

These findings are especially helpful if you or someone you love has undergone, or is undergoing mainstream treatments. Chemotherapy and radiation cause severe free-radical formation (oxidative stress) on the body. And while some oncologists have been concerned that antioxidant supplements may interfere with this type of cancer treatment, this has not been proven to be the case. Antioxidant supplements can help the body recover from the effects of cancer treatment as well as helping to prevent the recurrence of cancer.

Acetyl-L-Carnitine (ALC) is an amino-acid with antioxidant properties. ALC helps turn the nutrients in our food into energy for our cells. It can help you overcome fatigue and improves the function of the brain and nervous system. This can be very helpful for those recovering from cancer. It's also helpful to those suffering the effects of mainstream cancer therapies, such as the notorious "chemo-brain." ALC has also been studied for its potential to help enhance the effects of traditional chemotherapy. A generally recommended dose would be 1,000 mg per day.

Alpha Lipoic Acid (ALA) is an essential fatty acid that is critical for the body. ALA supports energy production inside the cells and is a powerful antioxidant. But it also has the unique ability to extend the life of other antioxidants like vitamins C and E—making it an antioxidant of antioxidants. This powerful antioxidant also happens to be both water- and fat-soluble. This means it can reach all parts of the body to help fight free radicals. Alpha-lipoic acid has been shown to have anticancer effects by activating glutathione peroxidase (another potent antioxidant in the body) and decreasing oxidative stress in cancer patients. One recent study found that ALA could initiate cell death in lung cancer cells.

ALA is found primarily in animal sources, including red meat, liver, heart, and kidney. The most abundant plant sources include spinach, broccoli, tomatoes, Brussels sprouts, potatoes, peas, and rice bran. It has also been suggested that food intake reduces the bioavailability of ALA. So when supplementing, it is recommended that ALA be taken 30 min before or 2 hours after eating. A generally recommended dose would be 300 mg per day.

Coenzyme Q10 is found in every cell in the body and is a powerful antioxidant. It plays a critical role in the process of turning food into energy for the cells. In the laboratory, coenzyme Q10 has been shown to prevent cancer and reduce cancer cell growth. It can also improve white blood cell and immune system function. One recent study has shown that coenzyme Q10 may provide much-needed protection to the heart when undergoing chemotherapy. In a recent pilot study, researchers found that supplementing with coenzyme Q10 and additional antioxidant vitamins (vitamin C, selenium, folic acid, and others) could extend survival time in patients with end-stage cancer. A generally recommended dose would be 150 mg per day.

Selenium is a powerful antioxidant, which means it helps protect against oxidative stress and free-radical damage. It is thought to work particularly well in partnership with vitamin E. Selenium also supports your immune system, helping to protect against infection. It also plays a part in human growth and development. Several studies show that the level of selenium in the food supply of a given population is related to their rate of cancer. The lower the selenium, the higher the risk of cancer.

In fact, I had the opportunity of serving as the principal co-investigator on a cancer prevention study using selenium in a county in China. This particular county (Qidong County, Jiangsu Province) had a particularly high incidence of liver cancer. We found that the areas that had low levels of selenium in the blood or in the locally available grains had a higher rate of liver cancer—and that by giving selenium supplements it is possible to raise selenium in blood to levels that prevent cancer.

Dietary selenium supplementation has also been shown to be effective in blocking the formation of chemically-induced tumors in the gastrointestinal tract, liver, breast, skin, and pancreas in laboratory animals. And in human clinical trials, dietary selenium supplementation has been shown to prevent skin cancer and lower the risk of other cancers.

Other studies have clearly shown protective effects of this trace element even when given after carcinogen exposure. Such results suggest that selenium owes at least part of its effects to a decrease in the spread of any cancer cells that form.

Remember to use caution when it comes to dosage

As I have warned before regarding recommended allowances, the cancer protection offered by selenium is generally observed at concentrations greater than those known to meet the requirements for normal growth and metabolic activity (i.e. the RDA). And, as observed with other nutrients, continuous intake of selenium is necessary for maximum inhibition of cancer.

However, while selenium toxicity is rare, it is a real concern. To avoid side effects and potential toxicity, it's best to keep selenium intake at or below 400 mcg per day. Organic forms of selenium, such as selenomethionine, are absorbed as well as sodium selenite salt, but can persist in the body longer and thus theoretically pose a higher risk of toxicity.

Chapter 5

Immune surveillance:
Detecting cancer before it strikes

Mainstream science bureaucrats continue to pour money into surgery, radiation, and chemotherapy. But the past still holds many promising answers. Better answers.

Fortunately, others outside the NCI science bureaucracy have embraced the possibilities. Many private institutions and independent scientists have provided a considerable amount of research on more positive approaches. These approaches are based on ancient knowledge and wisdom. But now, we are able to apply innovative, cutting-edge knowledge of how cells grow. This approach is actually way ahead of the curve when it comes to a new understanding of how the body works.

I have outlined a "triple-play" approach to fighting cancer. It focuses on three proven alternatives to the toxic triple approach of chemotherapy, radiation, and surgery. These proven approaches can help prevent and treat cancer, as well as improve the condition of cancer survivors. So far you've read about the power of anti-angiogenesis, and antioxidants. In this chapter, I will talk about the importance of immunity in fighting cancer.

In the 1960s, a leading group of researchers discovered a critical connection between the immune system and cancer. They found that strengthening the immune system can help prevent and fight cancer. This is now a cornerstone of a natural approach. (As opposed to standard cancer treatments that are actually harmful to the immune system and to other healthy human cells.)

Cancer cells are actually formed continuously throughout the body due to the presence of free-radical ions that damage our cells. A healthy immune system can actually recognize these abnormal cancer cells. Once an abnormal cell is spotted, the immune system sends out "Natural Killer" cells (NK cells). These NK cells eliminate the cancer cells before they can grow into actual tumors.

Pro-immune effects of natural products include both enhancing the immune system's immune surveillance system (like a "distant early warning" defense system) as well as stimulating the Natural Killer cells that eliminate cancer cells as they form in the body.

Following are some of the most important nutrients for supporting the immune system and fulfilling the need for immune surveillance in the fight against cancer. Of course, there are many, many more. But these are most readily available and have the research to support them as well. Many of these may also act in other ways, but their overall impact on immune health is substantial, and it's essential they not be overlooked.

Vitamin C (ascorbic acid) is one of the most effective antioxidants. However, research has shown it may have an overall profound effect on the immune system. This was apparent even in the early cancer research uncovered by my colleague at the NIH (as noted above). Where it was not only shown to help cut off the power source of the tumors, but actually stops the formation of unhealthy cells. But unfortunately, thanks to the complete misdirection of the NIH, the research on all the potential mechanisms of action of vitamin C is still lacking.

Epidemiological evidence shows that populations who eat diets high in vitamin C have a lowered risk for some cancers. This may be because of the antioxidant function of vitamin C and its ability to block the formation of N-nitrosamines (cancer-causing substances formed in the stomach from certain foods). A strong epidemiological finding has been the association between high intakes of foods rich in vitamin C and a reduced risk of stomach cancer. There is a weaker link to a decreased risk of cervical cancer in smokers. In other research, it may also help counteract the toxicity of some conventional cancer treatments while enhancing the cell-killing effect of others.

A protective effect of ascorbic acid in colorectal cancer could exist by its prevention of fecal nitrosamines or against other fecal mutagens. In addition, a mechanism has been proposed whereby vitamin C inhibits DNA synthesis and spread of preneoplastic cells. Administration of ascorbic acid has been shown to produce a 30—40% increase in protective enzymes.

Studies of rectal polyps among patients with a family history, support the possibility of a protective effect of vitamin C in polyp formation and thus possibly in colorectal cancer. With 400 mg of vitamins C and E administered to patients following polypectomy, after 2 years, the recurrence data rate was reduced approximately 20%.

Ascorbic acid is generally tolerated well, but at high doses it may cause stomach irritation, heart-burn, nausea, vomiting, drowsiness, and headaches. Some oncologists are concerned that high-dose vitamin C may alter the absorption and excretion of some drugs used in the treatment of cancer, and may interfere with radiation therapy. However, there are no clinical studies documenting such effects. In adults, there is significant anecdotal evidence that vitamin C is safe at dosages of 1,000 mg per day and very minimal toxicity has been reported even at much higher dosages. However, there are few controlled studies of the toxicity of vitamin C.

Major proponents of high-dose vitamin C for cancer treatment included the late Nobel laureate Dr. Linus Pauling and Dr. Ewan Cameron. And while their research would need to be confirmed by more rigorous studies, they did provide a number of observational reports, case studies, and pilot studies involving large numbers of advanced cancer patients. These patients were given high doses of vitamin C. They reported that it appeared to improve overall wellbeing and quality of life, as well as resulted in a significant increase in the survival of patients with various types of advanced cancer. High-dose vitamin C levels can be achieved through intravenous infusion under direct medical supervision, as well as oral administration.

For my last act, while serving as Executive Director of the Center for Integrative Medicine at Thomas Jefferson University Hospital, I fought and won through all the hospital professional, pharmacy, and safety committees to gain approval to offer high dose vitamin C infusions right in this major university hospital under direct medical supervision for patients recovering from cancer and cancer therapy.

A generally recommended dose is 750 mg per day, in combination with other "triple-play" nutrients (see Chapter 6) as a dietary supplement;

and high-dose IV under direct medical supervision.

Vitamins B1, B2, B3, B5, B6, B12. Most people have heard of B vitamins. But do you know what they can actually do for you? The B vitamins help optimize metabolism at the cellular level. Meaning, they are essential for energy of the cells. The B vitamins also play a role in many critical functions of the body. But they have also been shown to stimulate the immune system and inhibit cancer cell formation. Significant data suggest that a deficiency of vitamin B12 or folic acid may actually lead to increased tumor development. A study published in *Cancer Epidemiology Biomarkers & Prevention* in 1999 reported an association of low levels of B12 with breast cancer in postmenopausal women. Another study published in the *Annals of Internal Medicine* in 1998 has shown a protective effect of dietary folate against the development of colon cancer. A generally recommended dose of vitamins B1, B2, B3, B4, B5, and B6 is 100 mg of each per day. For B12, a generally recommended dose is 1 mg (or 1,000 mcg) per day in combination with other "triple-play" nutrients.

Zinc and calcium. Zinc, together with other minerals, like calcium, is thought to have a role in inhibiting cancer growth through enhancement of the immune system and/or by direct effects on the cells. Zinc, an essential constituent of numerous enzymes, functions in cell replication and tissue repair. Calcium plays an important role in many cell functions including the overall survival of the cell. It helps control cell proliferation and synthesis of DNA. Investigations found that supplementing with 1,250 mg of calcium per day significantly reduced cell proliferation in patients at high risk for large bowel cancer. Epidemiological studies support the hypothesis that a higher calcium intake may reduce risk for colon cancer. One large study showed that people who took calcium supplements of 1,200 mg per day showed a decreased risk of colorectal polyps. A generally recommended dose for zinc is 250 mg per day and for calcium it's 2,000 mg per day.

Lentinen and other mushroom extracts. Lentinen is a plant compound extracted from shiitake and other mushrooms. It has been shown to have potent anti-cancer properties, similar to other mushroom extracts. Mushrooms, such as shiitake, used for cancer in traditional Asian medicine, appear to contain a substance called polysaccharides. These polysaccharides appear to activate the immune system NK cells. In addition, some mushroom extracts have been shown in the laboratory to directly kill cancer cells, but leave normal cells alone. These observations have been made with mushrooms that are edible, such as shiitake, maitake, and gandoderma.

A study from Korea, including 272 patients, found that the higher the intake of mushrooms, the lower the prevalence of gastric cancer. In another study, 68 patients with advanced, non-small cell lung cancer were given a polysaccharide peptide mushroom isolate. This was a randomized, placebo-controlled, double-blind study. Patients in the intervention group showed stimulation of the immune system.

Some polysaccharides from mushrooms may also help protect bone marrow from the harmful effects of chemotherapy and may have clinical application in recovering from cancer. Clinical trials are under way in Japan evaluating the use of mushrooms as adjunctive therapy to chemotherapy. The National Cancer Center Research Institute of Japan conducted a 15-year epidemiological study from 1972 to 1986. They looked at the cancer rates in close to 175,000 people. They found that mushroom farmers had overall lower cancer death rates when compared to non-farmer populations (160.1 per 100,000 compared to 97.1 per 100,000).

A generally recommended dose of lentinen is 2,000 mcg (or 2 mg) from shiitake mushroom with a 4:1 extract of Lentinus edodes, caps and stems (equivalent to 8 mg of dried mushroom).

Vitamin D. A new research review looked at the results of 25 separate studies that measured vitamin D levels in 17,332 people at the time of their cancer diagnosis. Higher vitamin D levels were linked to significantly better survival rates for people with breast or colon cancer or lymphoma. There was also a positive effect for lung, stomach, prostate, and melanoma skin cancers, as well as leukemia.

In addition, a recent study that showed that women with breast cancer who had higher vitamin D levels had double the survival rate of women with lower levels.

And this result was in a population where the "high" vitamin D group of women actually just had "sufficient" levels of the vitamin. Imagine if all women were at the truly optimal levels shown by research to be most beneficial to their health?

I recommend a dose of 5,000 IU per day of vitamin D.

Chapter 6

COMBINED EFFECTS:
Double- and triple-plays with these fabulous five additional ingredients

In addition to all of the nutrients I discussed in the previous chapter, the following five additional ingredients have the unique power to address two or all three critical cancer-fighting effects. They provide **antioxidant protection, immune support, and have anti-angiogenesis** effects.

The yellow spice breakthrough: Curcumin (Curcuma longa)

Curcumin is the gold-colored curry spice commonly used in India. It has been used for centuries as a spice in foods (turmeric) and as an herbal remedy in India, Malaya, and Southeast Asia. But it has suddenly been "discovered" by modern science leading to a torrent of current research. Curcumin has been extensively researched as a treatment for cancer. Its antioxidant effects are 10 times stronger than that of vitamin E. And it has been shown to stop tumor growth.

In a review of over 728 curcumin analogs which covers the literature from 1815 to mid-2009, researchers showed that curcumin interfered with multiple cell signal pathways including the spread of cancer cells, angiogenesis, and inflammation. Therefore, among the national products shown to possess chemical preventive and anticancer properties, curcumin is one of the most potent.

Other recent research has shown that curcumin can help stop the spread of cancer (metastasis) by decreasing the invasiveness of cancer cells in a lung cancer model. It has also been shown to have a direct effect against cancer cells in colon cancer, chronic lymphocytic leukemia, liver cancer and ovarian cancer. And can slow the spread of melanoma, prostate cancer, multiple myeloma, lymphoma, and others.

In one recent study, curcumin was found to be lethal to human bladder cancer cells. It induced cell death and stopped the spread. The effect of curcumin was shown to be stronger than that of cisplatin (a common chemotherapy drug).

Curcumin has also been shown to have the unique ability to help enhance the effectiveness of chemotherapy when it may otherwise fail. Multidrug resistance to anticancer drugs is a major cause of chemotherapy failure for patients. Curcumin may be used as a chemo sensitizer to make tumor cells more sensitive to the effects of chemotherapy. Thus potentially lowering the effective dose of toxic chemotherapy—an example of true complementary medicine.

Studies have shown it to exhibit similar activities to those drugs that have been developed to block tumor necrosis factor, vascular endothelial cell growth factor, human epidermal growth factor, and HER2.

A generally recommended dose is 200 mg per day as a dietary supplement, although dietary intake can be higher when used as a food spice versus a supplement.

The pungent protector: Garlic (Allium sativa)

Unlike many other herbs, garlic, is also a biologically active food with presumed medicinal properties, including possible anti-cancer effects. Garlic has been found to possess over 100 constituent compounds. Some have been looked at individually, but one can't discount the potential importance of the benefits of the whole.

Clinical studies of garlic in humans address several areas including protective associations with cancer as well as clinical adverse effects. There are multiple clinical studies with promising but some conflicting results. Some data, primarily from case-control studies, suggest dietary garlic consumption is associated with decreased risk of laryngeal, gastric, colorectal, and endometrial cancer, and colon polyps.

Recent research has found that the allicin in garlic (the main ingredient in garlic that gives it its distinctive flavor) can stimulate cell death via various actions.

In a population-based, case-control study conducted in Shanghai,

China, investigators found a link between the intake of allium vegetables, including garlic, scallions, onions, chives, and leeks, and the risk of prostate cancer. Men in the highest of three intake categories of total allium vegetables (more than 10.0 grams per day) had a statistically significantly lower risk of prostate cancer than those in the lowest category (less than 2.2 grams per day). Similar comparisons between categories showed reductions in risk for men in the highest intake categories for garlic and scallions.

You can increase your garlic intake by adding it to your taste to any vegetable, fish, or meat dish. One to two cloves per day is recommended. If supplementing with a garlic extract, a generally recommended dose is 200-400 mg, two to three times per day.

The "back from the brink" cancer weapon: Sutherlandia frutescens ("Cancer Bush")

In my explorations of the silent cures of South Africa, Sutherlandia frutescens is regarded as one of the most potent. It has had a long but hidden history of use as a safe and effective remedy for various health conditions by all cultures in the region. It has long been used as a supportive treatment in cancer, hence one of its common names— "Cancer Bush." It is called *Kankerbos* in Afrikaans, a dialect of the Dutch settlers. And in the indigenous *Tswana* tongue, as in Botswana, it is called *"Phetola"* which means "it changes." And indeed the plant changes the course of many illnesses for the better.

Sutherlandia has traditionally been used for enhancing wellbeing, immune support, longevity, stress, depression and anxiety. It was one of the few treatments found useful during the deadly global "Spanish Flu" epidemic after WW I that killed 20 million people worldwide during 1918-19. It works by helping the body heal and restore a normal state of health (or homeostasis) by mobilizing its own resources to overcome many physical and mental stresses. Research studies show that is works broadly among the body systems. This indicates that it functions as an *adaptogen*, as well as an immune stimulant. Studies also indicate significant antioxidant activity, another important anti-cancer property.

Cancer bush contains a substance called *L-canavanine*. This potent compound has been shown to stop pancreatic cancer cells in their tracks. Cancer bush also contains GABA, which has been shown to stamp a "cease and desist" on tumor cells. And clinical trials are now underway testing it against the immune system's ultimate enemy, the AIDS virus.

But beyond the technical aspects of this wonder-find, there lies a mysterious aspect that could make it the "back from the brink" cancer weapon patients have been praying for. And that's the ability of the cancer bush to halt the deadly "wasting" process that so many terminally ill patients experience. This wasting away is called *cachexia*.

The presence of cachexia in cancer patients has long been understood to mean that cancer is a metabolic disorder, systemically throughout the body, rather than being just the presence of a malignant tumor. Therefore, a natural product like Sutherlandia, which also acts as an adaptogen, can show potential benefits over an approach to just killing cancer cells. Accordingly, it functions as an appetite stimulant in wasted patients, but not in healthy people. Dr. Credo Mutwa, one of South Africa's most respected healers, has seen patients who weighed as little as 57 lbs turn the tides and reach 100 lbs. in just 7 months.

A generally recommended dose is 600 mg per day of *Sutherlandia frutescens* leaf extract.

The Mother's Day cancer crusher: Chrysanthemum

Chinese medicine also offers complex mixtures of active herbal remedies for cancer. One interesting and important ingredient is Chrysanthemum. Chrysanthemum is better known in the West as a simple decorative, hardy flowering plant. But the chrysanthemum itself is full of at least 15 different active and potent phytochemicals. Many of these phytochemicals act as pesticides to discourage predators, so it's not surprising that it would contain compounds that have anti-cancer properties. It is also a hardy plant, well known for its ability to withstand cold and continue to bloom even after other plants have closed down for the autumn and winter.

Chrysanthemum is a powerful symbol in Chinese and Japanese culture. It is often used as a tea in ceremonial occasions. Often a plant that is revered for its symbolic or iconic significance also has constituents that are very powerful herbal remedies. I recognized this common property of medicinal plants early in the development of medical anthropology in the early 1980's.

Scientifically, Chrysanthemum morifloriam flowers have demonstrated various anti-cancer effects specifically against prostate cancer. In Chinese medicine it is used for prostate cancer and prostate health together with reishi mushroom (*Ganoderma*), licorice root (*Glycyrrihiza glabra*), saw palmetto (*Serenoa repens*), and the adaptogen Sanchi Ginseng (*Panax pseudoginseng*).

Chrysanthemum and seven other active natural products were once available in the traditional Chinese combination remedy known as PC-SPES. In one of their rare, but still misguided, attempts to test a truly innovative approach to cancer, the NIH unwittingly used contaminated PC-SPES and had to halt their study, wasting more taxpayer dollars and a golden opportunity to expand the cancer treatment frontier. As a result of the contamination of the PC-SPES being tested, it was pulled off the market and is no longer available. Which is a shame, considering it was exceptionally effective. Particularly for re-differentiation, or returning cancerous cells back to a normal, healthy state.

However, similar, equally promising formulations made by different companies are now available. Chrysanthemum is included in a formulation called PC-CARE.

Treatment with PC-CARE or similar formulations should be individually monitored and sought from a qualified and knowledgeable traditional Chinese medical practitioner. Such practitioners may be found in Chinatowns in major urban areas and even some modern university hospital settings in the U.S.

The Middle-Eastern marvel: Black cumin (Nigella sativa)

Black cumin (*Nigella sativa*) is an annual flowering plant found in

South and Southwest Asia. It is also called fennel flower, nutmeg flower, Roman coriander, black caraway seed, or black coriander, and sometimes onion seed or black seed. It is regarded as one of the greatest of all medicinal herbs in Islam. Modern research is actively investigating its anti-cancer properties. An extract has recently been found to be effective against pancreatic cancer in the laboratory. Pancreatic cancer is a notoriously difficult cancer to treat. So the potential of black cumin is giving researchers hope in finally finding an effective natural remedy.

Researchers at the Kimmel Cancer Cancer at Thomas Jefferson University in Philadelphia, with whom I used to work, have found that thymoquinone, an extract of nigella sativa seed oil, blocked pancreatic cancer cell growth and killed the cells by enhancing the process of programmed cell death. Using a human pancreatic cancer cell line, researchers found that adding thymoquinone killed approximately 80 percent of the cancer cells, but presumably without the toxic side effects of chemotherapy.

Black cumin seed supplements are available in some natural food stores, vitamin shops, and from online supplement retailers. A good general dose is 500 mg per day.

Chapter 7

The business of cancer: How more cancer screenings and the uptick in diagnoses are doing more harm than good

Few things in life are more frightening than a cancer diagnosis. Just hearing the words, "You have cancer," can throw a person into a devastating tailspin—taking their loved ones along with them.

So imagine hearing those words when they're not actually true. Imagine having your life turned upside-down and facing mortality eye-to-eye, only to find out what you have isn't really cancer… it's a case of *mistaken identity*, or **false labeling**.

That's just what's happening to countless people around the country every day. They are receiving the shocking and demoralizing news that they have cancer—a life-threatening illness—when they actually have something that has no chance of ever killing them.

Not all "cancer" is created equal

So how is this happening? It all comes down to what you call things, and our medical establishment has taken to calling things "cancer" even when they're not.

In dermatology, for instance, pathologists have long observed relatively benign tumors as only "Grade ½" based on the benign appearance of the cells. Normally cancer cells are graded on a scale of one to four, so a half-grade is meant to register that cells don't really look like cancer—and they don't behave like it either.

But instead of just removing these skin growths and letting their patients go on with their day, dermatologists put the fear of death in them by calling them cancer. (As it is, they already get a lot of practice putting the fear of death into their patients when it comes to the sun). The truth is most skin cancers are relatively benign growths and do not cause long-term problems if they're removed. So why call these growths that don't even meet the pathological requirements for the lowest level—Grade 1—cancer?

Even the National Cancer Institute (NCI) is starting to wake up to this problem. A working group they recently sanctioned just advised the medical community that the "use of the term *cancer* should be reserved for describing lesions with a reasonable likelihood of lethal progression if left untreated."

Translation? If it can't kill a person, STOP calling it cancer!

The far-reaching effects of cancer scares

These unnecessary cancer diagnoses have effects far beyond the initial scare. Many cancers are being treated that don't need to be. And as we all know, treatment isn't benign in itself.

For those "Grade ½" skin lesions, treatment is simple (removal with local anesthetic, if that). But for other so-called "cancers," people are put through major surgery, toxic chemotherapy, and/or radiation.

Take prostate cancer, the most common cancer in men. As men get older, they become more likely to develop an "occult cancer" of the prostate. But in most cases, this "cancer" is so slow-growing and silent that it never causes problems. In fact, if it's not discovered by overeager screening, it probably will go unnoticed—unless it shows up as an "incidental" finding at an autopsy of a man who has died in advanced old age of some other cause. If such a cancer is caught, however, you can count on aggressive, invasive and unnecessary treatment, not to mention mental anguish.

Cancer treatments remain among the most toxic, dangerous treatments still practiced anywhere since the Middle Ages—with many side effects of their own. They can even cause secondary cancers. *So the cancer you went in for won't kill you, but here's another one that probably will!*

When I was a medical resident, my next-door neighbor in Philadelphia was a retired fireman who came down with lymphoma.

He was treated with a new "miracle" cancer drug, Adriamycin (a chemotherapeutic agent originally developed from algae in the Adriatic Sea). He was cured of the cancer, but the Adriamycin destroyed his heart muscle and he quickly died—albeit "cancer-free." Knowing what we now know, I suspect the drug totally destroyed the cellular respiration function in the mitochondria, causing the heart to go first.

That's just one story, but there are lots more like it. And beyond its effects on individuals like my neighbor, this "over-diagnosis/over-treatment crisis" makes us less healthy as a society.

Just think of the epidemic of vitamin D deficiency that has resulted from our being kept out of the sun for fear of skin cancers (91 percent of which don't really behave like cancer at all).

We now realize that lack of vitamin D can contribute to other, typically more serious, cancers (and heart disease, and respiratory diseases, and more). So again, we're trading a relatively minor health concern for a major one.

Of course, the over-diagnosis/ over-treatment crisis wouldn't be possible without another, equally problematic aspect of modern oncology.

Cancer screening paves the way for problems

The concept of cancer screening in the United States has become highly problematic over the past three decades. For example, the medical establishment pushes dangerous, expensive and overused procedures such as colonoscopy, while virtually ignoring screening for lung cancer which causes far more cancer deaths.

Then, added to that, screening is identifying more of what doctors have been calling "early cancers," but which we now realize are not cancers at all. From a distance, it looks like the system has been catching more cancers and preventing more deaths due to cancer. But these statistics are misleading if the additional cancers were not going to cause death in the first place. It's all part of the statistical trickery used to create the illusion of some progress in the "war on cancer."

This numbers game makes us think we're getting ahead of cancer. But all we are really doing is just diagnosing more "non-cancers" and calling it a success when they don't kill us.

Here's an example: Breast cancer screening has led to an overall increase in incidence of new "cases," because both cancers and non-cancers are being detected. So when cancer death rates stay the same or decrease, despite a supposed increase in incidence, it allows the government to claim a false sense of victory.

The same is happening with prostate cancer and others.

And all the while, the real goal—to reduce the rates of late-stage cancers and cancer deaths—remains elusive.

Screening practices and programs designed for that purpose have not met their goals. All we have done is to increase detection of "early-stage" cancer but without any decline in "late-stage" cancer. If cancer is defined as a disease that will lead to death if untreated, then detecting an "early" cancer that would have never led to death is not detecting cancer at all.

And we have accomplished nothing.

When does screening make sense?

We need to understand and appreciate the biology of different cancers. If a cancer is very *fast-growing*, then no screening can realistically be effective when it comes to the population as a whole. If it is *slower-growing*, as with colon polyps that take a long time (15 years on average) to develop into colon cancer, then less frequent screening can be effective.

If growth is *very slow* (for example, exceeding human life expectancy, such as "occult" cancer of prostate) then screening is actually harmful because it detects lesions that need not and *should not* be treated.

The one unqualified success story we've seen with screening is for cervical cancer. Cervical cancer used to be one of the top causes of cancer deaths in women. But from 1955 to 1992, the cancer death rate has declined by almost 70 percent—thanks to widespread, easy, and effective screening. No other cancer screening has shown anywhere near these kinds of positive results.

Given this sad state of affairs, what else is the NCI-approved panel I mentioned above proposing?

A common-sense solution

The practice of oncology in the United States is in serious need of a host of reforms to address the problems of over-diagnosis and over-treatment.

The advisory panel laid out a plan for dealing with this problem. First, as I mentioned earlier, it specifically advised that a number of "pre-malignant" conditions should no longer be called "cancer." This includes the common intra-ductal carcinoma of the breast (within the breast ducts) and even "high-grade" intraepithelial neoplasia of the prostate.

Instead, a different category of growth or tumor should be recognized and labeled appropriately as "non-cancer." Doesn't that sound less frightening? The panel suggests using such terms as "indolent lesions of epithelial origin" or IDLE.

A big part of the problem is all the medical sub-specialties involved in cancer. Each has its own terminology largely based upon the technologies they use, rather than a fundamental understanding of the biology of cancer. The use of new tools for diagnosing or treating diseases has driven the creation and practice of different medical specialties, each of which has developed exclusive uses of these technologies. This state of affairs calls to mind the admonition, "If your only tool is a hammer, then you see every problem as a nail."

Another result of medical sub-specialization is the different terminologies in use across the spectrum of pathology, radiology, surgery, and other medical specialties as well as the general community.

The panel has recommended that a body such as the Institute of Medicine determine what we should call these lesions now called cancer.

Then—in order to actually affect the rates of late-stage cancers and cancer deaths—all the other "pre-malignant" lesions must be tracked separately by government statisticians, instead of being lumped together with cancer. That's the only way we'll get an accurate view of what is and is not causing real cancer. This would vastly improve the quality of our cancer statistics, on which our national health policies are based.

Another proposal focuses on reducing over-diagnosis by reducing the use of low-yield diagnostic tests, reducing the frequency of screenings, focusing on high-risk populations, and raising requirements for taking a biopsy.

Finally, the panel recommended alternatives to treatment by focusing on the environment in which tumors arise. Strategies such as diet or chemoprevention (reducing the risk of cancer by specific micronutrient vitamins and minerals) may be as effective, and are less toxic, than traditional therapies.

Of course, given misplaced priorities for cancer research funding, the oncology community still has a long way to go before understanding the right doses, forms, and micronutrients to use. But some research is beginning to emerge that may point us in the right direction.

How the government could prevent 12,000 lung cancer deaths per year, but won't

One out of 10 smokers gets lung cancer. And those who smoke the most are most at risk.

But, two years ago, U.S. researchers found a simple way to prevent lung cancer among those highest at risk. And government science-bureaucrats refuse to acknowledge it.

Instead, we just hear the endless preaching about smoking cessation. But, in fact, most people who get lung cancer today are *former smokers*. They've already quit. But they're still getting lung cancer.

What do we tell them?

Plus, even as smoking goes down, people are still getting lung cancer. And the number of *non-smokers* with lung cancer is on the rise. In fact, one out of 100 non-smokers gets lung cancer, without ever taking a puff. But the government doesn't talk about these statistics. And you don't hear about this troubling fact in the news at all.

While driving through upstate New York last fall I heard a heartbreaking radio broadcast about a rally to raise public awareness for the 50,000 women with lung cancer in the U.S. who never smoked at all. They feel completely abandoned.

And what do we tell these women? They can't stop smoking because they never started. What causes their cancer? And how can they prevent it?

We stopped doing routine annual chest x-rays long ago because they really didn't detect new occurrences of cancer. And the risk of radiation was not worth it. Plus, x-rays have become old hat.

Instead, hospitals spend fortunes installing expensive, new imaging facilities. They even offer "open access" MRIs and CAT imaging equipment in freestanding, "walk-in" facilities—all to make more money.

Unfortunately, we give these expensive high-tech scans to folks with lower back pain—instead of to those at risk for lung cancer. The lower-back pain patients would be better off skipping the scan anyway. And going straight to physical therapy.

Meanwhile, the folks at risk for lung cancer are given nothing to believe in but the flimsy "smoke-and-mirrors" smoking cessation statistics.

And that's a crying shame, because preventative scans could clearly help reduce their risk...

Two years ago, the National Lung Cancer Screening Trial made this important discovery. The researchers found that screening high-risk smokers and ex-smokers with annual CAT scans would prevent 12,000 lung cancer deaths per year. These high-resolution x-rays can spot suspicious lung nodules.

One of the study authors told Reuters, "This is the first paper that attempts to assess the impact of screening on lung cancer cases nationally."

But why is this only the first paper on this huge health problem?

Why don't we screen for lung cancer?

My old colleague, Larry Kessler, studies the diagnostic value of screening and he recently published an editorial, which accompanied the new study in the journal *Cancer*. He said this new study is a "pivotal event that should have woken people up."

It should have, Larry. But it didn't.

The government and the medical profession prefer wagging politically correct fingers against smokers. And even against former smokers and non-smokers.

One-hundred-and-sixty thousand people die each year of lung cancer. That figure is higher than deaths caused by auto accidents, Vietnam, and most other cancers combined.

So, remind me again, why don't we screen for lung cancer?

But wait, the science bureaucrats in Bethesda have their reason why not.

The Division of Cancer Prevention at NCI—which hasn't gotten anything right in the last 30 years that I know about—says the numbers would not translate in the "real world" because those naughty smokers would not *want* to be screened!

Really—this is the *sole* reason why we don't screen them?

Can you hear those wagging fingers slicing through all the stifling hot air in Bethesda as you read this? Let's just keep punishing those naughty, politically incorrect smokers!

First of all, when are the political science creatures at NCI ever concerned with—or even aware of—the real world of average Americans? I doubt anyone gleefully schedules a colonoscopy or a Pap smear. But they do it because the NCI says they should.

The NCI also points to problems with screenings in general—such as costs and false positives—to discredit lung cancer screening. But those same problems apply to every single kind of screening. Mammograms. Pap Smears. Colonoscopies. They're all prone to the same problems. But the government still pushes them. Including many that are worthless, or worse.

What an incredibly, stupendously stupid comment from the agency that pushes cancer screening at every other opportunity! By the way, NCI gave up on finding cures for lung cancer long ago in favor of the anti-smoking mantra.

If you did not think that there is still gross, government-wide, politically correct discrimination against some people who get lung cancer— smokers and even the thousands of innocent, non-smokers—this should prove it to you.

Usually the government loves to find "victims" for everything. But the government has no love for victims of lung cancer. But remains happy to collect their cigarette taxes for this legal substance.

Unfortunately the government refuses to budge in their ignorance to real science. Because if they did, maybe they'd be clued in to the dangers of screenings they actually advocate for…like the ones you'll read about in the next chapters.

Ten medical procedures you may do better without!

Hundreds of thousands of Americans are injured, poisoned, and killed each year by modern medical technologies. Even the most respected medical journals and institutions have confirmed in various reports over the past 10 years the failures of American "modern medicine." Including deaths from unnecessary surgery, medication errors, clerical errors, hospital- acquired infections, and even from the "expected" negative side effects of drugs. All the while, health care costs are spiraling out of control and insurance companies are requiring patients to pay a greater share of the cost.

So despite all our breakthrough technology, American medicine often appears to be doing more harm than good. In fact, you may be surprised at what can be done without it!

It's time to rethink some of the medical myths and rituals that result in millions of useless tests, procedures, and "interventions" that appear to do more harm than good. Besides the huge waste of time and money they represent.

And now the American Board of Internal Medicine Foundation is doing just that with a new project called "Choosing Wisely." The foundation consists of doctors from nine of the top medical societies in the U.S. And the Choosing Wisely program has identified 45 different medical procedures that are of little or no value, from tests, to surgeries, and even commonly prescribed medications. Below I'll review the most commonly performed tests that are now considered inappropriate. Removing this kind of waste and abuse from the healthcare system could save billions of dollars a year.

Even the benefit of the routine yearly "checkup" is being questioned for most patients now. As reported in a New York Times article, back in 1979 a Canadian government task force recommended giving up the standard top-to-bottom annual physical exam.[75] They said it was "inefficient, nonspecific" and even "potentially harmful." That Canadian diagnosis was made the same year I graduated from a U.S. Ivy League medical school where we all sincerely believed the annual "checkup" was just practicing good medicine!

But the potential danger or harm of unneeded exams is that they may show "false positives," potentially lead to risky procedures and treatments, and/or more tests, which leads to more of the same. It's a vicious cycle. And every step along the way comes with the potential for harm. The controversy over the PSA test to try to detect prostate cancer is a good example.

But from the first day out of medical school, there remains a lot of simple inertia about what doctors expect they should be doing for their patients, and about what patients expect from their doctors. Not to mention all the economic incentives from the health care industry to provide more "care" whether needed or not.

There are also perverse incentives in medical research to discover more and more "biomarkers" for screening and "early detection" of diseases like cancer, despite the repeated abject failures of this approach for decades. And now, the new Director of the National Cancer Institute, Dr. Harold Varmus (a past director of the NIH) is back like a bad penny, poised for another jump over the precipice with an obsessive focus on finding ever more "biomarkers."

And, sad to say, there are many diseases where early detection, even if "biomarkers" are found, simply doesn't make any difference in the prognosis, management, or treatment of the disease. There are also many problems that may correct themselves over time due to the body's ability to heal itself without any need for dangerous tests, procedures, or treatments.

So, before you make your next doctor's appointment, be sure to consider the following very carefully. According to the American Board of Internal Medicine and National Physicians Alliance, these are the "top ten" most commonly performed tests you can actually omit:

1. **Annual physical exam:** On average for healthy adults, rather than detecting real problems, it is more likely to find false positives or meaningless results leading to useless and dangerous procedures and/or more tests that lead nowhere.

2. **Annual EKG:** On average for people without heart disease, it is more likely to mislead than to find early problems—leading to further needless and dangerous tests, drugs, and even surgery.

3. **Annual "blood panel" tests:** For people who feel well in the first place, it is more likely to lead to false positives than to detect new disease.

4. **Annual cholesterol test:** If cholesterol previously tested "normal" (although what is considered normal is constantly being manipulated by industry- motivated NIH "reviews"), this test is needed only once every five years.

5. **Annual Pap Smear:** Although this is one very important and successful test for early detection of cervical cancer, it is only needed every three years in women who have tested normal.

6. **Prostate Specific Antigen (PSA) to detect prostate cancer:** Experts from the U.S. Preventative Services Task Force no longer recommend this test, saying it causes more harm than benefit. The harm is not from this test itself but that it is frequently misleading, resulting in useless procedures and surgery that frequently cause permanent disability or even death. Studies show that patients not given the PSA test have no higher mortality than patients faithfully screened for prostate cancer by this test.

7. **Pre-operative chest x-ray:** Many hospitals still require a routine chest x-ray prior to surgery but it is a wasted effort unless the patient has heart or lung disease. The annual routine chest x-ray as part of a yearly physical exam was given up long ago, since the risk from radiation far exceeded any benefit at detection of lung cancer. Of course, now you can give up the annual physical as well.

8. **Bone scans in women under 65 years:** Efforts to detect osteoporosis in younger women have resulted in many women taking dangerous drugs with terrible side effects that are unnecessary (besides, if you wait until you're 65, Medicare will cover this test if medically necessary).

9. **Radiologic tests for low back pain:** If back pain is of short duration (less than 2—4 weeks), doing imaging studies add no benefit or improvement in outcome. And, as I've said before, the vast majority of patients with low back pain should be treated first with spinal manual therapy, provided by physical therapists and chiropractors, rather than drugs or surgery. And one hospital in Seattle is now doing just that with success.

10. **Radiologic tests for headaches:** The common headache is sufficiently diagnosed by taking a careful medical history and doing a comprehensive neurological exam. Find a doctor who still knows how to provide that.

These 10 recommendations are not just theoretical. They are already being tried with positive results.

Local health care providers and some insurers are already improving the system by treating their patients better by providing less care. Following are just a few examples as reported in an editorial in *The New York Times*

Premier Inc. is an alliance of hospitals around the country that has ceased doing useless blood tests and screenings. Over three years in 157 hospitals in 31 states they have saved almost 25,000 lives and reduced costs by almost $5 billion, saving 12 percent of their overall spending.

Virginia Mason Medical Center in Seattle stopped doing useless radiologic tests for headache and back pain, decreasing the use of CT scans by one-quarter. Also, in collaboration with Seattle-based Starbuck's and Aetna Insurance they stopped sending people with low back pain to expensive orthopedic specialists (who could only see them after lengthy and painful waits, and then order a costly CT scan before providing any therapy). Instead they sent back pain patients directly for spinal manual therapy to physical therapists on the same day. Most patients were pain free and back to work in less time than it would have taken them to wait to see a medical specialist. And they avoided dangerous drugs and surgery.

That's true healthcare reform.

So what are the most common regular tests you should get?

They are actually few and simple.

For women over 40 it is useful to get a mammogram every two years.

After much controversy about the risks of mammograms, the optimal screening interval and hundreds of millions of dollars spent on research, the data indicate that it's simply not necessary to get a yearly mammogram. Bi-annually is just fine. However, women should perform frequent breast self-examinations (while standing in the shower or otherwise). Breast cancer remains the leading cancer among women, while heart disease is the leading cause of death overall (as in men).

So for heart disease, getting your blood pressure checked regularly is the single most important step you can take to prevent or control your risk. Unfortunately, as I reported in my *Daily Dispatch*, the healthcare system is failing miserably to detect and treat high blood pressure—which is an extremely treatable condition.

It's time to give up on all the dangerous and wasteful testing and focus on the things that really make a difference—and can literally mean the difference between life and death.

If your doctor is recommending any of the other 10 tests above, it can't hurt to talk to him candidly about the real risks and benefits. You can refer to the "Choose Wisely" campaign of the American Board of Internal Medicine Foundation. And of course, you can always get a second opinion. And if he doesn't recommend these tests, before you argue to have them just because everyone else is…you may want to consider counting your blessings. Instead, focus on what's really needed to ensure optimal health for whatever area of concern you may have.

Chapter 8

The deadly mammogram myth

Mammograms are one of those "routine" cancer screenings I mentioned in the previous chapter that affect millions of patients. Older women, in particular. And the dangers are very real.

Data shows mammograms do a lot less than you might think to save actual lives. And they have caused a sweeping epidemic of overdiagnosis and overtreatment. Yet, when you suggest anyone skip this cancer screening, or simply use it less frequently, politically correct zealots act as if you're mounting a campaign against women's health.

Of course, this reaction has very little to do with science. Indeed, when it comes to cancer—and breast cancer, in particular—politics, emotion, and fear can completely overwhelm the facts.

You see, 50 years ago, one clinical trial examined mammography as a screening tool for breast cancer. And in the ensuing years, legions of doctors, technicians, medical device makers, public health professionals, and government bureaucrats helped parlay this often-ineffective tool into a multi-billion-dollar enterprise.

Today, tens of millions of women dutifully get annual mammograms. They believe the mantra "early detection saves lives." But the real data about this approach shows otherwise…

In fact, doctors at the Geisel School of Medicine at Dartmouth University recently gave us some startlingly grim data about mammograms.

According to their estimate, up to 3.2 women, but as few as 0.3 women, out of every 1,000 who get yearly mammograms over a decade will avoid dying of breast cancer. In other words, mammograms, at best, will save three out of every 1,000 women from dying of breast cancer over a decade. At worst, they will save no one.

But up to 67 percent of the women will have at least one false positive during those 10 years. Plus, for every 1,000 women screened over the decade, medical interventions will medically harm as many as 14 women with overdiagnosis and overtreatment.

Think about it this way…

According to this analysis, over a 10-year span, mammograms harm five times, and up to 50 times, as many women as they save. Plus, a majority of all these women will experience at least one traumatic "false-alarm" along the way.

Here's another problem with mammograms…

Aside from not preventing deaths any better than physical exams, they're also harmful. They may actually *increase* your risk of breast cancer by subjecting you to radiation—and by physically abusing breast tissue.

Over the past 25 years or so, the frequency of breast cancer has dramatically increased—from about 1 in 11 to now about 1 in 9 women. This past quarter-century is exactly the same time period of time that "everyone" has been getting mammograms.

So maybe we are "detecting" more small cancers, and maybe even causing some, with annual mammograms. But remember, we're not lowering the death rates of the population.

Plus, mammograms are highly inaccurate. In fact, according to the National Institutes of Health, 90 percent of "abnormal" findings turn out to be false positives for breast cancer.

Even the pink-ribboned Komen Foundation admits when women get all the mammograms they recommend, 50 to 60 percent of them will end up with a false positive. So the majority of women get at least one traumatic "cancer scare" during their lifetime. (Ironically, mammograms miss 17 percent of breast cancers that are really present.)

Why all the false positives?

Well, today, mammograms are more sensitive than ever. They detect very small lesions of cells that look suspicious. So the woman (and her family) has to go through the pain and stress of a biopsy. But once you put the cells under a microscope, we discover they aren't cancerous at all.

Even when we *do* classify these small lesions as "cancer," sometimes they *don't* really behave like cancer in the body. They will never cause illness or death. This is often true of ductal carcinomas of the breast. But they still get treated as real cancer. And we subject the women to the tortures and dangers of real cancer treatment.

In a recent interview with *Medscape* , my friend and colleague Dr. George Lundberg explained why it's important to assess each individual cancer carefully. He's the former editor-in-chief of the Journal of the American Medical Association. He said:

For a long time, it made sense to try to eradicate all cancers, as early and as completely as possible. Mass efforts were launched to find cancers wherever they were and destroy them. Since the earliest cancers seemed to evolve from some identifiable premalignant conditions, wouldn't it make sense to also nip those in the bud? Sounds logical.

But, as with many exuberant efforts, this one got out of control. Many lesions that were called "cancer" really were not cancers at all in behavior, and this fact began to be recognized in large numbers of patients. These unfortunate victims have experienced massive psychological and physical harm and costs without any clear benefits achieved by finding and treating their "non-cancers."

And here's the real kicker…

In the cases where a woman has a real, aggressive cancer, and the mammogram finds it, she still needs a biopsy. And that biopsy can end up spreading the cancer.

Overall, mammograms are ineffective for the population as a whole. And sometimes dangerous. They also contribute to the epidemic of over-diagnosis and over-treatment of cancers. This has helped feed the growing beast of today's cancer industry.

Having said all of this, there are of course individual examples of women who discover they have breast cancer through their annual mammogram. Presumably, they would not have found it otherwise. Ultimately, the early detection made a real difference in their treatment and survival. But, of course, we will never know what *would* have happened in any individual case if she had not gotten that mammogram. That's why we do research to learn more about the real benefits of early cancer detection.

As a reminder, these *real* risk factors for breast cancer are:

- Early age at menarche (early puberty)
- Late age at menopause
- Having few (or no) pregnancies
- Late age at first pregnancy (over 30 years old)
- Lack of breastfeeding
- Lack of being breastfed (as an infant)
- Taking certain birth control and hormone drugs
- Having one or more first degree relatives with breast cancer
- Genetic risk according to the "BRAC" gene test

Of course every woman is an individual. With individual risk and concerns. So—what are your options as an individual?

First, always consult with your trusted, qualified doctor to make a personalized plan. Look at whether you have any of the real risk factors for breast cancer I've mentioned above.

Secondly, consider thermography. It's an alternative screening test that uses no painful mechanical pressure or dangerous radiation. It's a form of thermal (infrared) imaging, so it doesn't damage the sensitive breast tissue as mammograms can. Plus, studies show it identifies precancerous or cancerous cells earlier. And it produces clear results, which cuts down on additional testing.

While mammograms do still have a role in the world of cancer screening (albeit a smaller, less frequent role than currently used by the mainstream), in the next chapter, I'll tell you about one common method of cancer screening that should really be eliminated altogether in favor of safer, simpler alternatives.

Chapter 9

The hidden, grisly dangers of "routine" colonoscopies

The U.S. is well-known for its massive expenditures on end-of-life care. On average, people here incur more medical costs during the last six months of life than during their entire life up until then. But it turns out the cost of ordinary care is nothing to sneeze at either.

"Routine" tests and exams add up to $2.7 trillion per year (even more than the federal government's annual deficit). Colonoscopies are a case in point.

Colonoscopy is—by far—the most expensive screening test that Americans are exhorted to undergo. But there are several reasons you should think twice before "bending over," when it comes again. In fact, skipping your next routine colonoscopy might actually save your life.

There are some serious dangers associated with this supposedly safe test you won't hear about from the public health "experts." Or the mainstream hype. There are also alternatives to colonoscopy that are just as effective—and much safer (not to mention less expensive). More on that in just a moment. But first, let me tell you why some real health experts are questioning whether it's truly worth it to get a colonoscopy once you hit a certain age...

"Too old" for a colonoscopy?

The minute you hit 50, your doctor probably started encouraging you to get regular colonoscopies.

But at this point in life, is a colonoscopy really worth it?

You see, the major purpose of routine colonoscopies is to detect polyps growing from the mucosal surface of the colon. But it takes, on average, 15 years for cancer within a polyp to develop into full-blown colon cancer.

Yes, some people have a specific genetic predisposition which can lead to multiple polyps and a higher risk of colon cancer. And these people should be followed and managed closely. But anyone can potentially develop a colon polyp. And in light of that 15-year lag time, how old is "too old" to go through this uncomfortable procedure and be subjected to its risks? This question is important because "routine" colonoscopy can be quite dangerous—even fatal.

Horror-film injuries from a "routine" test

Colonoscopy is portrayed as a benign, safe procedure for everyone. But in my forensic medicine practice I have seen case after case of perforated intestines and peritonitis (a potentially fatal inflammation of the abdominal lining), lacerated and punctured livers with massive bleeding, and other fatal complications. All from "routine" colonoscopies.

I even had one case in which the air pumped into the colon (to inflate it for easy examination) escaped into the patient's abdominal cavity. It put so much pressure on the liver that it cut off blood supply back to the heart. The patient died from shock.

To make matters worse, colonoscopies are often prescribed more frequently than medical guidelines recommend.

ACOG in the wheel

Ten years ago, apparently having run out of things to say on TV from one end, Katie Couric had her colonoscopy performed on the other end, live, on national TV. Patients began demanding them like the latest cosmetic procedure. Then, the American College of Gastroenterology (ACOG) successfully lobbied Congress to have the procedure covered by Medicare (in other words, us, the taxpayers).

So now, when you become eligible for Medicare at age 65, with the 15 year lag time for a polyp to become cancerous, this Medicare benefit can help you avoid coming down with colon cancer at age 80 years or older, on average. Just doing the math. But I digress…

The fact is, several much less expensive and less dangerous techniques are also effective. Yet specialist medical practitioners have (not surprisingly) picked the most expensive—and dangerous—option. Without any scientific data to support it. I know it sounds bizarre, given all the hype and increased recommendations for colonoscopy…but it's true.

In fact, according to a study published earlier this year in the *American Journal of Gastroenterology*, colonoscopy has never even been compared to other, much safer—and less expensive—screening methods head-to-head in randomized trials. This despite the continual call from mainstream medicine for ever more randomized, controlled, clinical trials—which are considered the "gold standard."

Until the last 10-15 years, colonoscopies were only performed in doctor's offices. And only on patients at high risk for colon cancer or who were experiencing intestinal bleeding.

Then doctors reported they could detect early cancers even in people who are not at high risk and don't have bleeding. But, according to an article published in the Journal of the *National Cancer Institute*, there is no compelling evidence that colonoscopy offers any additional benefit over the older, cheaper, safer tests.

And the bottom line is <u>no study has shown that colonoscopy prevents colon cancer incidence or mortality any more than the other safer, less expensive screening methods.</u>

Nonetheless, the ACOG unilaterally declared colonoscopy as the "preferred" approach to colon cancer prevention. It certainly was preferred when it came to collecting membership dues apparently.

Of course, colonoscopy has also become very lucrative. One analysis even reported colonoscopy is <u>the</u> reason the U.S. leads the world in health expenditures!

But some primary care doctors don't realize the costs of the tests and procedures they prescribe.

The most expensive hour you'll ever spend

A colleague of mine in Hartford, CT recently called the local hospital in order to price a colonoscopy. And even he couldn't get an answer.

Because this "routine" screening procedure can cost anywhere from $6,000 to nearly $20,000. For an outpatient procedure requiring less than an hour.

They are the most expensive screening tests that otherwise healthy Americans undergo. In fact, colonoscopies in the U.S. often cost more than childbirth or an appendectomy in most other developed countries.

But colonoscopies represent such a large financial burden because, unlike hip replacements, c-sections, or even nose spray, everybody gets them—or is supposed to, whether they need it or not.

The final "knock-out" blow

And on top of all this, there is the "wild west" of administering anesthesia during colonoscopies. Not only does anesthesia add to the procedure's risk, but this service is billed separately—and is all over the map.

For anesthesia during one surgical procedure, for the exact same service, one anesthesia group practice charges $6,970 from a large private health insurer, $5,208 from Blue Cross Blue Shield, $1,605 from Medicare, and $797 from Medicaid. *What* is the real cost of providing this service? Who knows!

A better question is: *Why* are anesthesiologists involved in colonoscopies at all?

Colonoscopy does not require general anesthesia. Moderate sedation—a drug like Valium, or another intravenous medicine that takes effect and wears off quickly—is all you really need. Both of which could technically be administered by any nurse in any doctor's office. There is no clinical benefit whatsoever from having anesthesiologists involved in this procedure. But it adds a further cost of $1.1 billon per year.

So, who is keeping the anesthesiologists where they don't belong? Our "friends" at the FDA. They refuse to modify the drug labels advising that moderate sedation must be performed in the presence of an anesthesiologist (a policy that the American Society of Anesthesiologists lobbies strongly to keep in place, of course).

So all of this leads us to the $1 billion question…

What are the alternatives?

Here we have yet another situation where the most expensive, most dangerous screening procedure has simply never been proven to be better than less expensive, safer procedures.

Three proven alternatives to colonoscopy are:

1. The long-established **hemoccult test** detects blood in the stool as a sign of intestinal bleeding. When there is bleeding in the lower intestinal tract it can be seen as bright red blood in the stool. But when the bleeding is higher up, the blood breaks down and becomes invisible, or "occult." Fecal occult blood testing can decrease the risk of death from colorectal cancer by 33 percent. Not bad for a test that is cheap, and completely safe, non-invasive, and that you can administer yourself in the privacy of your own bathroom.

2. To get an actual look inside the lower intestine, opt for a **sigmoidoscopy**. Unlike colonoscopy, which examines the entire colon, sigmoidoscopy only enters the lower large intestine, which is where most cancers occur. Several recent studies have shown that this screening method is as effective as colonoscopy—if not more so. In fact, according to one of these studies, getting just ONE sigmoidoscopy between the ages of 55-64 can reduce incidence of colon cancer by 31 percent and colon cancer mortality by 38 percent. A sigmoidoscopy can be done right in your doctor's office and doesn't require any sedation. Which makes it much less expensive—and also much safer—than colonoscopy.

3. A relatively recent development has been CT colonography, which involves doing CT scans to detect colon polyps. In general, CT colonography is done every five years, but radiologists have worked out several more specific guidelines for individual cases (including instances of positive fecal occult blood tests (FOBT), and to deal with the frequent problem of an "incomplete colonoscopy.")

Another new way to avoid costly, dangerous colonoscopies

This alternative to colonoscopies became available in November of 2014. And it's a boon to millions of people who prefer to avoid the discomfort, danger and expense of colonoscopies—and instead want to do their own colon cancer screening at home. The new test makes use of one of the long-awaited promises of biotech. It's the first to detect cancer-related DNA in stool. You can't get more precise than that.

This home procedure is a reliable test that doesn't require the painful preparations that interfere with your life. Nor does it carry the dangerous risks and awful complications that may cost you your life. There's no tortuous "prep," no scope, no anesthesia—and no risk to the procedure.

But, of course, the threatened colonoscopy industry is already trying to dump on this new test. They admit this simple, safe test will boost effective screening for colon cancer. But then they try to claim that it will lure people away from colonoscopies, which they say have been "shown" to save lives.

This test will certainly "lure" people away from the costs and disastrous consequences of colonoscopies. And it will certainly make it easier, safer and more palatable for more people to get effective screening for colon cancer.

But hold on—the dodgy claim that colonoscopies are better at "saving lives" has never been proven.

The fact is, we don't have any head-to-head, controlled clinical trial comparisons of using colonoscopy vs. alternatives test like the old standby fecal occult blood test or FIT (fecal immunochemical test). And there are no comparisons for the new test.

Even the National Cancer Institute (NCI) experts say the new test looks promising. (And this organization, as you'll recall, derided the new lung cancer screening test, largely based, as far as I can tell, on unethical and unscientific bias against lung cancer victims. Although the U.S. Centers for *Medicare* and Medicaid Services (*CMS*) finally just approved it for coverage under Medicare.)

The FDA approved the new colon cancer screening test in September 2014. And the world-respected Mayo Clinic, where it was developed, now offers the test. Exact Sciences Corp of Madison, WI will sell it under the name Cologuard®. And the Mayo Clinic will get royalties. (So it does not exactly sound like another big pharma venture.)

The idea and procedure itself are simple.

Patients obtain and send a stool sample to the lab where the test detects any blood (like the old home tests). The presence of blood could indicate the presence of a tumor. Plus, Cologuard detects the presence of mutated DNA, which could signal cancer or a precancerous growth called a polyp.

If the test is positive for cancer, then the patient undertakes additional diagnostic steps, such as a colonoscopy or sigmoidoscopy, to remove the growth or polyp. Sigmoidoscopy, which looks at the lower portion of the colon (where cancers most commonly occur) is a safer option and doesn't require sedation. In Europe, sigmoidoscopy is virtually the only "scoping" done.

Of course, the only real measure of the worth of any cancer screening procedure is whether it lowers the risk of cancer death. (As I have pointed out before, use of mainstream government-industrial-medical approaches to screening breast, prostate, and colon cancer have yet to specifically show to any clear benefits in actually reducing cancer death rates in the overall population.)

But this new Cologuard test *does* appear to lower the risk of cancer death...

In a large study, researchers compared Cologuard to one of the older tests for fecal blood. The Cologuard test detected 92 percent of colorectal cancers and 42 percent of precancerous growths (polyps). By comparison, the older fecal blood test only detected 74 percent of cancers and 24 percent of polyps.

Like any test, the increased sensitivity of Cologuard at detecting real cancers also leads to more false positives. In other words, the test can sometimes find evidence of a polyp or cancer where none is present. And it correctly rules out cancer 87 percent of the time (compared to 95 percent for the older blood test).

Critics complain this means 13 percent of patients may go on to get colonoscopies anyway who don't really need them. But, let's stop and think logically about this point for a moment. Do they really think it's better to make 100 percent of patients get colonoscopies whether they need them or not…or just 13 percent of them who really do need them?

Cologuard can avoid the costs, risks, and problems of colonoscopy 87 percent of the time. And that's a huge accomplishment.

Medicare jointly reviewed the Cologuard test with the FDA. (It was a rare example of sensible, federal bureaucratic coordination.) It will also pay for the test for Medicare patients, so the $599 cost should not be a barrier (especially when compared to the bloated costs of colonoscopies).

Now, keep these two things in mind…

First—it takes 15 years, on average, for a precancerous polyp to became a cancer. So there is time and opportunity to catch it with regular, non-invasive testing.

Second—you don't need any fancy test to detect rectal growths. Government statisticians certainly like to lump all "colo-rectal" cancers together to make their "survival" rates look better. But colon cancer is very different from rectal cancer. And doctors can easily detect rectal growths, polyps and cancers with the old fashioned, digital rectal exam, as part of a routine physical examination. (If doctors are given enough time to do it anymore, that is.)

All statistics aside, sensible cancer experts say the best colon cancer screening test is one that people will actually go and get. So if the torturous colonoscopy prep turns you off, ask your doctor about this new Cologuard test. It's yet another good alternative to dangerous colonoscopies.

Please don't misunderstand my intention. In no way am I downplaying the importance of colon cancer and effective screening for this potentially deadly disease. However, I and many others do take issue with the medical subspecialist's carte blanche recommendation of colonoscopy. The available science simply doesn't support it as the be-all, end-all of colon cancer screening. And, as always, when it comes to your health, it's absolutely critical to follow the science.

The fact is, there are serious risks associated with colonoscopy…and its superiority is unproven. But there ARE alternatives. Safer ones. That do a better (or, at the very least, safer) job of reducing mortality from this disease.

If you have your doubts about getting a colonoscopy, make sure to consult with your primary care physician regarding your family history, personal medical history, and any current health problems or symptoms, to find out whether starting with safer, less expensive options—a hemoccult test, a sigmoidoscopy, or the new CT colonography scan— may be right for you for colon cancer screening and prevention.

And remember, you can lower your risk of colon cancer in the first place (and any other form of cancer, as well as many other chronic diseases, for that matter) by following the diet, exercise, and supplement recommendations you'll find throughout your issues of *Insiders' Cures*.

$$****$$

There is more to consider when it comes to fighting cancer. You've read about some heavy-hitters here, but there are many other specific nutrients, plant compounds, as well as mind-body therapies that when combined can have added benefit.

In fact, mind-body therapies are very effective for cancer patients and cancer survivors as true complementary medicine. An important step is to determine which mind-body therapies will work for you, and it is important to learn your "emotional type" by taking my simple survey in my book with Mike Jawer, *Your Emotional Type* (available through www.DrMicozzi.com or at your local bookstore).

If you have cancer or are a cancer survivor, don't try to conquer cancer on your own. It requires support from friends, family, and knowledgeable health practitioners.

For more detailed information on complementary approaches to cancer, see my 700-page handbook geared toward practitioners, *Complementary & Integrative Medicine in Cancer Care and Prevention*, New York: Springer, 2007.

Chapter 10

Revealed: At least 80% of women diagnosed with breast cancer can skip aggressive treatments

My 4-step, natural approach to preventing DCIS in the first place

I often report that some conditions considered "pre-cancerous" typically never lead to cancer. For years, doctors and researchers have pointed out that these frequently innocuous health issues get treated as cancer precursors—even though they don't behave like cancer at all.

This practice has led to an epidemic of overdiagnosis and overtreatment of "cancer." And this overdiagnosis epidemic has created unnecessary costs, confusion, and worry. Not to mention very real, very negative side effects from unnecessary treatments.

This is particularly true for certain conditions related to the skin, thyroid, prostate, and breasts.

One of the biggest culprits is something called ductal carcinoma in situ (DCIS). Basically, DCIS is defined as "abnormal" cells discovered by a mammogram within a woman's breast ducts.

The American Cancer Society reports that about 60,000 women were diagnosed with DCIS in 2015, accounting for almost 20% of all new breast "cancer" cases.

Mainstream oncology calls DCIS the earliest sign of breast cancer, and typically treats it as a medical emergency. Oncologists will order a lumpectomy within two weeks after diagnosis, followed by radiation.

Cancer organizations say this aggressive treatment of DCIS saves thousands of lives. But a new study on more than 100,000 women found that DCIS was associated with only a 3.3% rate of breast cancer deaths after 20 years.

That's similar to what the American Cancer Society cites as the risk of an average woman dying of breast cancer. In other words, you're *no more likely* to die of breast cancer if you're diagnosed with DCIS than someone without this diagnosis.

And, considering a five-year survival rate is the typical benchmark for success in treating cancer, DCIS hardly qualifies as the medical emergency so many clinicians treat it as.

In fact, surgery and radiation does not appear to be necessary at all for the vast majority of women with DCIS. It is only warranted in a small number of cases.

Assessing your own DCIS risk profile

Researchers analyzed 108,000 cases of DCIS diagnosed from 1988 to 2011. As I mentioned above, they found that 20 years after a DCIS diagnosis, the average death rate from breast cancer was only 3.3%— which was somewhat lower than previous findings.

However, depending upon other risk factors, some women who are diagnosed with DCIS have a much higher chance of eventually dying from breast cancer.

For example, the researchers found that women under age 35 who were diagnosed with DCIS had a breast cancer death rate of 7.8%. That's likely because women that young typically have much more aggressive forms of cancer growth than do older women.

Looking at the characteristics of the breast tissue cells in DCIS is also important. Risk factors to watch include the cells' response to estrogen (estrogen receptor status), size, appearance (grade), and whether there's surrounding tissue death. Women with higher-grade DCIS cells were 1.9 times more likely to die compared to women with lower-grade cells.

Finally, the researchers noted that African-American women with DCIS also had a higher mortality rate—7%.

Overall, 20% of women with DCIS had one or more of these other characteristics that placed them at higher risk of eventually succumbing to breast cancer. These are the women whom researchers said probably should have lumpectomies and radiation if they're diagnosed with DCIS.

For the other 80% of women with DCIS, the researchers discovered something quite surprising.

Aggressive treatment doesn't improve chances of survival

The 80% of women in this category who had a lumpectomy plus radiation, or even a mastectomy, were *no less likely to die* from breast cancer than women who didn't have those surgeries and treatments.

The main goal behind aggressive DCIS treatment has always been to prevent the "cancer" from spreading within the same breast. Of course, if breast cancer becomes invasive, it dramatically increases the risk of death. For example, the researchers noted that the risk of dying was 18 times higher in women whose cancer had spread within the same breast.

The researchers found that, as expected, women with DCIS who had a lumpectomy plus radiation reduced their risk of abnormal cell recurrence after 10 years—from 4.9% for women who didn't have treatment to 2.5% for women who did have treatment.

But the researchers were surprised to discover lumpectomy and radiation didn't lower the women's chances of dying from breast cancer.

Even the more radical surgery of mastectomy didn't reduce breast cancer mortality.

In fact, the death rate among mastectomy patients was higher (1.3%) compared to lumpectomy patients (0.8%). The researchers believe that's because women who have mastectomies tended to have higher-grade cancers in the first place.

These findings all run counter to the dogma that DCIS is a precursor to cancer. And that more invasive cancer therapy leads to better outcomes.

To recap, the researchers found that 80% of DCIS diagnoses are low risk, and could be best treated by "prevention strategies."

My own personal experiences have shown me that an ounce of prevention is indeed worth a pound of "cure"— especially when it comes to cancer.

In 1977, my 82-year-old grandmother, a life-long resident of France, was diagnosed with DCIS.

She had never once in her life had surgery of any kind, and refused to have surgery then. Instead, doctors treated her with radiation to the chest. The cancer never spread and was "cured," but the radiation severely damaged her lung tissue. She developed respiratory failure and died in 1983.

I remember traveling to France after my grandmother's radiation treatments to try to find appropriate long-term care for her.

Shortly thereafter, I began professional research on risk factors for breast cancer, and eventually completed my Ph.D. dissertation on the topic. Even then, 30 years ago, the evidence pointed to nutrition, growth, and development during childhood, and reproductive factors during early adulthood, as the keys to whether a woman was likely to develop breast cancer. All of the attention at the National Cancer Institute on adult weight and dietary factors, such as fat intake, was completely misplaced.

Ironically, last summer, after 30 years and hundreds of millions of dollars in research funding, I read how a career cancer expert had just "discovered" we need to look at factors during childhood to control the breast cancer epidemic!

Noninvasive, effective steps you can take to lower your risk of breast cancer

It's clear that mainstream medicine has been way off in its approach to breast cancer—from useless mammography screenings, to mistaken assumptions about the dangers of DCIS, to largely ignoring childhood experiences, and the real dietary factors, and refusing to confront the reality of all the reproductive factors.

So what can you do to lower your risk of breast cancer? Here's my 4-step, evidence-based approach.

1. Load up on fruits and vegetables. A new study of 1,042 women found that carotenoids— alpha-carotene, beta-carotene, lycopene, lutein, and zeaxanthin— may help prevent breast cancer.[94] Not only are carotenoids powerful antioxidants that can protect against DNA damage, but the researchers noted that they may even help keep normal cells from mutating into cancerous cells.

Alpha-carotene is found in orange foods like pumpkin and carrots. Beta-carotene is also found in carrots, along with leafy greens and peppers. Lycopene is what makes foods like tomatoes, watermelon, and grapefruit red. And you can find high doses of lutein and zeaxanthin in leafy greens.

2. Take your daily vitamins. Of course, all of the fruits and vegetables I mentioned above are also high in B and C vitamins. But I also recommend taking a high-quality B-complex vitamin every day, along with 250 mg of C twice a day.

A variety of studies have shown that vitamin E can also help prevent breast cancer. I recommend 50 mg per day.

And it's no surprise that the wonder vitamin, D, has been shown in numerous studies to be protective against breast cancer. Or if you are diagnosed with breast cancer, a long-term study involving 4,443 women shows that taking higher levels of vitamin D improves quality of life and doubles your chances of survival.[95] I recommend 10,000 IU of D3 every day.

3. Eat calcium-rich foods. Research shows that calcium and vitamin D together are protective against breast cancer. It's essential you get calcium from your diet, as calcium supplements are ineffective and dangerous. So make sure to eat plenty of seafood and healthy meat and dairy.

4. Supplement with selenium. Research shows this mineral can help suppress a protein involved in tumor development, growth, and metastasis. In fact, an analysis of nine studies involving more than 150,000 people found that selenium supplementation cut the risk of all types of cancer by 24%.

I recommend 50-200 mcg of selenium each day.

Bottom line: If you have a breast biopsy that shows DCIS, be sure to consult with your doctor about *all* your options—not just invasive surgery and radiation. The new research shows that when it comes to treating breast cancer, for the vast majority of women, less is more.

Your 3-step DCIS risk-assessment checklist

To assess your own DCIS risk, answer the following questions:

1. Are you age 35 or younger? **YES / NO**

2. Are you African American? **YES / NO**

3. If you've been diagnosed with DCIS, are your DCIS cells higher-grade? (If you aren't sure, ask your oncologist) **YES / NO**

If you answered "YES" to any of these questions, more aggressive treatment may be warranted if you're diagnosed with DCIS. If not, chances are there's no harm in "watchful waiting."

Chapter 11

Vitamin D takes on the No. 1 cancer killer in America—and solves the single biggest shortcoming of mainstream medical treatments

If researchers really understood how vitamin D essentially functions as a hormone in every cell in the body, they would not be so surprised at finding its many other health benefits. In fact, a large new study shows that D can address the single biggest shortcoming of mainstream medical approaches and treatments.

I'm talking about solving the problem of lung cancer—the No. 1 cancer killer in America.

Real answers—beyond tobacco

I've reported before how real research on biology, prevention, screening, and treatment for lung cancer was stalled for decades in favor of pursuing the government's politically correct campaign against tobacco. Government bureaucrats touted smoking cessation as *the* (only) solution for stopping all lung cancers. The result of this misguided government initiative? Today, 60% of lung cancer victims are former smokers. And another 18% have *never* smoked at all.

That's 78% who already did the only thing the government has to offer—and got lung cancer anyway.

So what are these victims supposed to do?

Well, fortunately after decades of neglect, lung cancer screening and early detection is a reality again. There is, in fact, a safe and effective new MRI lung-cancer screening test that the government has finally approved. I recommend it for anyone—especially former smokers—who might be concerned they're still at risk for this deadly disease.

And even better, there's a simple way you can substantially reduce your chances of ever getting lung cancer.

All you have to do is take my recommended dose of 10,000 IU of vitamin D3 every day.

How the sunshine vitamin fights lung and other cancers

A new analysis of 12 studies involving nearly 300,000 men and women found that people who had the highest levels of vitamin D in their blood had 17% less risk of lung cancer compared to people with the lowest levels of D.

The researchers believe that vitamin D may not only help keep people from developing lung cancer, but it could also help prevent cancer cell metastasis and spread in those who already have lung cancer.

And that's not the only type of cancer this amazing vitamin can fight.

Another new study demonstrates that pancreatic cancer may well be linked to insufficient vitamin D.

The researchers analyzed the incidence of this often-fatal cancer in 107 countries. They found that people who live in areas with increased cloud cover and at higher latitudes (further away from equatorial sun) are *six times* more likely to be diagnosed with pancreatic cancer.

Why? Well, the more sunshine you can soak up every day, the more likely your body is to produce sufficient levels of vitamin D.

Interestingly, multiple sclerosis has also been observed to be more common in areas where there is less sun. I have long suspected that lack of vitamin D is a key factor in this disease as well.

D can help ensure a smooth and successful surgery

While I was analyzing the new vitamin D cancer studies, another research review caught my eye.

Scientists evaluated 31 studies on a total of 16,195 patients. They found that in a whopping 84% of the studies, people who had low levels of vitamin D in their blood had at least one adverse outcome after having major surgery.

For instance, in one of the studies the researchers reviewed, people who had pre-surgery vitamin D levels lower than 30 ng/ml were three to four times more likely to get an infection of their incision sites while they were in the hospital. (For optimum health—whether or not you're having surgery—I recommend the D levels in your blood be at least 30 ng/ml).

Another study reported that people who had a kidney transplant had an 8% higher risk of cancer for each ngl/mL decrease in their vitamin D level. And yet another study found that lung transplant patients with low D levels at the time of surgery, and for one year afterwards, had a death rate nearly *five times higher* compared to people with normal vitamin D status.

The authors of this study noted today's widespread deficiencies of D—due to the perfect storm of poor diet, lack of supplementation, and avid sun avoidance. They recommended that anyone about to have surgery boost their vitamin D intake.

So why are healthy D levels so important when you go under the knife? Well, surgery is a major stress on the body. And the more vitamin D you have circulating in your blood, the better your body is equipped to meet the demands of trauma and the requirements for healing.

Can you overdose on vitamin D?

Despite all of the evidence, some mainstream doctors and researchers cling to the myth that vitamin D may be toxic since it is fat soluble. The argument is that, unlike vitamins B and C, which can be excreted in your urine, if you have more D than your body can use, too much could theoretically build up to toxic levels in your body's fat and liver stores.

This concern is laughable given the actual data, and compared to the toxicities of the modern drugs that are doled out. And biologically, the reason the body stores vitamin D because it needs it!

Hopefully a big new Mayo Clinic study has finally put the mythical concerns about vitamin D safety to rest once and for all.

The researchers analyzed 20,308 vitamin D tests collected from patients over a 10-year period. Eight percent of those people had D levels that were considered high—over 50 ng/ml. Less than 1% had even higher levels over 80 ng/ml.

For years it was rumored that too much vitamin D in your blood can lead to a condition called hypercalcemia, or high blood calcium. Hypercalcemia has been associated with some cardiovascular diseases. (Which is one of the reasons why I recommend you never take calcium supplements. But rather get optimal levels of this vital mineral from foods like butter, eggs, meat, and seafood.)

But the Mayo Clinic researchers found there was no increased risk of hypercalcemia in any of the study participants—even the ones with high D levels.

In fact, out of the nearly 2,000 people with elevated vitamin D, only four of them had temporary, *mildly* elevated calcium levels within three months before and after testing.

This study just reinforces that vitamin D toxicity is one of the rarest of all observed medical conditions—and typically due to intentional intake of extremely high doses of vitamin D.

So how much D should you take? I recommend 10,000 IU of D3 a day.

If you live north of the latitude of Atlanta in the east, or Southern California in the west, the sun does not get strong enough to activate vitamin D synthesis in your body each year from November to March. So while I recommend supplementing with D3 year-round, it's particularly crucial not to miss your daily dose of D during winter months.

Chapter 12

Could this controversial South Pacific stress-reliever be a 21ˢᵗ century cancer miracle-in-the-making?

New research supports kava's striking comeback

When I was doing research fieldwork in the South Pacific in the late 1970s, I kept hearing about how effective a native pepper plant called kava was at fighting cancer.

And I wasn't the only one. In the 1980s, dozens of research studies emerged showing the anti-cancer benefits of regular kava consumption.

In fact, in 1985, *The Hawaii Medical Journal* published research showing that in Fiji, where many people drink kava tea every day, there were 75 incidences of lung cancer per 100,000 men.

Guess what the number was in Los Angeles? 307.

More than *four times* as many lung cancer diagnoses as Fiji.

As I continued studying populations in the Pacific during the 1980s and '90s, I actually found I knew many of the scientists involved in making these early anti-cancer kava discoveries.

And their research was so impressive, I began referring to kava as "The Tane Secret." Tane (pronounced "tah-neigh") is the Polynesian god of nature—and in an even broader sense, the god of all good.

I think it's a fitting name because, as you'll see, this natural wonder has been helping the peoples of the South Pacific for centuries—and is now astonishing scientists in the world's most modern laboratories.

I'll tell you more about this exciting new research in just a moment. But first, let me fill you in on why you may not have heard of kava's cancer-fighting potential before now.

Another natural cancer breakthrough derailed by flawed research

You see, despite the promising evidence that emerged some 30 years ago, not everyone embraced the Tane Secret. In fact, it had its traditional name dragged through the mud for years.

More than a decade ago, further research into this herb was <u>completely derailed</u>. All because of a false scare about the plant's effects on the liver.

I did my best to fight this ignorance. In 2003, I asked leading European researchers to prepare a review of scientific studies showing the absence of toxicity in kava. I published it in the premier volume of my scientific journal, *Reviews in Integrative Medicine*.

That research review found that prescription drugs—*not* kava—were responsible for the liver problems.

It took others longer to make this realization, but they finally saw the light. Kava's supposed liver toxicity has now been debunked.

A ban on the herb was finally lifted in Germany. And research into kava's anti-cancer benefits continues.

The results have been impressive, to say the least.

Studies show The Tane Secret puts 7 different kinds of cancer in the crosshairs

Past research results has shown kava root extract to prevent lung tumors in *99 percent* of lab mice.

And other recent research is showing that kava may be effective at preventing breast, bladder, bone, colon, uterine, and prostate cancer as well.

Here's closer look at the evidence showing how this simple plant may be able to fight cancer naturally. *And* how the government-industrial-medical complex is preventing you from finding that out.

Why you don't hear about natural cancer fighters

The sad truth is, there are many natural products hiding in plain sight that appear to be effective at preventing and treating cancer. But they're ignored by the mainstream since they can't be patented as drugs. And because they often act by modifying the growth of cancerous cells and tumors, instead of outright killing them.

You see, when government cancer experts screen natural products for anti-cancer activity, they look only for the ability to kill cancer cells. What they don't take into account is that if something can kill cancer cells, it can and will also kill your normal cells. Which, of course, results in tragic and unnecessary side effects like you find with chemotherapy.

But government science bureaucrats simply ignore other important kinds of anti-cancer activity. Like preventing new blood vessels from supporting the growth of cancerous tumors, or starving cancer cells (instead of feeding them like typical oncology regimens). Other proven (but ignored) mechanisms include boosting the immune system to naturally eliminate cancer cells and transforming cancer cells back to "normal" cells.

Because of this scientific and economic bias in the cancer industry, natural products that are found to be effective at fighting cancer in laboratory studies just don't make it into hugely expensive human cancer treatment trials. And thus into mainstream cancer-fighting regimens.

That's why most kava studies are done on animals. Take, for example, the lung cancer study I mentioned earlier.

Mice were given a kava dietary supplement on a daily basis. The researchers then tried to chemically induce lung tumors in the mice. But they failed 99 percent of the time.

Think about that: 99 percent. A prevention rate that high is unprecedented among cancer studies using nutrients and natural products.

In fact, for any substance—natural or pharmacological—to qualify for funding for human studies, National Cancer Institute experts are thrilled if it can reduce cancer by four times, three times, or even two times (like the typical range of many vitamins and minerals).

But they ignore a finding that reduces cancer by 99 times. Unbelievable.

How much kava do you need?

Of course, when it comes to any health effect—including anti-cancer effects—the potency of a nutrient or herb (or drug, for that matter) is directly related to its ability to enter the body's tissues.

And because there has been so little human research into kava, there's a big question about just how well it does that. Consequently, scientists aren't really sure how much of the herb our bodies need to help prevent cancer.

South Pacific islanders are known to consume as much as 10 grams of kava a day. That's more than *30 times* the typical supplement dose. And as you see from the accompanying table, the more kava, the lower the cancer rates.

So how do the Polynesians ingest so much kava?

Well, they drink their kava rather than take it in pill form. In fact, the traditional method is to brew fresh or dried kava roots into a tea made with <u>local water</u>.

I'm not talking about Fiji Water—that expensive bottled stuff that is shipped 10,000 miles overseas (talk about a carbon footprint).

I'm talking about the water actually drunk in Fiji. As we learn more about the health properties of the water itself, and its interactions with the natural constituents in kava, I suspect it will prove to play a key role in the disease-fighting effects of the traditional kava drink of Fiji and the South Pacific. Because when it comes to winning the "war on cancer," the South Pacific may hold the key—just as it did in ultimately winning World War II.

In the meantime, it's not a big mental stretch to <u>imagine a beverage sold in the U.S. that mimics the effective dose of a traditional Fiji kava tea.</u>

Until that happens, though, you have a few different options when it comes to supplementing with kava for its traditional use as a relaxant and stress-reliever.

First there are capsules. The recommend dose is 400 mg a day (in the evening).

You can also find ground kava root powder, which can be mixed directly into water or juice. Like coffee, kava powders can be course- or fine-ground. If you opt for course-ground, it needs to be strained prior to drinking it.

Similarly, dried kava root is also available, and can be steeped in water, then strained.

Regardless of which form you choose, make sure it's organic.

Here are a couple of online sources to consider:

- **Herbal Island** (herbal-island.com)—This Utah-based company imports its kava products from Fiji, and offers a good variety of products.

- **Kona Kava Farm** (konakavafarm.com)—This company grows its kava in Hawaii (where climate is similar to the South Pacific) and adheres to strict FDA-compliant good manufacturing practices (GMP). They also offer a wide variety of kava products.

Keep in mind, most people report that kava doesn't have a pleasant flavor. It can also cause some numbness in the lips and tongue in some people. However, these effects are typically mild and temporary. Most people find the resulting relaxing effects on the body and mind very enjoyable.

Of course, quality and effects appear to vary greatly among sources, so it's important to look at existing feedback from other customers—and share your own about any products you decide to try.

There is more that kava can do...

Kava has been proven to tackle health issues beyond cancer. In fact, the herb has long been used in Hawaii, Fiji, Samoa, Vanuatu, and other exotic Polynesian locations as an effective anti-anxiety agent. Maybe that's why U.S. presidents from Lyndon Johnson to Bill Clinton sampled kava drinks during their election-year trips to American Samoa.

Earlier research on the muscle and nerve-relaxing benefits of kava focused on a specific compound: kavalactones.

Kavalactones are bound to lactic acid, which plays a prominent role in alternative energy-producing metabolic pathways in muscles and other tissues when they run out of oxygen (a process called anaerobic respiration).

This ability to produce energy without using oxygen probably harkens back to the biological equipment we inherited from aquatic cells— before oxygen accumulated in the atmosphere and life emerged from the oceans about 300 million years ago.

Accordingly, muscles are tissues in our bodies that are well-adapted to using alternate anaerobic respiration. They have an extraordinary ability to store lactic acid until it can eventually be eliminated from the body.

Because kavalactones are bound to lactic acid, I believe they can also be stored in muscles. And that helps produce kava's remarkable relaxing, anti-anxiety properties.

Chapter 13

Five foods to beat breast cancer

There are plenty of things you can do right now to reduce your breast cancer risk—and to improve your survival rate if you *do* get breast cancer.

In fact, time and again, research shows women have a much lower risk of developing breast cancer (as well as most other cancers) if they eat more of five key foods.

1. Broccoli

We have known about the ability of broccoli and other cruciferous vegetables to reduce cancer risk, especially breast cancer risk, for nearly 100 years. In fact, this knowledge first came to light during the British Empire Cancer Campaign studies in the 1920s.

But when the National Cancer Institute (NCI) finally started studying diet and cancer 60 years later, in the 1980s, they first chose to focus on carotenoids—specifically beta-carotene—as *the* "magic bullet" for cancer without any real evidence. And we all know how that turned out.

I started in another direction and analyzed the nutrient composition of broccoli with the USDA Human Nutrition Research Lab to first find out what nutrients are actually in cancer-preventive foods. Since I previously worked in forensic pathology as a Medical Examiner, I knew I should first get the evidence before jumping to conclusions! Sure enough, we found that broccoli is rich in many vitamins and phytonutrients, including carotenoids—but just not beta-carotene.

But the NCI persisted in barking up the wrong tree about beta-carotene, even trying to suppress publication of my research. As soon as I left the NCI to become an associate medical director at Walter Reed, I published the research and, in fact, received the "Young Investigator" Award at Walter Reed for doing it.

However, the NCI continued to ignore the USDA evidence and many other similar studies that followed. Arguably, they set back diet and cancer prevention research by dozens of years and millions of dollars.

Today, most experts (even at NCI) understand broccoli is a potent anti-cancer agent. But it's not enough to know broccoli protects you against cancer. They want to know *how* and *why* it works.

Well, while these scientists continue to spend time and money hashing out exactly why and how eating broccoli works…you can take the direct route…and just eat more of it.

I recommend eating broccoli and other cruciferous vegetables several times a week. They're delicious steamed with any fish or meat dish. You can also sauté broccoli with garlic and olive oil for a delicious stand-alone dish. It's also delicious served cold after cooking dressed with some olive oil and/or vinegar.

2. Garlic

Garlic contains numerous compounds that appear to prevent cancer by slowing the formation and growth of tumors, and interfering with cancer cells. In Eastern and Southern Europe—and in many parts of Asia and South America—people regularly incorporate garlic into their traditional cuisine. In European folk medicine, it is used as a remedy for treating early onset colds and flus. Lab studies show many benefits for the blood, heart and immune system as well.

Of course, you can add garlic for flavor in many dishes. You can insert garlic cloves into any meat before roasting. You can also add it raw in smaller amounts to salads.

Try this: Cut a garlic clove and rub it over the lid of the cooking pan, or run it around the inside of a salad bowl.

I see a lot of garlic salt on grocery store shelves. And manufacturers sell a lot of garlic supplements. But it's always better to stick with the fresh garlic. And it's easy to do.

Fresh garlic naturally retains its potency and flavor. In fact, until you "peel" or open it, the garlic clove will stay potent for months at a time. Always store whole cloves in open air—such as in a basket or ventilated clay pot—at room temperature away from direct sunlight.

3. Olive oil

Olive oil also gets a lot of attention for its anti-cancer activity. Scientists speculate that olive oil's "antioxidant" properties also contribute to its other benefits, such as reducing cardiovascular diseases and preventing heart attacks and strokes. Of course, it helps balance blood lipids (blood fats) as well, which could possibly help account for heart and other benefits.

I recommend using olive oil liberally in cooking and in salads. Always store it in a dark place at room temperature. Keep just enough on hand at a time to last about three months, so it will always stay fresh.

4. Salmon

Salmon comes up on my list because it promotes healthy cell growth and helps prevent breast cancer. Of course, it also has many other health benefits. It contains the all-important omega-3 fatty acids, which play a critical role in supporting the brain, heart and immune system. Plus, like other healthy fish and meat, it has high levels of bioavailable B vitamins and vitamin D, which are very difficult to get from even the healthiest vegetables.

Always make sure to buy wild-caught salmon. Farm-raised salmon can have as little as one-tenth of the key nutrients. Plus, they often contain high levels of heavy metals such as mercury and other toxins.

Unfortunately, virtually all Atlantic salmon today are farm-raised, whether from Scotland or Nova Scotia. So, ignore the crazy color-coding at places like Whole Foods and just make sure your salmon comes from the Pacific.

5. Turmeric (Curcumin)

With each passing year, we learn more and more about the role this ancient spice turmeric (curcumin) can play in preventing and treating breast cancer. One study from Southeast Asia shows women who eat more turmeric have a lower risk of metastatic breast cancer.

But remember—as I mentioned earlier with broccoli—scientists today don't just accept that something works. They want to know how and why it works. Fortunately, we are making good progress in that area of research on turmeric.

In fact, according to a comprehensive report from 2013 in the *Journal of Breast Cancer*, we now know turmeric incites cell death and inhibits tumor cell growth. It also inhibits the movement of breast cancer cells along known pathways in the body. Of course turmeric is also known for its potent anti-inflammatory activity. (Indeed, it's also a key component what I call the "ABCs of Joint Health".)

I should probably also mention three foods many so-called experts tout as cancer-busters. But really—you may be better off avoiding them…

First, there's green tea. Experts always seem to put it on the list for anti-cancer benefits. And many lab studies do show epigallocatechin gallate (EGCG) in tea has anti-cancer activities. But I wonder whether these experts have done the calculations to translate the lab research to real everyday people and drinking habits.

You would have to drink 16 cups per day of green tea to get active doses of EGCG. Plus, even if you *could* drink that much every day, at that point you get exposed to acids and oxalates that can cause GI problems and kidney stones. Not to mention the toxins in the paper and plastics used for "tea bags" and filters. Also, recent studies show we can attribute Asian women's increased longevity and health to other dietary factors besides green tea, such as hot chili peppers.

Cow's milk is the second anti-cancer dud. Some experts tell you milk protects women from breast cancer, perhaps because it's relatively high in vitamin D. But remember, manufacturers artificially add that vitamin D to cow's milk. Plus, research links cow's milk consumption during infancy and childhood to *greater* long-term risks of breast and other cancers. I uncovered this startling fact doing my Ph.D. dissertation research.

So skip the milk. But keep the vitamin D.

You may do this by spending 15 minutes in the sun every day without sunscreen between April and October to boost your vitamin D stores. Also—supplement daily with 10,000 IU of vitamin D all year long.

And finally, some experts still make woefully misguided claims about the benefits of soy. But don't buy into it. The processed soy found in products like soy milk and veggie burgers contains phytoestrogens, which can disrupt hormonal balance in both women and men. Also, virtually all soybeans grown in the U.S. today are genetically modified (GM), which is a disaster for ecology and the environment.

So now you know which foods to keep on the menu. And which foods to leave off.

Chapter 14

"Frat-boy diet" discovery leads to
ultimate prostate protection

I've written before about the government's failed campaign to promote beta-carotene as an anti-cancer solution. The more my colleagues at USDA's Beltsville Human Nutrition Research Center and I delved into the research, the clearer it became: There was no correlation between dietary or blood levels of beta-carotene and cancer.

In other words, beta-carotene was not the cancer savior the National Cancer Institute promoted it to be.

But something good did come out of the research my colleagues and I conducted some 25 years ago…

We found that while beta-carotene doesn't protect against cancer, other carotenoids—such as lutein and lycopene—*do*.

At the time, no one had ever heard of these carotenoids before. Of course, since then they've become much more well-known. In fact, lycopene has taken center stage for being highly protective against prostate cancer. And it really should be at the top of every man's prostate cancer prevention priority list—followed by a few other specific nutrients. There's also one very important step you should take when supplementing with these nutrients to ensure you get their full protective benefits.

I'll give you all the details in just a moment. But first, let's take a closer look at lycopene.

Pizza, burgers, fries…and healthy prostates?

When we performed our original study on dietary consumption and blood levels of carotenoids, we were initially amazed at the high levels of lycopene among young college students from our local state school, the University of Maryland.

When we broke this down further, we found the students had very high consumption of some seemingly "unhealthy" foods— like pizza, hamburgers, and French fries. But all of these foods had one thing in common: tomatoes.

The pizza, of course, was topped with thick tomato sauce. And the burgers and fries were typically doused with a hefty serving of ketchup.

In nature, of course, tomatoes are the primary abundant food source of lycopene. And when they're heated and concentrated during the manufacturing process to produce ketchup, tomato sauce, or other tomato-based products, the natural lycopene actually becomes more concentrated and remains bio-available.

Contadina tomato paste was famous for getting "eight great tomatoes in that little, bitty can." And tomato paste is essentially like a concentrated lycopene supplement.

Even lycopene's "side effects" are benefits

Since our discovery of lycopene at the USDA, numerous studies have demonstrated that this nutrient not only reduces prostate cancer risk, but also heart and circulatory disorders, immunologic dysfunction, and general inflammation.

Granted, not all the studies on lycopene have been positive. But this probably represents differences between using a therapeutic "dose" and an ineffective level of consumption.

For example, population studies show that a minimum daily intake is essential for disease prevention. Some studies have seen positive results with doses as low as 3-5 mg per day. But others have shown more promising results with daily consumption of 10-12 mg.

The most recent study, published in the journal *Neurology* showed a decreased risk in stroke with just 10 mg of lycopene per day. More than 50 percent decreased risk, to be precise. A truly remarkable feat.

Especially when you consider how easy it is to get 10 mg of lycopene. Even without supplements. A wedge of watermelon, for example, has about 12 mg of lycopene. And a cup of tomato juice has even more, of course, at 22 mg of lycopene.

Even the most effective drugs hardly come close to this magnitude of benefit. And they're usually associated with negative side effects.

Meanwhile, the "side effects" of lycopene are a simply more benefits. For example, studies completed at the University of Kentucky show that elderly individuals consuming 30 mg of lycopene had significantly enhanced preservation of memory.

And lycopene was enough to keep a substantial segment of the population free-living and independent—without requiring an extended-care facility. Such a simple step would result in substantial savings in health care costs. Not to mention a great improvement in the quality of life for senior citizens.

In other studies, eyesight problems, including macular degeneration, were significantly decreased by the consumption of lycopene.

Lycopene even appears to offer some "anti-aging" and cosmetic benefits. The consumption of lycopene has been shown to decrease the development of wrinkles. And it may be able to diminish your reaction to sunburn.

So this simple nutrient can protect you from harmful UV rays without toxic and dangerous "sun blocks." As an added benefit, it still allows you to get enough sun for healthy vitamin D levels. And getting optimal vitamin D is important for cancer prevention, including prostate cancer.

Four more nutrients to round out perfect prostate support

Speaking of nutrients to support prostate health, here is the complete list of my specific recommendations:

Lycopene: 5 to 15 mg
Selenium: 100 mcg
Vitamin D: 2,000 IU
Vitamin E: 50 IU

One important note: All of these nutrients are fat-soluble—which means taking them <u>with</u> an oil increases their absorption and their effectiveness.

So I also recommend taking a fish oil supplement, 1-2 grams per day. If you absolutely can't bring yourself to take fish oil, at the very least, you should opt for some other source of omega-3 fatty acids. And don't forget to eat plenty of fish, tomatoes, and other food sources of the above nutrients. See the box below for a list of good options.

Remember, people eat foods, not nutrients. Tomatoes, and other foods with lycopene also have an extensive array of other antioxidants and phytonutrients. It is important to remember that other carotenoids and flavonoids in foods often have synergistic benefits.

Of course, how foods are grown is also important to preserve their nutrient content, as well as their taste.

Prostate protection on your plate	
Nutrient	Food source
Lycopene	Tomatoes, tomato products (ketchup, tomato sauce, tomato paste, tomato juice), guava, watermelon, pink grapefruit, cherries
Vitamin D	Swordfish, salmon, tuna, sardines, liver, egg yolk
Selenium	Brazil nuts, tuna, halibut, sardines, shrimp, ham
Vitamin E	Sunflower seeds, almonds, hazelnuts, peanut butter
Omega-3 fatty acids	Fish oil, salmon, mackerel, cauliflower, chia seeds, flax seeds, walnuts

Harvesting your health

I admit that I'm more than a little skeptical of the so-called "organic" movement—at least since big government and big industry have stepped in.

And a recent study from Stanford University Center for Health Policy has cast more doubt on "organic" farming. Researchers examined data from 237 previous studies. They found that when it comes to certain nutrients, there is not much difference between organic and conventionally grown foods.

However, studies have shown that the levels of lycopene in organic tomatoes are at least double those in conventional tomatoes.

These days, it's easy to substantially improve your health with in-season consumption of locally grown tomatoes and other brightly colored fruits and vegetables. They not only taste better, but will yield long-term health benefits.

The surprising origin of this Italian staple

Tomatoes were originally called *tomatl* and cultivated among the Aztec in MesoAmerica (modern central Mexico). When the Spanish brought them back to europe in the 1500s, they were initially considered poisonous as a member of the *Solinacea* family which includes other plants such as "deadly nightshade." Believe it or not, tomatoes did not appear on an Italian menu until the 1700s. But by the time mass immigration of Italians to the U.S. occurred in the later 1800's, tomato sauce had been firmly established as an "Italian American" dish.

PART 2

HEALING PAIN INSTEAD OF TREATING PAIN

Chapter 15

The problem with pain:
Another reason the government
is literally a pain in the neck...
(and back, and head, etc.)

In the history of American medicine, alleviating pain has been one of the two central tenants of "rational medicine." (Preventing death was the other). Unfortunately, there's nothing rational about the way mainstream medicine handles pain relief these days.

From the arid mountains of Afghanistan, to the jungles of Honduras, from the gritty urban streets of New York, to the fruited plains of Nebraska, the government is hard at work protecting you from pain... medications.

You see, we live in an era where another misguided government "war"— this one on drugs—is intimidating competent and honest doctors and nurses. Keeping them from prescribing and administering adequate pain medication in effective doses. Even for those on their deathbeds, who often must suffer their last moments on earth in debilitating pain.

All under the guise of "protecting" the public from becoming addicted to pain killers.

If the situation sounds bleak, well...in many ways, it is. But before you give up hope, there is good news.

The fact is, there are many alternatives that can offer you *real relief*. For just about any type of pain. Ones you won't hear about from the government medical bureaucracy. (Whose agenda has nothing to do with actually helping those who are suffering.)

So let me tell you a bit about why the "War on Drugs" has turned into a "War on People in Pain."

The best painkiller on earth that the government is desperate to keep out of your hands

Despite its potential for misuse, the opium poppy (*Papaver somniferum*) has been one of nature's best gifts to humankind. It is, without a doubt, the world's most effective pain medicine. Opium is the source of morphine and all its various modern derivatives.

And to this day, even in our era of modern pharmaceuticals, morphine and morphine derivatives still have unmatched pain relieving and other healing properties. And they remain in widespread use throughout the world.

The reason they're so effective is that our brains and central nervous systems have built-in receptors for the opiates in these medications. It's a match made in pain-relief heaven.

But, unfortunately, like many good things, opium also has a history of abuse. And that's where the focus has been for centuries.

So although morphine, hydromorphone, oxycodone, and codeine remain the gold standard opioid analgesics, the ham-fisted prosecution of drug wars has made many good doctors afraid to prescribe them. And as a result, the pharmaceutical industry has put out a slew of rival analgesics. These rival pain meds are less restricted than the opioids. The problem is, they're also typically less effective. And more toxic.

53 years of useless—and dangerous— "relief"

For example, until recently, roughly 10 million Americans were taking the painkilling drug propoxyphene (sold as Darvon and Darvocet). But in November 2010, the FDA pulled it from the market because of serious heart risks. But here's the really interesting part of the Darvon story…

While it is classified by the DEA and FDA as a narcotic, it has <u>never</u> been shown in controlled studies to be even a **weak** analgesic.

In other words, it has all of the stimulating, addictive effects of opioids. But *none* of the pain-relieving benefits. Yet the FDA approved it for that very use back in the 1950s. Putting millions of people at risk for addiction, heart complications, and who knows what else for 53 years. Risk with absolutely no "reward" in the form of relief.

Then, to add insult to injury, the FDA recommended doctors switch patients to other painkillers, notably Extra Strength Tylenol (acetaminophen).

Take that advice and you trade in risk of heart problems for liver failure.

That's right. This common, over-the-counter painkiller—found in nearly every medicine cabinet in America—causes hundreds of deaths each year due to liver toxicity. But until now (there was finally a class action suit filed in 2012) nobody talked about it.

It's yet another example of major medical mismanagement spawned by ill-informed politicians and misbegotten government regulatory agencies.

But, again, just because the government denies citizens access to one form of effective pain relief doesn't mean you have to suffer. In fact, there are many other effective, natural options for alleviating pain.

The whole-body approach to pain relief

Conventional medicine is always focused on suppressing symptoms. And it frequently assumes that the location of pain is also the site of its cause and origin. Thus, knee pain is generally assumed to be a knee problem, shoulder pain is assumed to be a shoulder problem, and so forth.

This pain-centered diagnostic logic frequently leads to increasingly sophisticated and invasive diagnostic and therapeutic procedures. For example, if physical examination of the knee fails to define the problem clearly, the knee is x-rayed. If the x-ray film fails to offer adequate clarification, magnetic resonance imaging (MRI) of the knee is performed, and in some cases a surgical procedure follows.

All the while, this search for knee pain may be missing the obvious fact that the pain is caused by misalignment of the hip at the pelvis.

We should all remember the song from our childhood: "The knee bone's connected to the hip bone, the hip bone's connected to the back bone...."

The chiropractic approach to musculoskeletal pain involves evaluating the site of pain in a both regional and whole-body context.

Although shoulder, elbow, and wrist problems can be caused by injuries or pathologies in these areas, pain in and around each of the shoulder, elbow, and wrist joints can also have as its source segmental dysfunction (subluxation) in the cervical spine.

Similarly, symptoms in the hip, knee, and ankle can also originate at the site of the pain, but in many cases the source lies in the lumbar spine or sacroiliac joints. Pain in the knee might come from the knee itself, but tracing the nerve pathways between the knee and the spine reveals possible areas of causation in and around the hip, in the deep muscles of the buttocks or pelvis, in the sacroiliac joints, or in the lumbar spine.

Of course, chiropractors also use diagnostic tools such as radiography and MRI. The point isn't to disregard these technologies completely, but to present an alternative diagnostic model.

After all, it happens all too frequently where a patient undergoes this entire high-tech diagnostic scenario. After suffering through it waiting for a "diagnosis," the poor patient finally stumbles into the chiropractor (if he or she can still walk!). And finally, his or her knee problem is discovered to be a compensation for a mechanical disorder in the lower back.

Of course, even despite months of needless suffering, patients are still fortunate if they find the chiropractor before they agree to surgery.

The point here is that chiropractic SMT can provide effective relief even for pain that doesn't seem to have anything to do with your back or spine. Research shows it can be effective for neck pain, leg pain, headaches, and more.

Chapter 16

Chronic back pain wiped out with a surgery-free treatment

I always stress the importance of your gait (or how well you walk) as a key to health and longevity, especially as you get older. But it's not about *how much you walk*. It's about *how well you walk*. And indeed, it's the ability to walk upright that sets humans apart—but it's also what sets up for a lot of pain as well.

Walking has been a key factor in the ability of humans to survive. In fact, the ability to walk upright on two legs is a distinctly human trait. And throughout human history, this trait has freed the hands so that, together with larger brains, humans could express their creativity and productivity to build our modern, "man-made" world.

One important trade-off is that in order to walk (and run) more effectively, the legs needed to be placed more narrowly together than they are on other, four-footed mammals. This effect results in a narrower pelvis, especially at the hips.

However, humans have developed very large brains. So women need to have wider hips to allow infants to pass safely through the birth canal. (*Interesting side note:* Humans are the only animals who have such potentially difficult delivery, which is why we call it "labor.")

But since you can't walk effectively if the hips are <u>too</u> wide, human infants were born at earlier and earlier stages of development, while the brain is still immature.

So human young are the most immature creatures in the universe, and require a prolonged period of dependency—with implications for nuclear family, extended family, post-reproductive grandparents, and human social organization as a whole.

Consider it a grand evolutionary biological compromise between upright posture, freeing the hands, and having bigger brains.

But there's another tremendous impact that walking upright has had on humans. One that millions of people struggle with every day—back pain.

From discomfort to disability

The spine provides structure to the entire body and helps protect the vital organs. It also provides the protective conduit for the "wiring" that runs to all the parts of the body—the spinal cord and the spinal nerves.

In animals that walk on all fours, the natural design of the spine is like a simple suspension bridge. But over time (millions of years, probably), humans began to stand erect. And the shape of the spine converted from a suspension bridge to a shallow S-shaped (or sigmoid) curve... to provide balance, structural support, and some "suspension" as well as "shock absorption."

But as you can imagine, pounding away against hard surfaces while walking not only affects the joints of the legs, but the shock waves work their way up through the pelvis to the spinal column and the individual vertebrae. The result is degenerative arthritis, or osteoarthritis in the spine.

And just like in other joints, osteoarthritis of the spinal vertebrae can lead to stiffness. As well as contribute to bony outgrowths that can impact and irritate the spinal nerves that branch out from the spinal cord. These kinds of irritations are common in the arms and the legs ("pinched nerves"). And on a chronic basis, they can cause the familiar condition of "sciatica."

In the spine itself, the middle 12 vertebra are held relatively rigid by the ribs, but the seven cervical vertebrae in the neck, and the five lumbar vertebrae of the lower back have more degrees of freedom, and less support. Which is why lower back pain is such a universal source of discomfort in humans.

Of course, when there is a sudden rupture of a spinal disc (or cushion), or even a traumatic fracture of a portion of a vertebra, there can be sudden debilitating pain.

However, even without a sudden rupture or traumatic fracture, low back pain can be disabling. In fact, it's the most common cause of disability in working Americans (those who still have work).

Why back surgery should be your last resort

Low back pain may be an unavoidable consequence of walking upright. But living with it doesn't need to be.

And there are treatments for back pain that are much safer—not to mention more effective—than dangerous painkilling drugs and potentially disastrous back surgery.

In fact, surgery should be your absolute last resort. The results can be debilitating. And there's no "going back" from surgery.

Back surgery has become such a problem that is has actually spawned a new medical condition, called "failed back" syndrome. And there are doctors who specialize in treating people with it. It's become a kind of "crisis." But as I said to Pennsylvania Governor Ed Rendell at a U.S. Congressional Field Hearing in Pennsylvania in February 2003, perhaps this crisis is a blessing in disguise. Because it should finally help open the door for the effective, non-surgical treatments that can help the vast majority of people with back pain.

To his great credit (on this and many other public policy issues), Governor Rendell was genuinely concerned and refreshingly open-minded. And a few weeks later, he contacted me to provide all the details on these alternatives to his office in Harrisburg.

That information included overwhelming evidence about one particular—and *completely non-invasive*—treatment that works for almost every person who tries it...

Surgery-free pain relief

Spinal manual therapy (SMT), is the most effective and cost-effective treatment for most patients with low back pain. SMT is a technique for adjusting the alignment of the spinal vertebrae and other joints. Many believe that in addition to aligning the body adjustment balances the energy flow through the body similar to the concepts of many

Asian medical therapies. SMT is the primary treatment provided by chiropractors.

Chiropractors have historically emphasized the intimate relations in the body between **structure and function**, the mediating role of the **nervous system**, and the need for restoration and maintenance of structural and functional **balance** of the spine and musculoskeletal system. From this perspective, balance is the key—and the presence or absence of pain is incidental. For patients, however, pain is almost always the primary concern.

In recent years, the mainstreaming of chiropractic has taken many forms. Low back guidelines from government agencies in the United States, Great Britain, Australia, New Zealand, Denmark and Sweden have recognized spinal manipulation as one of a very small number of effective treatment methods for lower back pain.

In fact, a decade ago the former U.S. Agency for Health Care Policy & Research conducted a review and found SMT to be the most safe and effective treatment. Unlike the NIH, this agency was focused on using research and science to help guide rational medical practices. Things that would actually benefit the public.

Of course, their recommendation for SMT outraged orthopedic surgeons. So much so that they attempted to have the agency shut down. When that didn't work, they tried to have it de-funded. Eventually, they managed to at least get the office reorganized. (Today it's known as the Agency for Health Care Quality, and has little power to actually influence medical practice compared to the "medical mandarins" at NIH, or the federal purse strings controlled by Health Care Finance Administration and the Center for Medicare and Medicaid Services.)

But I digress…

At about this same time—during 2002-2003—I received a grant from the US Health Resources and Services Administration (another rare honest broker) to review all the studies on low back pain that had been done worldwide.

I worked with the Palmer College Research Consortium and a dozen other universities and scores of scientists around the country. And found—no matter how you sliced it—that spinal manual therapy (SMT) is indeed a safe and effective treatment for low back pain.

And, even better—it's easy to access. There are over 50,000 practicing chiropractors in the US (all of them from accredited schools). They are licensed in every state. But if you can't find a chiropractor near you for some reason, physical therapists also provide effective SMT.

Other useful therapies for low back pain include massage and acupuncture. But with the overwhelming evidence for and easy availability of SMT, most people should try it first.

Three herbal pain soothers worth a try

While they're not a substitute for effective spinal manual therapies, there are several herbs that can help relieve pain. They include:
- Boswellia serratta extract (gum)—400 -500 mg/day
- Curcuma longa (root) (Tumeric)—200 mg/day
- Withania somnifera (root extract) (Ashwaganda)—500 mg/day

Chapter 17

Managing migraines without drugs

Headache is probably the single most common cause of pain experienced regularly by most people. And the most difficult type of headache to treat is the migraine. But, again, there are very effective natural treatments. Ones that can actually keep migraines from occurring in the first place. And if you've ever had a migraine, you know that an ounce of prevention is definitely worth a pound of cure.

But before I get to the natural solutions for treating and preventing migraines, let's back up a step and talk about the onset of these often-debilitating headaches.

Too quick to pull the migraine trigger?

If you suffer from migraines, you may think chocolate or bright lights trigger your headaches. So you avoid these triggers at all costs. But that cause-and-effect relationship may not be as strong as you think.

In fact, Dutch scientists recently took a close look at two classic migraine triggers: exercise and bright light. The scientists wanted to know if exposure to classic triggers always results in migraine attacks. And are migraine "triggers" as strong as patients believe?

For the study, a team of researchers led by Anders Hougaard, M.D. recruited 27 migraine sufferers. Each of the patients said that bright or flickering lights or strenuous activity triggered their migraines. So, the researchers tried to *provoke* migraines in the patients using these reported triggers.

They exposed the patients to bright lights, strenuous activity, or a combination of both triggers. Only three patients (11 percent) actually had migraine attacks with aura following these provocative tests. Three other patients reported migraines but without aura. The researchers discovered that exercise proved a stronger trigger than light exposure.

Dr. Hougaard suggested that these results could benefit migraine patients. "Migraine patients are usually advised to identify triggers and try and avoid them," he told *Medscape Medical News*. "But our research suggests that this may be limiting people's lives and causing unnecessary stress in trying to avoid a wide range of factors which may turn out not to be triggers after all."

In fact, Dr. Hougaard warns migraine patients to carefully evaluate whether or not something is an actual trigger. He said, "Patients need to try to identify triggers but they need to establish that they are true triggers before cutting them out of their lives. So I would advise that they allow several exposures before defining a trigger."

So if you suffer from migraines, be very careful before you blindly cut out all "classic" triggers. Especially since many purported triggers—such as sunlight, exercise, wine, coffee, chocolate, and cheese—are actually *good* for you in moderation!

Plus, many other factors affect your threshold for a migraine attack. In fact, your fatigue, your hormone levels, and even the time of day can make you more vulnerable to an attack. For instance, how tired were you when you drank that glass of wine? Or were certain hormones high when you went for that three-mile run in the bright morning light?

In addition, you may confuse migraine "triggers" with cravings or certain behaviors. We know that feelings of tiredness, excitement, and depression, or food cravings often *precede* migraines. So, you may think eating chocolate triggers the migraine. But it's really a warning signal. Doctors call it a "premonitory symptom."

For example, you may crave chocolate one afternoon, so you eat a small piece of a candy bar. By dinnertime, you have a migraine. You kick yourself and think the chocolate triggered the migraine. But chocolate wasn't really the trigger. The craving was actually part of the onset of the migraine itself.

My former colleague, Stephen D. Silberstein, M.D., is a Professor of Neurology and Director of the headache center at Thomas Jefferson University. He agrees that avoiding triggers may be flawed advice. He says, "If migraine is a disorder of habituation of the brain to ordinary sensory signals, should one try to train the brain to habituate rather than avoid the trigger?"

That may explain why biofeedback helps so many migraine sufferers. With biofeedback, you learn to control your body's functions. You watch or listen to a monitor. And you learn by trial and error to control your heart rate, temperature, even your brain wave patterns. With biofeedback, can you may even be able to train your brain to handle exposure to so-called triggers, as my colleague suggests.

If you suffer from migraines, I recommend investigating biofeedback along with other "mind-body" therapies. You should choose these therapies based on your emotional "type." I explain all about this in my book *Your Emotional Type*.

But there are several other natural ways to manage migraines in addition to biofeedback.

Feverfew is probably the most well-known natural migraine remedy. This herb is a short, bushy flowering plant that grows in fields and along roadsides and blooms from July to October. The leaves have been used for all sorts of medicinal purposes since the ancient Greek and Roman physicians. Recently, though, it was approved for treating migraine headaches in both the United Kingdom and Canada.

A dried feverfew leaf preparation containing a minimum of 0.2% parthenolide (the active ingredient) is effective for preventing migraines. You'll need at least 125 mg per day.

Although it's most commonly used to improve cognitive function, **Ginkgo biloba** may also help ward off migraines. The effective dose is 120-240 mg per day.

And anyone who experiences regular migraines should be taking 200-600 milligrams of magnesium per day. Low levels of **magnesium** can contribute to migraines.

Food allergy may also be a problem for some migraine sufferers. The most common allergens (in decreasing order) include wheat (gluten), orange, egg, coffee/tea, milk, chocolate, corn, sugar, yeast, mushrooms, and peas. A small proportion of migraine sufferers may also react to the presence of tyramine in foods such as aged cheeses, yogurt, beer, wine, liver and organ meats.

If you use the above remedies and for some reason still find yourself battling a migraine at some point, there are a couple of reports that ginger may help them go away sooner. Mix 500-600 mg ginger powder with water and drink it every 4 hours until the migraine subsides (for up to four days—but hopefully not that long!).

Another, lesser-known herb—**butterbur**—made history in 2012 by gaining recognition from the American Academy of Neurology (AAN) as an effective migraine therapy.

In 2012, the AAN reviewed all the studies for alternative migraine treatments published between June 1999 and May 2007. Butterbur (*Petasites hybridis*) stood out as an effective alternative to prescription drugs. And, given all the clinical research on butterbur, the AAN's announcement is well-deserved.

Several clinical trials published over the last 10 years prove that butterbur can help patients who get migraines on a regular basis. In fact, in many of these trials, patients who took butterbur root extract reduced the frequency of their migraines by up to 50 percent.

Beyond butterbur extracts, experts reviewed other alternatives such as Co-enzyme Q10, magnesium, and hyperbaric oxygen as treatments. In addition, they reviewed Papaverine (a derivative of the opium poppy, Papaver somniferum). Papaverine affects blood circulation in the brain, which is a key factor in migraine headaches. Not surprisingly, Papaverine also works extremely well as a pain reliever.

In the AAN report, the neurologists acknowledged that non-prescription drugs are important for many migraine patients.

This is a big step for the AAN. It's important to migraine sufferers too because standard migraine drugs can cause serious side effects. And, in too many cases, the drugs just don't help! In fact, in severe cases, the very drugs prescribed to treat the migraine can *lead to chronic, unremitting headaches that never go away*.

But the good news is, there are many healthy alternatives to help!

Chapter 18

Why those tired, old natural arthritis "fixes" don't work

Plus, the long-forgotten ancient remedies that DO

Far too many people think glucosamine and chondroitin are a one-stop solution to arthritis pain.

If glucosamine and chondroitin were truly the wonder nutrient supplements that marketers claim they are, we wouldn't still be talking about arthritis. In fact, with all the "solutions" that have been dumped onto the public for decades, joint pain should have gone the way of the dinosaurs years ago.

Yet, as long as there have been joints, there has been joint pain.

Historians tell us that, unlike many common diseases that have become more prevalent in our modern industrialized era (think cancer and heart disease), arthritis has been afflicting humans since prehistoric times. In fact, paleopathologists estimate almost half of early humans—as far back as Neanderthal man—suffered some sort of joint condition.

Unfortunately, the best- documented health problem in human history is plaguing us still. And it will for generations to come—if we keep putting faith in supplements that get it all wrong.

But the good news is when an ailment has this much history, we have the benefit of millennia of trial and error before us.

And our ancestors—from many cultures around the world—have left us clues that point us to real solutions for joint pain.

I've spent years investigating history's clues, and I've found alternatives to glucosamine and chondroitin that actually work.

So let's get down to the real cause of this problem first.

The REAL cause of joint pain is
something glucosamine can't touch

Joint pain fits into one of four categories:

1. Osteoarthritis. Deterioration from "wear-and-tear" on joints that leads to painful inflammation.

2. Rheumatoid arthritis. The immune system itself attacks joints, causing pain and deterioration.

3. Degeneration of the discs. The discs between the vertebrae in the spine wear down, causing neck and back pain.

4. Pains of undetermined nature. These may be linked to mind-body-immune system connections, as explained in my book with Mike Jawer, *Your Emotional Type* (www.drmicozzi. com).

But while there are different types of joint pain, they ultimately have one thing in common—inflammation.

So if we can treat inflammation, we can do away with these ailments. Simple, right?

But here's the thing: glucosamine and chondroitin—the most common natural products used to treat joint deterioration and pain do not have the power to correct inflammation in the joints.

Joint remedies that actually do the job need to address the cause of joint damage. And the fact is that inflammation plays a central role.

Here's what you need to know about joints and bones, and why you can't treat joint pain effectively without treating inflammation:

• Our body is constantly absorbing and replacing old bone with new, healthy bone.

• Where one bone meets another, the bones are covered in cushioning called cartilage. This keeps bones from rubbing against each other.

- Cartilage is nourished by fluid called synovial fluid, which fills the spaces in the joints, between the bones.

- When the joints are inflamed, cartilage can't get the nourishment it needs from the synovial fluid. So inflammation destroys normal cartilage tissue and gets in the way of new, healthy cartilage being formed.

- If inflammation is controlled, the body can again begin forming and nourishing new, healthy cartilage. The result? Normal, healthy, comfortable joints.

In some cases of joint pain, such as rheumatoid arthritis, inflammation comes first and destroys cartilage and—if left unchecked—bone.

In other cases, like osteoarthritis, the "wear and tear" destruction of cartilage leads to inflammation in the joint tissues. Either way, what results is a vicious cycle that can only be interrupted in one way: by controlling inflammation.

Here's why that's so important: once you control inflammation, the damaged joints and underlying bones can begin to heal themselves. This self-healing ability of bones and joints is the basis of all natural healing in all tissues of the body. No matter how many so-called bone-supporting nutrients you pour into the system (assuming they even make it into your joints), they won't work if you don't stop the inflammation cycle.

Can your body even use glucosamine and chondroitin?

Many doctors and medical scientists have questioned for decades whether glucosamine (a sugar amine) is even sufficiently absorbed into the joint tissues, believing that it is destroyed in the gastrointestinal tract and/or the bloodstream before it can even enter the joints.

It is, after all, a combination of glucose or sugar (which is readily metabolized for energy) and an amine, which like most protein constituents, are broken apart by digestion and enzymes.

Chondroitin comes with its own list of issues. Concerns have been raised about the source it comes from and how well the body can actually absorb it, and to what extent. It seems like most all the "new" discoveries over the years when it comes to chondroitin have to do with some new, exotic species or location from which this common natural substance is harvested. This has made for some putatively attractive marketing pitches...but not evidence that it is absorbed into the body and actually works for joint pain. That's why chondroitin has become widely regarded in the medical community as worthless.

Side effects of glucosamine include digestive complaints such as abdominal pain, poor appetite, nausea, heartburn, constipation, diarrhea, and vomiting. Which makes sense for something that is not being absorbed properly in the gastrointestinal tract.

History holds the secret to joint relief

Modern science is proving what our ancestors knew: Natural remedies can curb inflammation and promote bone and joint health.

Do you remember what the wise men brought as gifts to celebrate the birth of Jesus? Gold, frankincense, and myrrh. Believe it or not, all three of those are proven arthritis remedies (and you can trust men who just walked halfway around the world to know what soothes achy joints!). No wonder they were so valuable.

Gold injected into the joints actually does help arthritis, but its expense puts it out of reach for most of us. Frankincense and myrrh, on the other hand, have a long history in supporting joints—and new research continues to support their use.

Frankincense, also known as **Boswellia**, is best known in the West as a potent incense that fills churches with a familiar fragrance. But far beyond smelling good, frankincense is valued for its medicinal properties. In fact, it has held an important place in Asian medicine for millennia. Ayurvedic practitioners have known for ages that Boswellia is a key treatment for joints. And the reason it works: It stops inflammation.

And, again, that allows your cartilage to rebuild itself. Like most natural healing, rebuilding healthy bone and cartilage to a permanent solution is a slow and steady process that takes time. But if you take care of the inflammation in the meantime, it helps stop the pain and increases mobility, while allowing the joint to repair itself over time.

Myrrh, found in abundance in the Middle East, is valued for its anti-inflammatory effects too. In fact, it's held in such high esteem that it was one of the gifts the Queen of Sheba brought to King Solomon.

Vitamin C (500 mg/day), **vitamin D** (2,000 IU/day), and **vitamin E** (400 to 600 IU/day—see page 106 for further explanation on dosage information) are always important for bone and joint health. And yes, you need all three to work best together.

Capsicum frutescens (**cayenne pepper**). You generally see capsaicin as an ingredient in topical creams (usually in 0.025% and 0.075% strengths). They can be very effective for relieving joint pain. However eating red chili peppers (if you like spicy food) can also have remarkably beneficial effects.

Curcuma longa (**turmeric**) The active ingredient, curcumin, of this commonly used spice has anti-inflammatory and lipid-lowering effects. It is one of the three common components of traditional curry spice (together with coriander and cumin, and sometimes red chili pepper). Curcumin's lipid-lowering effects observed in animal experiments are attributed to changes in fatty acid metabolism and facilitating the conversion of cholesterol to bile acids. There are also reports of its benefit in patients with osteoarthritis. The benefit of turmeric is not conclusively proven but its use as a spice in an overall healthy diet is appropriate. Curcumin supplements are widely available in natural food stores and online supplement retailers. A good general dose is 200 mg per day.

Withania somnifera (**winter cherry**). Basic science studies suggest that this herb may have anti-inflammatory, antioxidant, immune-modulatory and anti-aging properties. It might also have a positive influence on the endocrine and central nervous systems. The mechanisms of these proposed actions require additional clarification. Several observational and randomized studies have reported its usefulness in the treatment of arthritic conditions

Zingiber officinale (**ginger**). Ginger is widely used in Asia, most commonly for control of nausea and osteoarthritis pain. Several randomized trials have shown its benefit in controlling nausea associated with pregnancy, motion sickness and anesthesia, and some studies have demonstrated its usefulness in the treatment of osteoarthritis.

Omega-3 fatty acids. The essential fatty acids in fish oil are another tremendous natural anti-inflammatory. However, to get as much as you need—3 to 10 grams per day—you'll likely need to increase the amount of omega-3 containing foods you eat (like salmon, sardines, and walnuts) and take a fish oil supplement as well. Fish oil supplements are widely available. Just be sure to look for one that contains both the DHA and EPA fatty acids.

It should be mentioned that the methodology and quality of many studies aimed at determining the effectiveness of various herbs are less than satisfactory. Also, many studies involve the use of preparations which contain several herbs and other nutrients, which is quite common in herbal practice. While such trials are useful, they do not, in and of themselves, identify and discern the beneficial effects of specific herbs. In one such trial involving a combination preparation of Withiania somnifera, Bosweillia serrata, Curcuma longa, and zinc, osteoarthritis patients reported a significant reduction in their level of pain compared to those in the control group.

If you're looking for a joint supplement, you'd do well to find one that has these potent herbal anti-inflammatories, as well as some specific nutrients whose effectiveness is proven by modern science.

Chapter 19

Rheumatoid arthritis:
One of medicine's most agonizing
mysteries—UNRAVELED!

Modern medicine botches a lot of things. But the way it treats rheumatoid arthritis may be one of the worst examples.

For centuries, rheumatoid arthritis (RA) has largely been a mystery. A very painful one at that.

The problem is, once again, that western medicine only focuses on ONE aspect of the disease.

Modern medicine has classified RA as an auto-immune disease. Of course, when I was in training during the 1970s, that's what the experts ended up calling a lot of diseases they simply didn't understand.

Today, we know there is indeed an immune component involved in rheumatoid arthritis (RA). But, as is the case in many other auto-immune disorders, there's also a strong mind- body connection. And, more recently, yet another factor has come to light—the nervous system connection.

Finding real relief from this mysterious chronic condition requires treating all three aspects. Unfortunately, most doctors simply aren't.

That said, make no mistake: RA is a dangerous systemic condition that requires management by a competent rheumatologist. And the good news is, more and more doctors are recognizing that there are also complementary approaches that can help soothe RA. More on that in just a minute. First, it's important to understand how it all ties together.

It's all connected

I talk a lot about the mind-body connection in my *Insiders' Cures* newsletter. But I have to—because western science separated the two long ago. And that was—and is—a huge mistake. Other ethno-medical traditions in Asia and around the world never separated them. This is one reason these other medical traditions appear more "wholistic" to us today.

But even based on modern science, growing evidence shows the mind and body are linked—or "married." For better or worse, in sickness and in health.

It boils down to three inter- connected components:

1. "Psycho"—the mind/brain connection

2. "Neuro"—the nervous system connection

3. "Immunology"—the immune system connection

In fact, today there's an entire field of medicine called "psycho-neuro-immunology." Which provides a tangible scientific approach, a physiologic model, and a growing body of data proving the mind-body connections.

Here's how each component works…

For the "psycho" component, we know that the mind-brain is connected through thoughts, emotional feelings, and levels of consciousness to influence the body. But it's not just a one-way street. The biochemicals, called neuro-peptides, that we associate as being in the brain, such as neurotransmitters, are actually present throughout the body. In fact, neurotransmitters are found in even greater quantities in the gut, for example, than they are in the nervous system.

Further, the production of specific hormones (which occurs throughout the body in the thyroid, pancreas, adrenal glands, and ovaries or testes) is controlled by specific neuro- peptides released by the pituitary gland of the brain. These hormones are released into the circulatory system and carried to all parts of the body in the blood.

For the "neuro" part of the equation, the nervous system originates in the brain and spinal cord as well. Nerves also travel to all parts of the body, both sensing and influencing all tissues at both voluntary (conscious) and involuntary (unconscious) levels.

But now there's a third piece being added to the puzzle—"immunology."

Like neuro-peptides and nerves, the immune system is also present throughout the body. Immune cells (white blood cells) travel throughout the blood. And there are specialized concentrations of these cells in the adenoids, tonsils, spleen, appendix, and throughout the gastrointestinal tract (without fully understanding their role, 20th century surgeons considered them all to be expendable). They are also concentrated in the thymus gland during childhood.

When you look at how each of these three components impacts the body from head-to-toe on their own…it's not hard to see how they are all inter-related as well. The psycho-neuro-immunology- connection becomes quite apparent.

So what causes rheumatoid arthritis?

One way the immune system works is by making antibodies that match to antigens on invading bacteria and viruses. Antigens are foreign substances that stimulate the immune system. The antibodies attack the antigens and then white blood cells can destroy the microbes.

These microbial antigens are often made up of proteins and/or polysaccharides that are commonly found in nature. These are some of the same proteins and polysaccharides that exist in normal, healthy biological substances as well. Unfortunately, when the immune system can get out of synch, some of the antibodies it makes against microbes get confused and cross-react with certain normal tissues. Thus, the immune system can attack our own bodies—causing an "auto" immune disease.

RA is the result of your immune system attacking the cartilage in your joints. This confusion can stem from a true bacterial infection, like "rheumatic fever." Or it can appear more mysteriously from a stress-related immune imbalance—this is the mind-body-immune connection.

While there is accordingly a mind-body component, caution must be exercised with rheumatoid arthritis. It causes real, physical damage with serious complications that require experienced medical management.

The best thing you can do is to consult a rheumatologist who can help determine which of the drugs for RA appear to be safe, effective, and appropriate for you. And whether there older ones that are more reliable (as in the case with blood pressure medications).

That said, doctors and patients alike are realizing that there are also natural approaches you can take to help alleviate RA. Especially when it comes to addressing the mind- body connection.

True "complements" to RA treatment

A wide range of "mind-body" approaches can reduce the stress that inevitably accompanies the pain with which RA patients struggle on a daily basis. For those best suited to your emotional type take the short quiz featured on www.drmicozzi.com, or in my book with Michael Jawer *Your Emotional Type*.

Gentle movements—as in traditional yoga or tai chi—can also be helpful. Likewise, swimming can provide just the right kind of low-stress movement and physical exercise. Light massage, low-impact exercise, and just getting outdoors (walking, riding a bike, or light gardening) can also be good.

For the pain itself, acupuncture can often work wonders.

In China and India, rheumatic conditions are associated with "cold and damp." So while the inflammation may seem hot, it actually helps to seek warmth and avoid cold and damp circumstances and climates. In fact, one ancient Ayurvedic treatment involves immersing the joints in warm sand.

This can easily be accomplished on a sunny beach (while also providing you, and your bones and joints, with some much-needed vitamin D).

Whatever complementary therapy you decide to try, don't go it alone. The best way to ensure you get the most relief is to work with a rheumatologist who can recommend the best complementary therapies for your particular needs.

Chapter 20

What you need to know about NSAIDs

Obviously, for mainstream medicine, figuring out how to effectively treat pain can be a real…pain.

This is especially true when doctors persist in ignoring all of the natural approaches for pain management, and slavishly comply with all of the political prohibitions placed on effective pain relievers by big government regulators and armed law enforcement. Suddenly, these doctors find they don't have many good options left. So it's no surprise that their desperate patients turn to over-the-counter pain remedies. But there are some important things you need to know about these pain relievers.

The common painkiller you should avoid at all costs

Fortunately, there are some over-the-counter drug and herbal remedies that are effective—and *safe*—anti-inflammatory agents. But you may be surprised to learn that Tylenol (acetaminophen) is not among them.

Also known as paracetamol, acetaminophen was originally an industrial chemical developed in Germany. Since then, it has caused more pain than it has cured. In fact, it has become the leading cause of acute liver failure in the United States.

Tylenol was actually one of the first drugs for which we developed protocols to monitor therapeutic and toxic blood levels when I worked with a technical team at McDonnell Douglas (now Boeing) on instrumentation from the manned space program.

Our job was to adapt analytical technology from the NASA space exploration program to everyday clinical use. We were also looking at other potent and potentially dangerous drugs, like anticonvulsants, amphetamines, barbiturates and psychoactive drugs. That's right: All of these dangerous toxic potential killers were treated in the same category as a common household pain-reliever.

I have known otherwise intelligent people who kept taking more and more Tylenol until their knee pain went away…just so they could keep their appointments to play handball or basketball. They may have won the match, but at what cost? I guarantee you they won't be thinking about those victories when they're diagnosed with liver failure.

Acetaminophen found worthless for pain besides being highly toxic

Well, now doctors have come out with a second opinion about acetaminophen (Tylenol). For years, everyone has admitted it is the leading cause of liver toxicity and fatal liver failure in the US today. Now they have a second opinion; it's also worthless for pain!

An important new study found the use of acetaminophen for the most common cause of pain and disability in working Americans was no more effective than placebo, or taking a sugar pill. The drug was worthless whether it was taken regularly three times every day (3,990 mg total, or nearly 4 grams—more like a food quantity than a drug), or only taken when needed.

Patients taking this drug, whether on the 4 gram per day regular schedule or only as needed, suffered an average of 17 days before recovering from a bout of disabling back pain.

But patients taking a sugar pill took only 16 days to recover!

The drug actually made patients spend an extra day in pain and disabled, missing work, or school, or daily activities. To someone suffering from back pain spending that 17th day in pain by taking Tylenol can seem like an eternity.

So, that's what you get for your trouble and expense, not to mention risking liver failure. You get to spend an extra day in pain before recovering.

Since Tylenol is a metabolic poison, I suspect it actually interferes with your body's normal ability to heal naturally and safely—and delays your healing by one day while doing nothing to help you.

This group of researchers from Australia had previously conducted an analysis of prior studies that found no benefits to the use of this drug. To further their analysis of this gap, they enlisted 1,643 participants of average age 45 years from 235 pain centers in Australia in the Paracetamol for Low Back Pain (PACE) trial. Note: Acetaminophen is known as Paracetamol outside the US (like a criminal fugitive, it goes by aliases, perhaps for the same reason).

There were no benefits to the drug in any of the studies. The researchers did provide good quality advice and reassurance to all study participants, a feature that is often absent from usual care.

The scandal is that universal medical practice guidelines for management of low back pain call for the first-line use of this toxic drug. You have to wonder where that idea came from?

The researchers point out, that despite the "universal" acceptance for the first use of Tylenol , there was <u>never</u> any good evidence for it—leading to their review analysis and then to their clinical trial.

So, what was all that about the importance of so-called "evidence-based" medical practice? What a painful scandal.

The mainstream management of low back pain was never any good—at least when left in the hands of drugs or surgeries.

And acetaminophen was never a good drug based on its toxicity alone. The new evidence that it doesn't even work; makes this drug a big "less-than-zero" as far its therapeutic index of benefits versus risks.

A safer way to find OTC pain relief

While I urge you never to take Tylenol, I have found ibuprofen drugs like Advil and Motrin to be effective pain relievers when nothing else works.

The key is to be vigilant against these drugs' alarming side effects, and to carefully monitor your dosages.

Ibuprofen, along with aspirin, naproxen (Aleve), and a whole host of prescription drugs, is part of a class of pain relievers known as NSAIDs (non-steroidal anti-inflammatory drugs). Many of these drugs came onto the scene during the 1980s and were quickly accepted by people seeking pain relief.

However, NSAIDS are associated with dangerous side effects in the gastrointestinal tract, including ulcers, bleeding, and colon perforations. These drugs can wreak havoc all the way through the average 26-foot length of the GI tract. That's a lot of territory for damage to occur.

Alarmingly, these problems are not rare. In fact, about 1 to 2 percent of routine NSAID users experience GI complications that are so severe, they have to be hospitalized. And if you're older than 65, have a history of peptic ulcers, take NSAIDS and anticoagulants at the same time, or pop an NSAID when you're taking a daily aspirin, you may be particularly susceptible to these complications.

The good news is, at recommended doses, ibuprofen is the least likely of the NSAIDs to cause these side effects. But while you don't want to take too much of this painkiller, you also don't want to take too little.

Ibuprofen is still available as a prescription pain reliever, and an effective dose is considered to be one or two 800 mg tablets. Compare that to the puny 200 mg in the Advil or Motrin tablets you buy at the drug store. I've found that when ibuprofen does not provide fast, effective pain relief, it's often because the doses in these over-the-counter products are simply too low.

Of course, I always recommend trying natural pain relievers first. But if you choose to use NSAIDs, make sure to let your doctor know. You should also keep an eye out for signs of GI bleeding, including dark stools or blood in your toilet.

Chapter 21

Let the "Koop Pain Technique" change your life like it did mine

I've never been in favor of steroid injections for relief of any type of pain—neck, back, or joints.

Under the best of circumstances, steroids only provide a quick fix and don't do anything to remedy the long-term problem that's causing the pain. At worst, I've seen hundreds of cases of contaminated steroid preparations that have caused fatal fungal brain infections in unsuspecting people.

As I discuss in my report *The Insider's Ultimate Guide to Pill-Free Pain Cures*, and in my best-selling learning program: ***Dr. Micozzi's Arthritis Relief and Reversal Protocol: A Drug-Free Plan for Easing and Elimination Arthritis Pain***, there are many natural alternatives to steroids for managing pain. And for joint pain specifically, new research shows that manual and physical therapies and another little-known natural treatment—prolotherapy—are just as effective as steroid injections. But without any of the risks.

I refer to it as the "Koop Pain Technique" after my late colleague and mentor, Attorney General C. Everett Koop, who used it to cure his own nagging knee pain.

Let's take a look at this natural therapy and the compelling new research that shows how it can end your joint pain—*forever*.

A simple sugar shot soothes 10 years of knee pain

Ten years ago, I was preparing a medical textbook on natural therapies for pain with my colleague, Mike Weintraub, MD, professor of neurology at New York Medical College. He suggested we include a chapter on prolotherapy. But back then it was not easy to find practitioners of this little-known pain treatment.

We searched high and low until finally locating Donna Alderman, DO, of Hemwall Family Medical Centers in California.

As one of the few prolotherapy practitioners in the state, Dr. Alderman commuted between Hemwall's San Francisco and Los Angeles area clinics. On Fridays, she was at her clinic in Glendale, where my brother and his family live.

In 2007, I went out to visit my brother during "spring break", and I ended up getting prolotherapy from Dr. Alderman for my right knee. The knee had been bothering me ever since I had injured it in 1997 and then took to a long airplane trip, and a long drive, to visit Dr. Larry Dossey near Santa Fe, New Mexico.

My brief, painless prolotherapy treatments worked like a charm. Afterwards, I was able to drive and sit in airplanes without any pain—which I hadn't been able to do for 10 years.

Prolotherapy is based on the premise that chronic joint pain at least partially results from inadequate repair of connective tissues around the joints. Prolotherapy practitioners inject minute amounts of substances such as cornstarch, sugar, or a cod liver oil mixture into those connective tissues.

The body reacts by promoting tissue repair and growth—like tiny, cellular "micro-sutures" that tighten up the tissues without surgery. Taking vitamin C before and after prolotherapy treatments also helps lay down the collagen that cross-links the new connective tissues to make them strong.

You have to wonder why such a simple, effective, safe, and inexpensive treatment for something as common as joint pain remained hidden for so long? Of course, it probably has something to do with the fact that prolotherapy doesn't require expensive (yet often ineffective) surgery—and repeat surgery—by the burgeoning orthopedic industry.

The good news is, prolotherapy has recently been attracting more interest from researchers. And they are reporting fantastic results.

For instance, a new study looked at 38 adults who had at least three months of osteoarthritis-related knee pain. During the first, fifth, and ninth weeks of the study, the participants were given prolotherapy injections containing dextrose (a sugar) in the connective tissues surrounding their knees. More injections were given to those who needed them at 13 and 17 weeks.

The researchers concluded that these prolotherapy treatments resulted in significant levels of safe, sustained improvement in mild to severe knee pain, function, and stiffness. And there were no adverse effects.

In addition, at the end of the study, *91 percent* of the people who had the prolotherapy treatments said they would recommend them to others with painful knee osteoarthritis.

If you'd like to try prolotherapy yourself, it's much easier today to find a practitioner than it was a decade ago. In fact, there's an entire website, www.getprolo.com, listing practitioners throughout the United States.

Considering the proven effectiveness and safety of prolotherapy and physical therapy for joint pain, there is truly no need for you to ever have steroid injections. And, certainly, never consider surgery until you have tried these much safer and more cost-effective alternatives first.

Chapter 22

The (pain) killer in your medicine cabinet

Pain may be a part of life, but lucky for us, pain relief is a part of nature. Which is why a natural approach should reign supreme.

For as long as humans have existed, they've experienced pain…and turned to plants for relief. Which is only natural. After all, plants pre-dated animals—dinosaurs and humans alike. This is why animals are "pre-adapted" to use plants as a source of nutrition and medicine.

And through the millennia, the plants we've turned to are those that either reduce inflammation, or pain sensations. These sensations are felt by the nerves and perceived by the brain and central nervous system.

Plants pack a powerful punch

The most powerful pain relievers of all come from the opium poppy (*Papaver somniferum*). The poppy contains morphine and related plant alkaloids. These plant chemicals deaden the brain and the central nervous system's perception of pain, and makes the patient indifferent to pain sensations.

Other plant chemicals such as cocaine (from the coca plant) are used as local anesthetics. These include related drugs procaine and novocaine. Cocaine was once used routinely as a local anesthetic for ear, nose and throat surgery. It even appeared in popular beverages and tonics for a quick "pick-me-up" during the 19th century.

Indeed cocaine can affect the body in many ways. Native Americans of the Andes chew the coca leaf to help digest complex carbohydrates, for energy. And probably to even help thin the blood. The blood can become thick and "sludgy" at their high altitude.

In comes the strong arm of the law

Of course morphine and the opiates (such as the synthetic opiate diacetyl-morphine, or heroin), as well as cocaine, are all either illegal or highly regulated as controlled substances by the federal Drug Enforcement Administration (DEA).

And in case you didn't know, the power of the DEA far exceeds that of the Food and Drug Administration (FDA). And thanks to the government's ineffective "war on drugs," many physicians are outright restricted from prescribing the most effective drugs in many cases. Or, are intimidated by the DEA and afraid to prescribe what actually works. And laws on prescription narcotic pain relievers just keep getting tougher.

In the meantime, an over-the-counter pain reliever—one that I can almost guarantee is in your medicine cabinet—has long been proven to cause liver failure. But it still gets the green light from the government!?! I'll explain more on that shortly. But first...

Is inflammation the cause?

Narcotics work by interfering with pain signals and perception. But many pain relievers work by controlling or reducing inflammation. Redness, heat and swelling are the cardinal signs of inflammation. But what causes these symptoms in the first place?

When a tissue, body cavity or joint space is inflamed, blood flow increases, fluids accumulate, swelling occurs, and immune cells rush into the area. The immune cells release histamines, enzymes and other biochemicals. All these effects aggravate sensitive pain fibers. These fibers send signals through the spinal cord to the brain...indicating all is not well. Those signals are discomfort, irritation and pain.

Steering away from steroids

The most potent (and dangerous) anti-inflammatory agents are corticosteroids. But here's something you may not realize—steroid hormones are actually produced naturally by the body.

The center of the adrenal gland produces the "fight or flight" hormone adrenalin, or epinephrine. While the outer core produces steroid hormones.

The steroid hormones have a wide range of important physiologic effects. Including causing growth and "body-building," reacting to stress, balancing fluids and electrolytes, playing a part in reproductive and other metabolic functions, as well as influencing inflammation and pain.

Problems can arise, however, when steroids are used as drugs. They can be given as injections directly into painful areas, applied topically to irritated skin or taken internally as prescription medication. And while they may work, steroid medications have serious side effects.

Steroid drugs circulating in the blood stop the normal metabolic production of steroid hormones. This means that when the course of drug treatment is finished, the patient must be slowly weaned off—cutting back on the dose a little each day to give the body a chance to restore normal metabolic function. Otherwise the consequences are dangerous...even deadly.

So you can probably see why I advise avoiding steroids if at all possible.

Take two of these and call the doctor in the morning (for a liver transplant)

Fortunately, there are some over-the-counter drug and herbal remedies that are effective—and *safe*—anti-inflammatory agents. But you may be surprised to learn that Tylenol (acetaminophen) is not among them.

Also known as paracetamol, acetaminophen was originally an industrial chemical developed in Germany. Since then, it has caused more pain than it has cured. In fact, it has become the leading cause of acute liver failure in the United States.

Tylenol was actually one of the first drugs for which we developed protocols to monitor therapeutic and toxic blood levels when I worked with a technical team at McDonnell Douglas (now Boeing) on instrumentation from the manned space program.

Our job was to adapt analytical technology from the NASA space exploration program to everyday clinical use. We were also looking at other potent and potentially dangerous drugs, like anticonvulsants, amphetamines, barbiturates and psychoactive drugs. That's right: All of these dangerous toxic potential killers were treated in the same category as a common household pain-reliever.

I have known otherwise intelligent people who kept taking more and more Tylenol until their knee pain went away…just so they could keep their appointments to play handball or basketball.

They may have won the match, but at what cost? I guarantee you they won't be thinking about those victories when they're diagnosed with liver failure.

Don't get a headache over aspirin

Aspirin has seen its share of controversy. But it still has its merits when used appropriately.

This remarkable product of nature (acetyl salicylic acid) originally came from the white willow tree (Salix alba).

It was well known to Native Americans. They used it to reduce fevers among other things. Salicylates are prominent in nature, also occurring in wintergreen. They are also used in many digestive aids and in topical pain relievers.

Aspirin is indeed the "granddaddy" of all over-the-counter pain relievers. It was grandfathered into approved use by the FDA, since it was already in common use before the FDA was created in 1906.

But some argue that the gastrointestinal irritation and bleeding it causes (it is an acid, after all) would prevent it from being approved by the FDA today.

Taken in low doses long-term, aspirin has been found to lower the risk of heart disease (perhaps by inhibiting blood clots). And recent research shows it lowers the risk of cancer.

People who are taking blood thinners or who have a certain type of age-related macular degeneration (of the eye) should consult with their doctors before taking aspirin (or other pain relievers).

Avoid "sugar" coating

There's another debate surrounding aspirin related to a commonly used coating on the tablets. This is done to theoretically protect the stomach. However, some question whether or not these coatings make a difference. And they may in fact obscure the benefits, leading doctors to prescribe more expensive prescription drugs. This is according to a recent study published in the journal *Circulation*.

The conclusion about coated aspirin was only one finding in the study. The main goal was to test the hotly disputed idea that aspirin does not really help prevent heart attacks or stroke in some people.

For more than a decade, cardiologists and drug researchers have speculated that anywhere from 5 to 40 percent of the population is "aspirin resistant." But some prominent doctors say drug makers with a commercial interest in disproving aspirin's benefits have exaggerated the prevalence of aspirin resistance.

In fact, the new study did not find a single case of true aspirin resistance among the 400 healthy people who were examined. They claim the coating on aspirin interfered with the way that the drug entered the body, making it appear that the drug was not working.

The study was partly financed by Bayer, the world's largest manufacturer of brand-name aspirin, much of which is coated.

And, aside from whether coating aspirin conceals its heart benefits in some people, there is little evidence that it protects the stomach better than uncoated aspirin.

A rare modern therapeutic breakthrough

I had the opportunity to witness the development of a true breakthrough pain reliever when ibuprofen (Motrin) came on the market while I was still in training.

Many patients with a variety of conditions from arthritis to menstrual pains who could never find relief suddenly were swearing by Ibuprofen.

Initially, it was available only by prescription in 800 mg tablets, but later the generic form (Advil) became available in 200 mg tablets.

Ibuprofen is one of the original "non-steriodal anti-inflammatory agents" or NSAIDs. This approach to pain relief did represent a rare, therapeutic breakthrough. It provided pain relief with something other than aspirin. And without having to resort to potent and metabolically disruptive steroids. (Of course, effective narcotic pain relievers were already off the list due to government political agendas.)

Then, in the late 1990s and early 2000s, "cox-2" inhibitors became the new pain relievers *du jour*. They work by preventing formation of certain prostaglandin hormones (originally discovered in the prostate gland) that cause pain. There was a rush to market these new drugs, but their side effects have been so intense that one of them—Vioxx— was quickly taken off the market in 2004 because of its toxic effects on the heart.

So, in short, Ibuprofen is the only over-the-counter (OTC) pain reliever I would recommend, in addition to aspirin. Though, you may need to take the full 800 mg dose, since the OTC 200 mg dose may not be effective.

I would steer clear of ALL other OTC pain relievers. And if aspirin and Ibuprofen don't work, you need to talk to your doctor about other options, including natural approaches.

Effective natural remedies

Luckily there are a number of safe, effective anti-inflammatory compounds that appear to function as natural cox-2 inhibitors but without the dangers.

- **Curcumin** (*Curcuma longa*), or turmeric, is the spice that gives curry its bright yellow color. It is also an ancient Ayurvedic remedy that appears effective at a dose of 200 mg per day.

- **Omega-3 fatty acids** also appear to be cox-2 inhibitors and can reduce pain and inflammation, while providing a host of other health benefits.

- **Capsaicin**, an active ingredient in hot peppers, is also an effective pain reliever. It is generally used in topical creams and ointments. But it is also taken orally, including as a staple of several traditional cuisines worldwide.

- **Resveratrol** also appears to have these activities. It is a prominent constituent of red wine, among other natural sources. The moderate levels of alcohol in wine, of course, are also well known as an effective pain reliever.

- A traditional Chinese herbal remedy known as **Thunder God vine** also appears effective.

- A number of **flavonoids** and **phenolic** compounds, which are prominent components of many fruits and vegetables, are also being investigated for these effects.

- **Boswellia** (the ancient fragrant incense known as frankincense) is another traditional Ayurvedic remedy with potent anti- inflammatory and pain-relieving effects (400—500 mg per day).

- Winter cherry (*Withania somnifera*, 500 mg per day), also known as **Ashwaganda root**, is another Ayurvedic remedy with potent anti- inflammatory and pain-relieving effects. It is also considered an "adaptogen" like Chinese ginseng, or South African *Sutherlandia frutescens*.

Beyond oral pain-relievers

Since pain has its origins in the body, many therapies that work directly on the body, or through "mind-body," are also very effective for pain. For example, spinal manual therapy is the most effective and cost-effective remedy for back pain, which is the most common cause of pain and disability in working Americans.

The good news

As I've described, nature has provided us with countless ways to reduce inflammation and control pain. So there's no reason at all you should need to turn to the dangerous pain killers on pharmacy shelves. And remember: Pain is a signal that something is wrong in the body. So rather than masking it, pay attention to the pain and allow time for your body to heal.

Chapter 23

6 safe options to make pain go away

You probably remember a time when your family doctor gave this stand-by advice for pain: "Take two aspirin, and call me in the morning."

But somewhere along the line, Tylenol (acetaminophen) took aspirin's place. Today, it's the most common pain reliever in the U.S. And doctors and hospitals widely recommend it instead of aspirin for everyday aches and pains.

But I hope you know by now to never take Tylenol for anything. Ever. Period.

First of all, Tylenol doesn't even work at all for lower back pain, the most common cause of pain and disability in working Americans. In fact, it prolonged pain by a full day compared to doing nothing. In another study, researchers found it's useless for shoulder pain, another common problem.

Second, a recent British study found long-term acetaminophen use increases the risk of high blood pressure, heart attack, stroke, kidney disease, and GI bleeding.

Ironically, they told us to switch to acetaminophen because of the risk of GI bleeding with aspirin. At least aspirin lowers your risks of heart disease. It also lowers your risk of colon cancer and cervical cancer.

Third, Tylenol is also the leading cause of toxic liver failure in the U.S. And it increases the risk of premature death by 60 percent.

Overall, Tylenol is a metabolic poison that interferes with production of glutathione, a vital antioxidant throughout cells of the body. The antioxidants present in blueberries and grapeseed, for example, can help protect you against Tylenol. But nothing can fully overcome this metabolic poisoning.

Fortunately, you have six safe, natural, and time-honored ways to make pain go away.

Your first option is **Boswellia serrata,** a resin from the gum trees of South Asia and the Middle East. It's an ancient Ayurvedic remedy for pain that made its way into European use during the Crusades. (Although historic evidence suggests it was known even to the ancient Greeks and Romans, probably from the Spice Route.) The common name Frankincense comes from the Frankish King Frederick Barbarossa who led one of the most successful Crusades and probably brought some with him back to Europe. Boswellia helps ease the pain associated with both rheumatoid arthritis and degenerative arthritis. Look for it in better joint supplements. You can safely take 400 to 500 mg per day.

Capsaicin is a natural ingredient found in hot chili peppers. It effectively relieves joint pain, respiratory congestion, and sinus congestion. It works against pain by depleting your body's supply of substance P, a chemical involved in transmitting pain signals to your brain. Many people seem to think you can only apply it topically on painful joints to get relief. But, of course, you can also take it orally and get results. Indeed, in many countries around the world—such as Eastern Europe, Italy, Mexico, India, China, and Southeast Asia—they routinely incorporate hot chili peppers into cooking.

Curcumin is the bright yellow active compound found in the common spice turmeric. You combine curcumin, coriander, cumin, and, sometimes, red chili pepper to make curry flavoring. Of course, each curry spice on its own has pain-relieving properties. But curcumin reduces pain *and* joint inflammation. In fact, it reduces inflammation as effectively as the potent prescription drug phenylbutazone (Butazolidine). Plus, according to some natural medicine experts, the right dose of curcumin is the most effective pain reliever available anywhere. Some studies suggest it reduces pain even when drugs are ineffective. In addition, it has potent activities against dementia, depression, and cancer. It also promotes healthy brain and gastrointestinal functions. A common dose is 500 mg per day.

Studies show **tart cherries** work as well for joint pain and inflammation as ibuprofen. You should eat at least 20 cherries per day to feel a difference. You can also take a 2,000 mg tart cherry extract. This remedy may also reduce the risk of colon and other cancers (as does aspirin). As an added benefit, tart cherries promote restful sleep.

The wild cherry known as **Ashwaganda** (also called winter cherry, or Withania somniferum) is another ancient Ayurvedic remedy for joint pain. I call Ashwaganda, together with Boswellia and Curcumin, the ABCs of effective joint pain relief and healing.

Willow bark contains salicin, a phytochemical similar to acetylsalicylic acid, or aspirin. Willow bark relieves pain and reduces inflammation. Plus, it may cause fewer side effects than non-steroidal anti-inflammatory (NSAID) drugs such as ibuprofen. In Europe, it's approved for the treatment of arthritis and headache. In the U.S., you can purchase it as an herbal extract, powder, or capsules. I recommend a daily dose of 120 to 240 mg per day depending on your pain level.

Chapter 24

A lifetime of pain relief in just three days

Concern about opioid pain drugs is reaching a fever pitch. These drugs are killing Americans of all stripes, whether prescription or non-prescription, accidental or intentional overdoses. So the scramble is on to find "new" alternatives.

Of course, the original, natural opium poppy was a much safer opioid. But long ago, big pharma "refined" it into concentrated, semi-synthetic and synthetic drugs, which can be sold for profit.

First there's morphine, which derives from the opium poppy. There is also Fentanyl, an impossibly powerful derivative that is 100 times more potent than morphine.

Once, a front page article in *The New York Times* reported a growing trend in overdose deaths related to Fentanyl. The total number of adverse drug reactions has jumped by nearly eight times in just two years between 2012 and 2014.

As a consulting forensic pathologist, I have seen many deaths caused by Fentanyl, both accidental and intentional, whenever patients apply more than one skin patch that dispenses this deadly drug.

Of course, it's not just Fentanyl causing problems. We have any number of prescription opioid drugs that lead to addiction, abuse, and overdose. In fact, a front page story in the *Boston Globe* published on the same day as the *Times* article on Fentanyl reported that opioid drug hospital admissions doubled over seven years between 2007 and 2014.

Tragically, with all these opioid drugs, the lines between accidental vs. suicidal overdose get blurry. And based upon what I have witnessed in my own practice, I believe the insurance industry keeps them blurry intentionally.

Mainstream continues to ignore
natural pain relief alternatives

The mainstream is desperate to find safe, effective alternatives. But it comes with a catch—they still want to profit from these alternatives. So ironically and tragically, they ignore the many safe, effective, and natural approaches to pain that I have been reporting about for years.

How desperate are they?

Well, big pharma is now looking at tarantula spider venom[9] to help fight pain as a "natural" approach. Of course, they're working on developing a synthetic, non-toxic version…one they can profit from.

But while big pharma continues to weave its web and trap pain patients in its next "advance" for pain treatment, I will continue to tell you about all the natural, proven, non-drug approaches for pain management hiding in plain sight.

Meditation turns off pain receptors

One of my favorite approaches to treating chronic pain is mindfulness meditation.

I recently came across another new study that shows meditation could replace opioid drugs for pain relief.

The new study came out of Wake Forest Baptist Medical Center, founded by my friend and colleague Dr. Kathi Kemper.

The study took a two-fold approach. First, the researchers reviewed the success of natural approaches to reduce pain, including cognitive-based approaches, acupuncture, hypnosis, distraction, and even placebo response. Other studies claim the success of these approaches must be due to a reductionist model whereby the body releases its own opioid-like molecules (endorphins, or endogenous opioids).

Second, the researchers investigated whether meditation has benefits for pain. And if it does, how does it work?

To begin, researchers divided 78 healthy study participants into two groups. They injected participants in one group with a drug called naloxone, which blocks the effects of endogenous opioids (opioids the body makes itself). They injected the second group with a saline solution placebo.

They then divided the groups again into a meditation treatment group or non-meditation. The meditation group (which included participants who received both the pain reliever and the placebo) practiced meditation over three days.

Next, they subjected all the participants to pain by using a hot probe at 120 degrees F. They asked participants to rate their pain using a sliding scale.

The key to pain relief may be "all in your head"

Results showed that those who meditated reported significantly less pain compared to those who did not meditate, whether they received naloxone or placebo. In fact, patients in the meditation group who received naloxone showed a 24 percent reduction in pain, even though the drug blocked any effect of endogenous opioids.

This research demonstrates meditation isn't simply like giving an opioid drug—or having the body release its own opioid-like endorphins... contrary to what the skeptics postulate.

The mind-body connection is much more complex than they can imagine. And meditation does something much more complex than just cause the body to release its own endorphins.

Furthermore, this research points out that non-drug approaches work well even in people who have developed tolerance to high levels of opioid pain drugs.

When it comes to understanding and using natural, non-drug approaches to safe and effective pain relief, once again, evidence shows that the "mind is a terrible thing to waste."

Chapter 25

ALERT: New research shows pain pills are creating a deadly epidemic

We're currently seeing an epidemic of abuse of narcotic pain-reliever prescription drugs in the U.S. This has led to calls by local, state, and federal governments to rapidly reduce people's dependence on these unsafe drugs, as well as tackle the many health and social hazards that result from this dependency.

How bad is this epidemic? Well, after a century of improving health and declining death rates among all Americans, the U.S. Urban Institute in Spring 2015 released a study showing *dramatically increasing* death rates among women ages 15 to 54.

The primary reason? Accidental overdoses of prescription pain-reliever drugs.

Perhaps even more shocking is data from the CDC and other sources, analyzed by the 2015 Nobel Laureate in Economics Dr. Angus Deaton and his wife, Dr. Anne Case, who is an economist at Princeton University.

In a study, Drs. Deaton and Case showed that death rates among middle-aged white people with no more than a high school education have increased half a percent per year over the past 15 years.

And guess what the No. 1 cause of those deaths was? Overdoses (either accidental or intentional) of narcotic drugs, as well as alcohol.

You may think a death rate that's only rising half a percent per year doesn't sound that bad. But consider this: The study reported that from 1978 to 1998, mortality rates for the same group of people *fell* 2% a year.

But starting in 1998, the death rate began steadily rising. And pain pill abuse and dependency has a big reason to do with it.

This sad truth is particularly upsetting because *no other group of people* in what Case and Deaton call "rich countries" has ever shown increases in death rates during our modern era. And historically, no population has had a comparable increase in death rates over just 15 years, unless there was a disease epidemic or ecological calamity.

And that's not the only bad news. Along with drug and alcohol overdoses and suicides, Deaton and Case say the other chief cause of the increase in middle-aged Americans' deaths is chronic liver disease and cirrhosis.

And while some of that is due to alcohol abuse, other liver problems can be attributed to pain pills as well.

As I've told you before, popular over-the-counter pain relievers like acetaminophen (Tylenol) have long been known to be the leading cause of fatal liver toxicity in the U.S. And to add insult to injury, recent research shows they are not even effective for back or other common pain.

Fortunately, there are safe, affordable alternatives to pain drugs that are readily available today. I divide them into two categories: supplements and mind-body techniques.

Natural, safe pain solutions that really do work

There are a variety of mind-body approaches that can help alleviate pain, including meditation, acupuncture, guided imagery, behavioral therapy and even yoga.

To learn which of these approaches will work best for you, it is important to understand a psychometric indicator developed over several decades at Tufts University Medical Center in Boston by the late Ernst Hartmann, MD. This indicator, called the personality boundary type, helps predict your susceptibility to various mind-body treatments.

You can use the personality boundary type in the book I co-authored with Michael Jawer, *Your Emotional Type* to determine your personality boundary type and the most effective treatments available for that type.

One of the most interesting mind-body approaches for pain relief is **guided imagery** (GI). This is a technique in which you are guided by a professional to form images in your "mind's eye" that literally overcome pain.

Guided imagery can work for everything from arthritis to surgical pain. In fact, it's now being used for pain relief after knee replacements—one of the most common, and problematic, orthopedic surgical procedures today. One new study found that most people who tried guided imagery after knee surgery had high levels of satisfaction.

Another natural mind-body powerhouse is **mindfulness meditation**, which includes mindfulness-based stress reduction (MBSR) for pain.

A new study demonstrated that only eight sessions of MBSR reduced pain and improved quality of life in people with chronic low back pain.

Of course, anxiety and depression often accompany chronic pain. In one new study, a group of chronic pain patients completed an eight-week program that consisted of an hour of mindfulness meditation training three days a week, and then an hour of meditation daily at home. Over the next year, the patients had significant improvement in anxiety, depression, and pain.

These studies involved formal, group meditation programs, but you can also get significant benefits meditating on your own. My book with Don McCown, *New World Mindfulness,* tells you all the tips for achieving mindfulness every day—no matter how busy your life.

The ABCs of pain supplements

Of course, another way busy people can alleviate pain is to take a tablet or capsule. But that oral pain medication doesn't have to be a prescription drug.

Especially when there are powerful and proven ancient natural remedies readily available for pain and inflammation in supplement form.

For centuries, traditional healers have known the secret to successful pain management includes tackling the inflammation that typically accompanies pain—something the drug companies just don't understand.

There are a variety of herbal supplements that can help reduce pain and inflammation, but I've found the most effective (especially for joint pain) is the pain-killer combo I call "the ABCs"—ashwagandha, boswellia, and curcumin.

These three pain powerhouses have come under increasing scientific scrutiny not only because of their benefits for pain and inflammation, but for a host of other health benefits as well.

One new study compared a **boswellia** extract to standard medical treatment (including pain drugs) for knee osteoarthritis symptoms. After 12 weeks, the people who were given boswellia had just as much reduction in pain and restoration of knee function as the group that got the standard treatment. In addition, the boswellia group was able to walk better than the other group, and had better overall emotional and social functions.

Curcumin's effectiveness at relieving pain has been well established in a wide range of inflammatory conditions. A new laboratory study used the novel approach of loading lipid (fat) nanoparticles into a curcumin supplement, which markedly improved pain and molecular measures of inflammation.

And in a new Belgian study, 820 people with osteoarthritis who took a curcumin extract had improved pain, mobility, and quality of life in just six weeks. The curcumin was so effective that more than half of the study participants were able to toss out their drugs for pain and inflammation.

Of course, I have long observed that the ABCs are even more potent when taken together, in the same supplement (I recommend products that contain 450 mg of boswellia gum extract, 500 mg of ashwagandha root extract, and 200 mg of curcumin.)

In a new study, researchers gave people who had painful tendon repair a boswellia-curcumin combo before and after surgery. The researchers found that the herbal duo alleviated the patients' pain better than a placebo.

Finally, **fish oil** is also well known as an anti-inflammatory and painkiller.

A major new clinical trial of fish oil for treatment of knee osteoarthritis showed a reduction in pain and improvement in walking ability. And another study found that these benefits are just as good with a lower dose compared to a higher dose of fish oil. I recommend 1-2 grams of high-quality fish oil a day.

So, as you can see, there is no reason to suffer in pain…And no reason to suffer from the potentially deadly hazards associated with mainstream pain drugs. There are a number of safe, natural alternatives that are just as effective as drugs—without the added risk.

Chapter 26

Three "hands-on" ways to get immediate relief from back pain

As far as I'm concerned, the science couldn't be clearer—the right treatment for back pain is a settled question. And it has nothing to do with drugs or surgery!

In fact, I was even invited to write an editorial about it that was published in the esteemed *Annals of Internal Medicine* nearly 15 years ago.

And from 2002 through 2007, I was principal co-investigator on one of the biggest studies on back pain ever conducted. It was funded by the U.S. Health Resources and Services Administration (HRSA). We gathered data from over 700 studies from around the world.

We organized a consortium of over a dozen accredited chiropractic colleges and medical schools, such as Harvard Medical School and Jefferson University Hospital, and had committees of dozens of clinical researchers to review the results. And we concluded the same thing that "hands-on" healers had concluded a century ago, and that modern research had even concluded a decade before:

Drugs and surgery should be your <u>last resort</u>!

There are much more effective strategies for relieving both acute and chronic back pain—no matter what the cause.

So, please, before you reach for that bottle of pain pills…before you subject yourself to an endless cycle of x-rays and MRIs…and certainly before you sign that consent to surgery—please, consider the "alternatives" FIRST.

I'll tell you more about them in just a moment. But first, it's helpful to know why back pain is such a common problem. And believe it or not, it's a problem that has evolved right along with mankind.

The great evolutionary trade-off

Your gait (or how well you walk) is a key to health and longevity, especially as you get older. But it's not about *how much* you walk. It's about *how well* you walk. And indeed, it's the ability to walk upright that sets humans apart—but it's also what sets us up for a lot of pain as well.

Walking has been a key factor in the ability of humans to survive. In fact, the ability to walk upright on two legs is a distinctly human trait. And throughout human history, this trait has freed the hands so that, together with larger brains, humans could express their creativity and productivity to build our modern, "man-made" world.

One important trade-off is that in order to walk (and run) more effectively, the legs needed to be placed more narrowly together than they are on other, four-footed mammals. This effect results in a narrower pelvis, especially at the hips.

However, humans have developed very large brains. So women need to have wider hips to allow infants to pass safely through the birth canal.

But since you can't walk effectively if the hips are too wide, human infants were born at earlier and earlier stages of development, while the brain is still immature. So human young are the most immature creatures in the universe, and require a prolonged period of dependency— with implications for nuclear family, extended family, and human social organization as a whole.

Consider it a grand evolutionary biological compromise between upright posture, freeing the hands, and having bigger brains. But there's another tremendous impact that walking upright has had on humans. One that millions of people struggle with every day—back pain.

From discomfort to disability

The spine provides structure to the entire body and helps protect the vital organs. It also provides the protective conduit for the "wiring" that runs to all the parts of the body—the spinal cord and the spinal nerves.

In animals that walk on all fours, the natural design of the spine is like a simple suspension bridge. But over time (millions of years, probably), humans began to stand erect. And the shape of the spine converted from a suspension bridge to a shallow S-shaped (or sigmoid) curve... to provide balance, structural support, and some "suspension" as well as "shock absorption."

But as you can imagine, pounding away against hard surfaces while walking not only affects the joints of the legs, but the shock waves work their way up through the pelvis to the spinal column and the individual vertebrae. The result is degenerative arthritis, or osteoarthritis in the spine.

And just like in other joints, osteoarthritis of the spinal vertebrae can lead to stiffness. As well as contribute to bony outgrowths that can impact and irritate the spinal nerves that branch out from the spinal cord. These kinds of irritations are common in the arms and the legs ("pinched nerves"). And on a chronic basis, they can cause the familiar condition of sciatica.

In the spine itself, the middle 12 vertebra are held relatively rigid by the ribs, but the seven cervical vertebrae in the neck, and the five lumbar vertebrae of the lower back have more degrees of freedom, and less support. Which is why lower back pain is such a universal source of discomfort in humans.

Of course, when there is a sudden rupture of a spinal disc (or cushion), or even a traumatic fracture of a portion of a vertebra, there can be sudden debilitating pain.

However, even without a sudden rupture or traumatic fracture, low back pain can be disabling. In fact, it's the most common cause of disability in working Americans.

But regardless of the origin of your pain, the treatments are the same.

The best ways to beat lower back pain, naturally

While it may seem counter-intuitive...one of the most important and simplest things to do when your back is sore is to actually keep moving!

Gentle exercising, such as walking and swimming, are good for your lower back, provided you have not developed a disabling condition. In fact, not moving *enough* contributes to developing the discomfort in the first place.

And a new study conducted at the University of Tel-Aviv in Israel shows that walking is as effective as clinic-run rehabilitation programs for back pain.[21]

And it only takes as little as 20 minutes twice a week.

In addition to walking, acupuncture is another extremely successful treatment for relieving low back pain. Sir William Osler, who was a leading physician at the University of Pennsylvania, Johns Hopkins, and then Oxford, during the late 19th and turn of the 20th century recommended acupuncture for the treatment of lumbago (lower back pain) through the 3rd edition of his classic textbook of medicine in 1910. (Unfortunately, all mention of acupuncture disappeared in subsequent editions of his textbook issued after his death.)

But the No. 1, proven treatment for relieving back pain and restoring function, based on decades of indisputable science and data is...

Spinal manual therapy—or an "adjustment" carried out by a chiropractor or a physical therapist.

The original "bone setters" helped pave the way for "drugless healing"

The problem of low back pain was primarily responsible for the success of two entirely new medical systems that arose in the American mid-west during the late 19th century. First osteopathic medicine and then chiropractic medicine sprang up in regions where there were fewer doctors practicing.

There had been a tradition in both European and Asian societies (whose members emigrated to the American west) of folk healers and "bone setters" that offered "adjustments." So osteopaths' and chiropractors' ability to "lay on hands" and physically manipulate the back and the body back into shape— and health—was a big attraction to suffering patients.

Another big attraction of these hands-on healers was that they promoted "drugless healing." Which allowed people to avoid taking the drugs of the time. Some of which contained toxic compounds like arsenic, lead, and mercury. So, seeing a chiropractor or osteopath wasn't just about getting effective physical treatments. Opting for osteopathic or chiropractic therapy saved people from dangerous, unpleasant, and less effective (or completely ineffective and even toxic) regular medical treatments. A good plan for our present day as well.

Unfortunately, despite the evidence, the benefits of chiropractic therapy got overshadowed by the supposed "breakthrough" of back surgery. Meantime, back surgeons got into a crisis of their own…

Don't wait until it's too late

About 10 years ago, the problem of "failed back" surgery had become so common that in some states, insurers were refusing to provide malpractice insurance to doctors who perform back surgery.

I attended Congressional field hearings in Pennsylvania to determine whether or not patients should be able to obtain back surgery in the state at all. Gov. Ed Rendell testified in these hearings. We had met before, when I opened the C. Everett Koop Community Health Education Center in Philadelphia in 1996, and we spoke afterward. He was quite open to the idea that most patients with back pain do not require surgery, and should not get back surgery. If only the medical community was as open-minded.

Of course, it wasn't a secret. In fact, it was known for a long time in the U.S. that acupuncturists, massage therapists, spinal manual therapists (chiropractors), and even herbalists were helping people with back pain.

Granted, it was usually <u>after</u> a patient had received an ineffective medical therapy. At which point it was often too late to be able to heal naturally.

And since the interpretation of all research tends to be that we still need more research, the problem of low back pain has continued to be studied. Long after the average doctor and patient should have had the results they needed to guide sensible and safe treatment.

But having to wait for more studies just prolongs the agony.

So if you suffer from low back pain, skip the expensive medical tests and surgery. And stay as far away from steroid injections as you can! You can get rapid relief from a licensed chiropractor, physical therapist, acupuncturist, or qualified massage therapist. And if you can, keep moving.

Three herbal pain soothers worth a try

While they're not a substitute for effective spinal manual therapies, there are several herbs that can help relieve pain. They include:
- Boswellia serratta extract (gum)—400 -500 mg/day
- Curcuma longa (root) (Tumeric)—200 mg/day
- Withania somnifera (root extract) (Ashwaganda)—500 mg/day

Chapter 27

A dozen ways to avoid Tylenol

I've written a lot about the dangers of Tylenol—from liver failure to having a child with behavioral problems. Of course, taking Tylenol doesn't automatically mean you'll die of liver failure. Nor does it automatically mean your children will suffer behavioral problems. It only means you have an increased risk of experiencing these adverse outcomes.

But many readers don't want to risk it. They want to know about safe alternatives to Tylenol. And I'll tell you about a dozen safe options in a moment. But first, remember this...

Always consult with your personal physician before trying ANY treatment. Even an over-the-counter (OTC) drug. Or a natural remedy. If you have a bleeding problem or take drugs that reduce blood clotting, the issues can be complex when it comes to pain relief.

That said, let's look at some potentially safe pain-relief options you can bring up with your doctor...

I highly recommend asking your doctor about **ibuprofen**. When this drug came on the market as a prescription in the early 1980s, it truly seemed like a rare therapeutic breakthrough. It seemed to work for just about everyone...from older people with arthritis pain to young women with menstrual pain.

Today, ibuprofen is available as an OTC remedy in doses of 200 mg. However, this dose is often too small to effectively relieve pain. But doctors can prescribe more effective 800 mg doses.

Some of my readers want to avoid all drugs. And I can understand that preference. I too prefer to avoid drugs whenever possible.

I have dedicated my career to determining the *real* natural alternatives to mainstream medical treatments. But I'll also tell you when the science falls short about a natural approach.

During the course of my research, I have found that virtually every folk medicine tradition includes natural and effective remedies for pain. But first, you need to know what type of pain you have. For example, some natural remedies work by reducing inflammation. Indeed, inflammation is a frequent source of pain. Other natural remedies work directly on the brain's perception of pain.

This first natural remedy, called **capsaicin**, comes from South America. And it reduces your brain's perception of pain. Derived from hot chili peppers, capsaicin is an effective, natural pain reliever most often applied topically over painful joints. But you can also take it internally.

Ginger is another natural pain-relief powerhouse. And it's been used in Asia for centuries, mainly for gastro-intestinal disorders. But ginger can also help with joint and muscle pain because it helps control inflammation.

Feverfew is an ancient European folk remedy used throughout history for everything from stomachaches to toothaches. Today, research suggests it's most useful for migraine headaches, especially when used together with the essential mineral **magnesium**.

You can also try these three ancient Indian remedies…

Turmeric can help alleviate pain by controlling inflammation. It's especially effective for reducing joint pain when combined with **Boswellia** (frankincense) and **Ashwagandha** (winter cherry). When inflammation is under control, joint cartilage can repair itself naturally and reduce pain and restore function in your joints.

In addition, Native-American Indians traditionally used **willow bark** (the original source of aspirin) to relieve their aches and pains.

Some natural remedies on the horizon are **ginseng** for fibromyalgia. **Kava kava** for tension headaches and neuropathic pain. And **valerian root** for muscle cramps and spasms.

Chapter 28

Get rid of pain permanently with new, non-invasive treatment

In an exciting study, Japanese researchers found an innovative, effective, and non-invasive way to help stroke victims cope with pain. The new technique doesn't involve drugs or surgery. In fact, it represents a whole, new approach for relieving pain, as I'll explain in moment. But first, let's look at why we even needed a whole, new approach for this common problem...

Mainstream medicine fails to treat pain effectively because it follows an old, simplistic model of the human body. They think all drugs, herbs, vitamins, and procedures interact in a physical-mechanical way with the body's cells. In other words, they think of our cells operate like old-fashioned "lock and key" mechanisms, based on 17th century Newtonian mechanics. Thus, they talk about receptors on/in cells that receive therapeutic substances like a docking station on the starship Enterprise. These receptors magically open doors to cells and cellular processes.

But for the past century, fundamental sciences—such as physics and quantum mechanics, biology, and ecology—have begun to look at *energetic* interactions. These energetic interactions form the common basis for health and healing. So, in this view, all the other therapies just access the body's energy in ways that influence health and healing.

With this new understanding about energy, the medicine of the future will learn to bypass invasive drugs and surgeries. They will go straight to the source of energetic healing.

But not everything has to await the future.

Transcranial magnetic stimulation (TMS) is already available now.

TMS is a non-invasive procedure that uses magnetic fields to stimulate nerve cells in the brain. Doctors use TMS to help treat depression, anxiety, migraines, and now—pain.

For the procedure itself, doctors place an electromagnetic coil against your scalp near your forehead. The electromagnet used in TMS creates electric currents that stimulate nerve cells in the region of your brain involved in pain.

The new study involved 18 patients who had experienced a blood clot or bleeding in one side of the brain, called unilateral ischemic or hemorrhagic strokes. Several weeks into recovery, patients began to experience severe hand or leg pain because of brain damage from the stroke. Indeed, stroke can cause severe pain sensations, such as uncomfortable numbness, prickling or tingling, as well as other pain.

All the patients in the study received repetitive TMS treatments—called rTMS—to the primary motor cortex for at least 12 weeks.

After 12 weeks of rTMS, 11 patients achieved satisfactory-to-excellent pain relief. (Researchers defined "satisfactory" relief when a patient achieved a 40 to 69 percent reduction in pain scores. They defined "excellent" relief when a patient achieved a 70 percent or greater pain reduction.) The six study patients who continued treatment for one year achieved *permanent* pain relief.

The researchers for this study urge neurologists and pain management specialists to take an interest in this effective method, which has minimal side effects. In fact, none of the 18 patients reported any serious side effects from the weekly sessions. And just two patients reported short, transient, and slight discomfort of the scalp.

I'm not surprised to see this important research come out of Japan. Since the 1990s, the country has been an active center for the study of electrical brain stimulation.

A growing body of research shows non-invasive electrical stimulation can even help improve physical rehabilitation after stroke. In fact, some experts believe electrical stimulation helps the brain form new neural connections to take over functions from damaged brain tissue.

Of course, acupuncture also helps support rehabilitation after stroke as well as manages pain. Essentially, acupuncture modulates energy, so these observations make sense. It also makes sense that Japanese researchers would take such a keen interest in TMS, since Chinese acupuncture also heavily influences the practice of medicine in Japan.

Unfortunately, these approaches get far less attention in the U.S.

When I ran the Jefferson Center for Integrative Medicine 10 years ago, we suspected you could achieve health and healing by going straight to the energetic sources. Of course, we knew the mainstream minions would never replace their drugs and surgeries with simple, safe, and energetic healing. But to my disappointment, many of the "alternative" practitioners didn't have much interest either in energetic healing. I suppose they weren't ready to give up their herbs, needles, potions, and procedures.

Of course, we are still learning how to use energy for healing.

PART 3

BRAIN-HEALERS FROM BEHIND THE CURTAIN

Chapter 29

The Insider's answer for dodging dementia

Brain deficiencies and disorders have been a mystery to medicine for centuries. In fact, scientists are just as puzzled about "mental health" and disease today as they were a hundred years ago. This is despite the efforts of our recent politically-designated "Decade of the Brain" (1990-1999). Unfortunately we've yet to overcome this century-long challenge despite the lavish funds poured into the usual academic-medical complex.

Years ago, many mental illnesses were thought to have an underlying disease (or pathology). If an underlying disease could be found, then a treatment could be developed. Sigmund Freud originally became a brain pathologist, searching for these organic causes. But when the brains of people with mental illnesses were found to be "normal" pathologically, he eventually switched courses. This is how he came to establish psychoanalysis as a different path to understanding mental health.

On the other side of the equation, brain disorders that, in fact, turned out to have an underlying pathological cause were mistakenly thought to be psychological illnesses. For example, "general paresis of the insane" turned out to be caused by tertiary syphilis, where the untreated syphilis organisms go on to destroy brain tissue.

Modern psychiatry still struggles with how to diagnose and classify brain disorders. Periodically they issue a new edition of the *Diagnostic and Statistical Manual* (DSM), the "bible of mental health." But lacking an understanding of the mechanisms of many disorders, we fall back on using statistical descriptions and characteristics.

In addition, the process for updating the DSM for 2012 has been fraught with conflict and dissension, as documented in the popular press. And of course, it's all due to the same problems we find throughout modern medical research: academic careerism, medicalization of life events and processes (which particularly have an impact on how people are "feeling"), limitations in research methodology, government interference with professional practices, politicization and political correctness, and the bias to replace psychotherapies with psychiatric drug therapies.

Another part of the problem is the large and powerful organization of professional psychologists.

While they do not use psychiatric drugs, they have been slow to embrace the kind of "mind-body" therapies that have been effective for problems that seem to cross the border between mind, body, and spirit (although they politely gave audiences to me and my colleagues, and our medical textbooks, at their annual meetings through the 2000's).

And of course all the while, research, development, and discovery of effective treatments for you slog on at a snail's pace.

So what, exactly, DO we know?

All confusion and debate aside, thankfully, there are some important fundamentals about how the brain works that are central to understanding the similarities and differences inherent in brain biology.

The brain is very metabolically active. Therefore, it needs a constant supply of a lot of blood to deliver oxygen and glucose to support brain metabolism. One-third of total blood volume flows to the brain. That means one-third of the blood cells, one-third of the oxygen, one-third of the blood sugar and other nutrients circulating in our blood is needed by the brain.

Accordingly, the brain is very sensitive to deprivation of oxygen, glucose, and nutrients. In fact, the brain will die if deprived of oxygen and glucose for only 2-3 minutes (loss of consciousness, coma, then death). This is a striking difference when compared to the needs of the lower body. For example, during surgery, when blood flow is clamped off below the kidneys, the legs can go without oxygen for hours and return to normal health as long as blood flow is eventually restored.

The brain is also very selective in what it allows to pass from the blood into the brain tissue. This is something we refer to as the "blood-brain barrier." While other tissues of the body are generally bathed in the same constituents that are carried in the blood, the brain carefully selects what is allowed to pass into the fluids that surround the brain (cerebro-spinal fluid). This property is fortunate because it keeps out a lot of toxins that would be harmful to the sensitive brain tissue.

This selective nature of the brain becomes critical when it comes to medications that are prescribed for mental health and disease.

At the same time, it's important to make sure any nutrients you may be taking are in forms that will make it across the highly selective blood-brain barrier.

7 simple tips for spotting early signs of Alzheimer's disease

As I've mentioned before, recent research indicates you are the best expert there is when it comes to early detection of Alzheimer's disease (AD).

And that's great news. Because early detection is crucial with AD. And the sooner you spot the problem, the sooner you can do something about it. In fact, keep reading and I'll tell you more about a natural powerhouse that can help prevent and slow the progression of Alzheimer's disease.

But first, take this short quiz. It will help you assess the difference between normal, age-related memory loss and cognitive decline due to Alzheimer's disease.

1. Are all new signs of memory lapses significant for dementia?

Answer: No.

It's very typical to forget names, dates, and appointments as you get older. These "signs" may be part of a lifelong pattern. These changes have more to do with neural organization than degeneration. But if you have to ask for the same information, over and over, that is not typical. Also, take note if you need to rely more heavily on memory aids. Or, do you frequently forget regular dates, like the day of the week the trash truck comes?

2. If I misplace objects more often, is that an early sign of dementia?

Answer: It depends.

Misplacing objects frequently is more likely due to distraction rather than dementia. But if you frequently have to <u>replace</u> missing eyeglasses, checkbooks, keys, jackets, etc. it's time to get a formal cognitive assessment. In addition, if you find lost objects in strange places, that can also signal cognitive decline. For example, if you find your car keys in the bathroom cabinet or in the dishwasher.

3. Which speech pattern is a sign of dementia?

a. speaking clearly and concisely
b. rambling on, frequently forgetting words or phrases
c. not recalling a word or two
d. all of the above

Answer: B.

Forgetting a word or searching for the right word is a typical part of everyday life. But consistently struggling with the same word or words repeatedly is a sign of cognitive decline.

4. Which is a sign of cognitive decline?

a. Taking a wrong turn in a familiar area
b. Getting lost driving in a new area using a map
c. Never having any idea where you are unless using a GPS device to tell you
d. Frequently getting lost in familiar areas

Answer: D.

Getting lost in familiar places while walking or driving is a strong sign of cognitive decline. But remember to check on the many cognitive side effects from drugs, which may be responsible and are reversible. This problem happens especially among older adults who take multiple drugs.

5. **I habitually miss bill payments and appointments. Does this mean I might have Alzheimer's disease?**

    Answer: Again, it depends.

Missing appointments and bill payments can happen to anyone at any age. But an increased pattern can signal a decline in cognitive function. However, these lapses can also happen with mood dysfunction. So, take this question to a deeper level…does it take you much longer to pay the bills or work on your budget? Or do you now have trouble adding a group of numbers accurately? These changes may indicate a problem with cognition.

6. **It takes me longer to complete routine tasks. Isn't this just normal aging?**

    Answer: Maybe not.

Studies show that when you multitask, you actually work more slowly. So don't try to balance your checkbook while watching TV and talking on the phone. It will take you longer. If you want to finish more quickly, focus your efforts on one activity at a time. If you still have trouble performing a single routine task like following a favorite recipe, it may signal more significant memory problems.

7. **I react to everyday stresses with greater anxiety, anger, depression, and/or mood swings than ever before. Is this a normal part of aging?**

    Answer: No.

Typically, we learn to handle emotions better as we age. But some people never learn. And in some, exaggerated emotional responses may indicate the onset of progressive cognitive decline. People with Alzheimer's disease rely on routines to go about their day. They may become irritable or uncomfortable when their routine changes for any reason. As a result, they may begin to withdraw from social experiences they once enjoyed.

If any of the scenarios above sound familiar, don't ignore them!

Talk about your concerns with friends and family. And the sooner you act, the better!

Neuro-nutritive nutrients for your body and mind

There are many approaches to maintaining health and managing diseases of the body using herbal and dietary supplements. However, when it comes to understanding and applying basic nutrition to enhancing and improving the normal mental functions and performance of the mind, there is still the "blood-brain barrier" to contend with. The good news is, it *can* be done.

Through the combination of cognitive science and nutritional medicine, science has developed dietary supplements and food products that can enhance basic brain and mental function and performance.

While there is much *talk* of "smart drugs," which may theoretically be taken by anyone to support improved mental performance, there is some *proof* of smart nutrients that cross the blood-brain barrier and help the brain do its basic job using safe and effective vitamins, minerals, and natural constituents.

Unfortunately, many of these natural "smart nutrients" are still clouded in controversy. Fielding heavy criticism from the modern medical-complex. So much so, that many "alternative" practitioners will even avoid the topic completely.

Even herbs that have been used effectively for decades—such as *ginkgo biloba* for dementia, *kava kava* for anxiety, *St John's wort* for mild-moderate depression, *valerian* for insomnia, and *feverfew* for migraine headache.

So you can imagine that when it comes to addressing something as serious, and confounding, as Alzheimer's disease, nearly everyone looks the other way. Which is tragic because currently, it's estimated that nearly 5 million Americans have Alzheimer's Disease (AD).

It's also the 8th leading cause of death in the United States. And once diagnosed, the average life span of an Alzheimer's patient is eight years.

The spectrum (and fearful specter) of age-related cognitive decline is a major neuropsychological area that has yet to be addressed by the pharmaceutical or the natural products industry.

But there are alternatives that may help.

And recently, the research behind one nutrient in particular is beginning to lead the pack…more on this breakthrough in just a moment.

Type III diabetes—the brand new, DEADLY epidemic no one saw coming

You've probably heard the old saying "bad things come in threes." And after nearly a century of research, it appears that may be the case with diabetes.

You're likely familiar with Type I and Type II diabetes. But now it looks like there's yet another form on the horizon—Type III diabetes. And it may be the most sinister, dangerous form of the disease yet.

A modern-day disaster 90 years in the making

For centuries diabetes had been known primarily as a condition of excess fluid loss through frequent urination, with sugar in the urine.

But in 1922, two researchers won a Nobel prize when they discovered that diabetes mellitus was a primary deficiency of insulin. Insulin is responsible for moving glucose (sugar) from the blood into the tissues. Without it, the tissues, including the brain, literally starve to death in a sea of plenty.

Since then, there have been many more discoveries regarding this condition. Like the difference between Type I and Type II diabetes.

The Nobel-prize winning researchers discovered what has come to be known as Type I (or "juvenile") diabetes. With Type I, from childhood, the pancreas simply does not make insulin. Type I diabetes is treatable by injecting synthetic insulin over regular time intervals.

But as the 20th century progressed, an initially mysterious new type of diabetes emerged. People with this form of the disease produce adequate insulin. But their tissues become resistant to the actions of that insulin. And, as a result, glucose can't enter the tissues. Instead, it accumulates in the blood.

This "insulin-resistant" diabetes became known as Type II diabetes.

Now, I believe we are witnessing a third form of the disease—Type III diabetes. And it may have been masquerading as the No. 1 medical mystery of our time—the modern misery of Alzheimer's Disease.

Elevated blood sugar shrinks your brain

A recent Australian study found that high blood sugar levels appear to actually cause the brain to shrink. Even in people who don't have Type I or Type II diabetes.

This study of 250 men and women showed that high blood sugar levels appear to damage the brain. Specifically, they cause the areas associated with memory, cognitive function, and emotional processing to shrink. And impairments in these areas are the hallmark symptoms of Alzheimer's dementia.

In fact, these researchers found that highly-educated people in their 60s, with even mildly elevated blood sugar, had the brains of unhealthy people in their 70s.

While prior studies have shown that diabetics have higher rates of dementia, this is the first study to show these effects even in people who are not diagnosed as having Type I or Type II diabetes.

So, are they suffering from Type III diabetes?

In non-Type I or -Type II diabetics, high blood sugar can result not only from consuming too much sugar in the diet, but from generally poor diet, lack of exercise, and chronic stress. So, blood sugar is a problem for everyone, not just diabetics. And now we're seeing just how significantly it can affect your brain (as well as other parts of your body).

I first heard about this link last September, and have been looking into it ever since. And, indeed, a large body of evidence is now suggesting that Alzheimer's is primarily a metabolic disease, just like diabetes. But different enough from the already well-known Types I and II to warrant its own classification. Type III diabetes.

Why your brain needs insulin

As I mentioned above, an association between Alzheimer's dementia and Type II diabetes is already long-established.

In fact, the risk of dementia among Type II diabetics is *two to three times higher* than in the general population. There are also associations between Alzheimer's and obesity, and Alzheimer's and metabolic syndrome (a pattern of diet- and metabolic- related disorders).

Some researchers first proposed that Alzheimer's was actually another form of diabetes back in 2005. The authors of these original studies investigated the brains of people who had died of dementia. They found that the levels of both insulin and insulin- like growth factors in the brains of Alzheimer's patients were sharply reduced.

And insulin levels were lowest in the parts of the brain that appeared most affected by dementia.

Insulin in the brain has a number of important functions in addition to glucose metabolism. It helps regulate transmission of signals from one neuron (nerve cell) to another. And it influences their growth as well as their ability to adapt to changes and survive.

Experiments conducted since then appear to support the link between diet and dementia. As ever, these observations show the biochemistry of dementia to be fantastically complex, involving inflammation, stress, oxidation, the accumulation of a certain brain protein and the transformation of another—among other factors.

This is one case where more research does, in fact, need to be done. And this is the kind of research that NIH should really be doing.

However, if current indications hold true, Alzheimer's disease could be yet another catastrophic impact of poor diets.

Perhaps one of the worst thus far

Around 35 million people suffer from Alzheimer's disease worldwide and based on current projections, with the rate at which the population is aging, this epidemic will rise to 100 million by 2050.

But if, as many scientists now believe, it is caused largely by the brain's impaired response to insulin, those numbers could rise much further. In the U.S., the percentage of the population with Type II diabetes has almost tripled in just 30 years.

If Alzheimer's dementia—Type III diabetes—acts the same way, the potential for more human suffering is immense.

But while U.S. government research on Alzheimer's flounders around, there are steps you can take to help protect yourself and your family now. In fact, there are some exceptionally effective tools for combating this burgeoning epidemic.

Starting with one that I'm particularly excited about.

The latest blood-sugar darling
tackles Alzheimer's, too

Berberine is quickly becoming one of the new "darlings" of the nutritional medicine world. And the "buzz" has focused largely on this herbal remedy's ability to balance blood sugar and combat diabetes. But the new research on berberine that caught my eye recently had nothing to do with blood sugar or diabetes—or so I initially thought.

Several new studies have shown impressive results using berberine for Alzheimer's.

But now that Alzheimer's is emerging as Type III diabetes, the link between these two fields of research on berberine makes perfect sense.

But berberine defends against Alzheimer's not only by helping to regulate blood sugar.

3-tiered brain protection
you won't find anywhere else

New experimental results have found that berberine protects the brain in at least three more distinct ways:

1. It can safeguard your brain from the dangerous oxidation damage that can "eat away" at brain tissue.

2. It targets and destroys memory-killing enzymes that have long been considered key in the development of Alzheimer's.

3. It promotes healthy blood flow directly to the brain—an essential element to conquering dementia.

Berberine also seems to be able to block certain nerve receptors, which may partly explain its anti-Alzheimer and neurotransmitter-modulating properties.

Add these specific actions to berberine's well-established blood sugar benefits and it appears that this herb may hold the key to preventing and even slowing the progression of Alzheimer's disease (Type III diabetes) like nothing before it.

I recommend 500 mg per day, taken over the course of two or three doses to achieve a steady state.

The first step in avoiding and managing
ANY type of diabetes

Of course, no discussion of metabolic disorders is complete without addressing the importance of diet.

The food industry engineers its products to bypass the neurological signals that would otherwise prompt people to stop eating. Filling them with unhealthy fats, sugars, and high fructose corn syrup. Essentially ensuring they're completely devoid of any real nutrients. Which makes processed, packaged foods a disaster not just for your waistline, but also for your blood sugar, your brain—and your health in general.

Cutting out overly processed foods should be the first step in avoiding—or treating—ANY disease, including diabetes (Types I, II, and III).

Three more common causes of dementia

Alzheimer's is just one form of devastating dementia. There are three other common neuro-degenerative problems afflicting the brain and mind. The common denominator in all dementia is neuro-degeneration, destruction and loss of neurons, or nerve cells in the brain.

Schizophrenia-related cognitive impairment. Today as many as 60 million people worldwide have schizophrenia. Most people with schizophrenia also suffer from cognitive impairment, although it is independent of the psychotic symptoms of the illness. In North America, it is estimated that more than two million people have schizophrenia. While there is an $18-billion drug business to treat the psychosis associated with schizophrenia, there are no approved drugs for treating the cognitive impairment.

Mild cognitive impairment from bypass surgery. Approximately 500,000 patients in the U.S. and 800,000 patients worldwide undergo coronary artery bypass graft (CABG) surgery every year. It has now been recognized that the changes in blood flow associated with the procedure bring about dementia in many patients. Currently there is no therapy available approved to ameliorate or treat the cognitive damage associated with artery bypass surgery.

Stroke. Every 45 seconds in the U.S., someone experiences a stroke. This fact translates into approximately 700,000 new or recurrent strokes in the U.S. each year. It is the second leading cause of mortality in the world, the third leading cause of death in the U.S., and is the leading cause of long-term disability. In spite of this, there has been failure to provide effective treatments.

Chapter 30

Berberine—the Alzheimer's answer no one will pay attention to

Berberine is a mental powerhouse that may have the ability on almost all fronts to provide greater cognitive support and protection. To dodge dementia before it stops you. And it's a solution you aren't likely to hear about elsewhere.

Berberine has long been used throughout history. It is still used today in Northern India, as a bright yellow coloring dye for leather, wood, and wool fabrics. In fact, if you have a woven Indian carpet on your floor, you have probably already noted the bright yellow color imparted by berberine. It also has a use in modern medicine and pathology because of its ability to stain certain tissue cells to show their appearance under the microscope.

Berberine is found in numerous plants worldwide, including the large plant family *Berberis*, or the barberries. It is also found in the important (and ecologically threatened) medicinal plant *Hydrastis canadensis* (Goldenseal), and the important Chinese herb *Rhizome coptidis* (Golden thread or *Huang-Lian*), among others. Berberine is usually found in the roots, stems, and bark. Chemically, it is an isoquinolone alkaloid, and the plant alkaloids are known to have a number of potent biological activities.

Indeed, typical of plant alkaloids, berberine has a number of health effects, throughout the body, including acting as a potent antibiotic (which can also overcome infections caused by bacteria that are resistant to drug antibiotics), anti-fungal, and anti-parasitic.

Hundreds of recent research studies (far too many to share in detail here) reveals this medical marvel can provide a host of additional health benefits. It's been shown to help lower cholesterol, improve blood sugar metabolism, and has anti-cancer properties.

And incredibly, new research shows berberine may also hold the key to preventing and even slowing the progression of Alzheimer's disease and other dementia, like nothing before it. In part, because berberine has been found to be able to penetrate the blood-brain barrier and effect cells of the central nervous system. And new experimental results have found that berberine works in three distinct ways:

1. It can safeguard your brain from the dangerous oxidation damage that can "eat away" at brain tissue.

2. It targets and destroys memory-killing enzymes that have long thought to be key in the development of Alzheimer's.

3. It promotes healthy blood flow directly to the brain—an essential element to conquering dementia.

Berberine also seems to be able to block certain nerve receptors, which may partly explain its anti-Alzheimer's and neurotransmitter modulating properties. Other experimental studies have shown berberine to increase neurotransmitter (noradrenaline and serotonin) levels in the brain. Berberine may also act in a manner comparable to some anti-depressant drugs by increasing available serotonin in the brain.

Results suggest benefits in patients with depression, bipolar affective disorder, schizophrenia, or related diseases in which cognitive capabilities are affected.

The half-life of berberine suggests administration of a daily dose of 500 mg, taken two or three times per day to achieve a steady state.

Chapter 31

Beyond berberine: Your nutrient toolbox for cognitive support

As mentioned above, there are several natural products that have been shown to help protect the brain. Following is a quick list of those least talked about in terms of brain function and mental health by both mainstream and alternative practitioners.

Creatine

Creatine is a beta-amino acid popularized in recent years by bodybuilders and other athletes for muscle development and repair of muscle tissue after exercise, as well as energy-enhancing properties. Some reports suggest that people over 60 do not make enough creatine to maintain muscle and strength.

But creatine is becoming more widely researched for its neuro-protective and neurogenesis benefits. For example, as an element for some alternative treatments for Amyotrophic Lateral Sclerosis (ALS) and Parkinson's disease. The dosages for such treatment would be at a higher, therapeutic level, and not the more typical recommended dose of between 1 and 2 grams. Accordingly, use of creatine should be individually tailored and monitored under supervision of a qualified health practitioner.

Lecithin

Lecithin is generally a mixture of glycolipids, triglycerides, and phospholipids (e.g. phosphatidylcholine, phosphatidylethanolamine, and phosphatidylinositol). Phospholipids are the major component of the membranes that encase every cell in the body. In the brain, phosphatidylcholine and phosphatidylinositol protect nerve cells by forming a protective sheath around them to insulate them, allowing nerve impulses to move more efficiently to and between cells. In addition, phosphatidylcholine is a precursor of acetylcholine, a neurotransmitter in the brain and muscles. An increase in acetylcholine may lead to more efficient nerve and muscle function and increased memory performance and capacity. Unfortunately, some medications can deplete acetylcholine. Supplementing with lecithin may help counter this drug side effect.

Some qualitative research on lecithin supplementation found that when a short-term or long-term memory deficit exists, a single therapeutic dose of lecithin can increase memory performance within 90 minutes. It may also help improve verbal and visual memory. And has neuro-protective effects related to Alzheimer's disease.

Lecithin is available in 1,000 mg supplement doses, but may require up to 25 grams (25,000 mg) daily, used in food quantities, to see the full benefits.

Royal Jelly

Royal jelly is an amino acid-rich gelatinous substance secreted by worker bees to feed queen bees. Since queen bees grow to be considerably larger than worker bees, and live much longer, it has been assumed by many enthusiasts to produce benefits for humans. The popularity of health products containing royal jelly has increased over the past years. While its anti-aging and energy-enhancing properties have been reputed for many decades, only recently has more rigorous research been performed to separate fact from folklore.

Modern research shows that royal jelly improves lipoprotein metabolism, promotes growth of neuronal stem cells and neurons, inhibits oxidation of lipids (as in brain tissue) and is a general antioxidant. A dose of 6 to 10 grams (6,000 to 10,000 mg) per day, essentially used in food quantities, is recommended.

Cocoa

Cocoa contains biologically active flavonols and polyphenols. Flavonols have recently been the subject of much research. They have been found to enhance vasodilation which in turn decreases blood pressure and increases peripheral blood flow to the muscles as well as to the brain. Cocoa has also been shown to improve lipid metabolism. And international researchers have recently uncovered even more healthy properties associated with the flavonol antioxidants found in cocoa beans.

Eighteen chocolate-centered studies—including investigations of how cocoa might affect blood pressure, heart disease, painful nerve disorders and cancer risk—were presented at the American Chemical Society's annual meeting in March 2012. These studies establish the biological plausibility of antioxidant effects of dark chocolate in small groups and even demonstrated the potential harm-reducing effects for smokers.

But don't look for health benefits from your favorite milk chocolate candy bar. Most of the studies used unsweetened regular cocoa powder. There are a couple of degrees of separation because when you make chocolate you add fat, in the form of cocoa butter and sugar. And nobody's going to eat a tablespoon of unsweetened cocoa. So the studies used cocoa-flavonoid compound supplements, with average doses of 400 to 500 milligrams. Which is equivalent to 32 bars of milk chocolate or eight to nine bars of dark chocolate. Too much for even the most die-hard chocoholic.

You can find cocoa flavonol extract supplements with up to 1,000 mg in natural supplement shops and from online supplement retailers.

Virgin Coconut Oil

Coconut oil, in its virgin state, is a tropical oil consisting of medium-chain fatty acids that convert readily into energy and are not stored in the body as fat. These kinds of essential fats are important for brain tissue cell membranes and neuronal sheaths.

A saturated fat, it has been maligned for several decades as a result of misinformation by the vegetable oil industry. Alternative health practitioners advocate coconut oil consumption for weight loss and maintenance regimens. Coconut oil is a rich source of lauric acid and monolaurin, known agents that are being explored by pharmaceutical companies for drug development potential. Coconut oil lowers lipoprotein cholesterol levels in the blood and tissues and lowers lipoprotein markers for heart attack.

A dosage of 20 grams (20,000 mg), essentially in food quantities, appears beneficial.

Taurine

Taurine is so named because it was initially isolated from ox bile (*Taurus, the bull*). It is a beta-amino acid gaining attention from researchers and supplement manufacturers for health-promoting and anti-aging properties.

Research has shown taurine plays a role in the function of skeletal muscles and the central nervous system, as well as regulating blood pressure and glucose levels. It's also being explored as an adaptogen and anti-anxiety agent. Taurine has been identified as an amino acid neurotransmitter.

A dose of 500 mg per day offers sufficient health benefits.

Lutein

Lutein is a prominent constituent of green, leafy vegetables. I helped discover its role in human metabolism and nutrition in the 1980's. Since then, it has developed a role in vision and eye health as a dietary supplement. Since the eye contains neurological tissue, this has led to current interest in its possible benefits for the brain. In addition to eating green leafy vegetables, a daily dose of 12 mg of lutein is recommended.

Going above and beyond for total protection

In addition to supplementation, staying active (mentally and physically) will help keep your brain fit as well as your body. Do the daily crossword puzzle and keep up with your monthly *Insiders' Cures* newsletter and *Daily Dispatch* emails.

A healthy diet and maintaining a healthy weight is also important. And controlling blood pressure and heart disease is key to maintaining healthy circulation and blood flow to the brain (and to avoiding strokes). Controlling diabetes is also critical as high blood sugar can destroy nerves and the blood vessels that supply them.

Chapter 32

Vitamin E outperforms drug
for Alzheimer's disease

All of the nutrients I've discussed so far are important for keeping your brain functioning as you age. But according to a new study, a simple vitamin may be the one of the biggest brain breakthroughs to come along in decades.

Researchers have found that people who have high levels of vitamin E tocotrienols in their blood have a lower risk of cognitive impairment—including Alzheimer's disease.

In fact, in a new study, men and women with AD who took this vitamin significantly delayed the progress of their disease. They lived longer overall.[6] Plus, perhaps more importantly, they lived longer *independently*.

Here's another interesting point about this study…

Researchers compared the vitamin to a drug commonly prescribed to treat moderate-to-severe AD patients. And the vitamin **outperformed** the drug!

For this study, published in the *Journal of the American Medical Association* (JAMA), researchers recruited 613 patients with mild-to-moderate Alzheimer's disease. Most of the participants attended 14 various Veteran's Affairs medical centers around the country. Researchers randomly divided them into four groups.

The first group took 2,000 IU of vitamin E each day for a little over two years, on average. Vitamin E is a fat-soluble vitamin that acts as an antioxidant. It can slow down processes that damage cells in the brain and elsewhere.

The second group took 20 mg of Memantine, a commonly prescribed AD drug. The third group took *both* vitamin E and Memantine. And the fourth group took a placebo.

Researchers found that the vitamin E group had significantly slower "functional" decline compared to the placebo group. This means they lived longer independently. They continued to do their own cooking, washing, and shopping. And they required less caregiver time and attention compared to the other three groups.

Overall, the researchers saw a "delay in clinical progression of 19 percent per year" in the vitamin E group compared to the placebo group.

Interestingly, neither the Memantine drug group nor the combined Memantine-vitamin E group showed any clinical benefits. Researchers think Memantine must interfere with how the body metabolizes vitamin E. It's a sad state of affairs, indeed, when a mainstream AD treatment not only doesn't work, but negates the effects of a basic nutrient that *does* work!

Vitamin E showed other benefits as well. The annual death rate in the vitamin E group was only 7.3 percent. But the groups that didn't take vitamin E had an annual death rate of 9.4 percent.

This study shows used a daily dose of 2,000 IU of natural mixed vitamin E. A level which has struck some awestruck observers as "high"—but only because RDA's are so ridiculously low to begin with.

Tocotrienols also appear to help prevent cancer (including prostate cancer), as well as cardiovascular disease.

All it takes is some real knowledge of human diet and nutrition to make sense of the isolated bits and pieces from today's often incoherent medical research.

Just don't look to the FDA or the mainstream government-industrial-medical complex to provide that knowledge or guidance.

My advice?

While we continue to wait for more useful results to come in, you can't go wrong taking 50 IU per day of vitamin E (as d-alpha tocopheryl acetate). If you are actually struggling with dementia, check with your doctor about upping your dose of vitamin E. Hopefully he or she is not still following the misguided, outdated research from 10 years ago.

Yes, in this study, Alzheimer's disease patients took 2,000 IU of vitamin E daily. And their symptoms improved.

But remember, when you take a vitamin to <u>treat</u> a disease, it will most likely require much higher doses than when you take one for general health. Unfortunately, most researchers don't get this right when they study nutrients for chronic diseases. Instead, they use low-ball doses that can't reverse a disease that took a lifetime to develop.

But when you use vitamins primarily to support general health, you must consider many different factors, such as:

1. **How much of the nutrient do multivitamins or once-a-day vitamins contain?** When I make dosage recommendations for individual nutrients, such as vitamin E, I must consider that many people probably already take a daily multivitamin. And when recommending a specific dosage, I allow for the amount many already get in the daily multivitamin. In this case, typical multivitamins contain 100 IU of vitamin E. So, when I recommend taking 50 IU of vitamin E, it takes into account that many already get 100 IU from multivitamins.

2. **How much is the Daily Recommended Allowance?** I also consider the USDA's Daily Recommended Allowance (RDA). While RDA's are by no means the basis of my recommendations, and they are wholly inadequate for reversing chronic diseases, I certainly don't ignore the standard. In this case, the RDA for vitamin E is only 22 IU. However, the RDA goes on to state a "safe upper limit" of 1500 IU.

3. **How much of the nutrient can we assume an average healthy adult already gets through diet?** Remember, the purpose of dietary of supplements is to "supplement" what is already in your diet. For general health, your goal should be to get most of your nutrition from the whole foods you eat. And I assume if you're interested in supplementing with vitamin E, you're also highly educated about good nutrition. And probably eating better than average to begin with. You also get large amounts of vitamin E by eating green, leafy vegetables, healthy oils, eggs, nuts, and seafood. So, when

I recommend supplementing with vitamin E, I take these dietary sources of vitamin E into account.

4. **What other supplements do you take?** Manufacturers often add vitamin E to their "custom" supplements. So starting with 50 IU gives you room to get vitamin E from these other supplements as well as from dietary sources.

All things considered, 50 IU of vitamin E is a safe place to start for anyone and everyone who wants to support their general health. Now, as I said, if you want to treat a specific disease, like Alzheimer's disease, you will likely need a higher dose. But in that case, as with the management of any medical condition, a qualified doctor should closely supervise your regimen.

I often look with alarm at some of the dosages I see in typical, "run-of-the-mill" dietary supplements. It seems to me that much of the supplement industry just throws in "mega" doses and "super" doses. But they don't have any real science to support these excessive doses in the general population.

Maybe they think it looks more impressive. But *excess does not equal success*. That's just not how a healthy, balanced approach works.

My mentor, the late C. Everett Koop, former U.S. Surgeon General, used to quote, "the least medicine that works is the best medicine."

Let's keep working with the right doses, not just the largest.

In addition, make sure to get plenty of all the B vitamins. Folic acid is especially important. It helps reduce homocysteine levels, which sharply increase your risk of developing AD and heart disease. In one European study, a daily dose of 800 micrograms of folic acid significantly lowered homocysteine. It also improved cognitive function and memory in middle-aged and older adults.

Chapter 33

Meat and fish help you stay lucid longer

The nutrient combo that can reduce brain aging by 40 percent

We all know there are rarely "magic bullet" solutions to health and healing—whether a single drug or even a single nutrient.

No nutrient works in isolation from other nutrients. In fact, an important new study shows that a good way to protect against age-related brain wasting and dementia is to ensure you get enough B vitamins *and* omega-3s—at the same time.

This nutrient combo is so effective, it slowed down brain atrophy in people with mild cognitive impairment by an average of *40 percent*.

I'll tell you more about this exciting study in a minute, but first, let's examine why so many doctors and researchers still seem to act like nutrients operate in a void in our bodies and brains, independent of other nutrients.

Why you don't take nutrients one at a time

Of course, it's very complex to analyze the interactive effects of different nutrients in a single study. As I point out earlier, one of the biggest failings of the National Cancer Institute's diet and cancer research program 30 years ago was the insistence by an old-time surgeon, Dr. Jonathan Rhoads, (who was chairman of the National Cancer Advisory Board) that nutrients must be studied only one at a time.

Nothing in the human body works by Dr. Rhoads' ridiculous "one-at-a-time" rule—but rather in a series of balanced, synergistic, and synchronized actions. We tried to get around this old doctor's ill-informed dictum by developing a design for cancer studies so that several different nutrients could be analyzed at once. But our approach was used more in theory than in practice.

While the mainstream still fumbles along trying to understand the importance of balanced nutrients for cancer and other chronic diseases, it has equally big problems understanding nutrition and the brain.

For example, we all know the importance of B vitamins for general health and for the brain and nervous tissue. In Europe, they call B vitamins "neuro-vitamins." Likewise, we all know the importance of omega-3 essential fats (typically from fish oil) for heart health, immune function, and brain and nervous tissue.

But we didn't know precisely how these two key nutrients work together in the brain. Which leads me to the new study.

A one-two nutrient punch against dementia

Researchers from Oxford University analyzed data from 168 people age 70 or older. All of the study participants had mild cognitive impairment.

The researchers found that the people who took daily vitamin B supplements (B6, B12, and folate) only had a reduction in brain wasting if they also had high omega-3 blood levels.

On the other hand, the people with low levels of omega-3s showed *no* brain benefits from taking B vitamins.

Researchers suggested that one way B vitamins and omega-3s together may benefit the brain is by lowering levels of a key amino acid known as homocysteine. Interestingly, this is the same way B vitamins help protect our hearts and blood vessels as well.

Optimum ways to get your Bs and 3s

The best way to get the healthiest balance of vitamins, minerals, and other nutrients is through both your diet and dietary supplements.

For Bs, that means eating eggs, fish and other seafood, and meat at least twice a week. And taking a high-quality B-complex supplement that includes at least 50 mg each of thiamine, riboflavin (B2), niacin/niacinamide (B6), and pantothenic acid, plus at least 200 mcg of folic acid/folate, 12 mcg of B12, and 100 mcg of biotin.

Eating two servings of fish a week will also give you omega-3s. And I recommend 1 to 2 grams of fish oil supplements per day as well.

Chapter 34

The surprising secret for shaving decades off your brain's age

There is a constant flow of research showing more and more health benefits for chocolate. Now, studies are reporting that this tasty treat can actually *reverse* cognitive decline in older adults. And reduce blood pressure and insulin sensitivity.

An Italian clinical trial called the Cocoa Cognition and Aging Study is the first scientific examination of how consumption of cocoa flavonols can affect cognition in older people. Cocoa flavonols are the ingredients that give chocolate its healthy properties.

The study included 90 people, ages 65 to 85, who had mild cognitive impairment but not dementia. The participants who consumed a drink with the most cocoa flavonols daily for eight weeks had notably better scores on cognition and verbal fluency tests.

In addition, the people who drank the cocoa beverage with a high or intermediate amount of cocoa flavonols had lower blood pressure and insulin resistance than the people who consumed the least flavonols.

A recent follow-up to that study found that cocoa flavonols can do even more for our brains. The researchers found that daily consumption of a cocoa flavonol beverage substantially reversed age-related memory decline in healthy people ages 50 to 69.

"If a participant had the memory of a typical 60-year-old at the beginning of the study, after three months that person on average had the memory of a typical 30- or 40-year-old," said lead study author Dr. Scott Small of the Columbia University Medical Center.

Keep in mind these studies used specially formulated cocoa flavonol-containing drinks. You can get the same effects from eating chocolate, but you need to be careful. Unfortunately, many methods of processing cocoa remove a lot of the flavonols found in the raw plant.

Bitter is better (and why you might like it more than you think)

The best approach for getting the benefits of cocoa flavonols is to consume moderate amounts of dark chocolate with as little added sugar as possible. Or you can drink hot or cold dark-chocolate beverages. After all, the Mayans traditionally consumed chocolate as a beverage, as did the Spanish who "discovered" it in the 16th century. Solid chocolates were not widely available until the late 18th century.

Either way, you're better off avoiding the less-nutritious milk chocolate or white chocolate.

You may think you won't like dark chocolate because it does not have as much sugar and milk as "milk chocolate." But you may be surprised. A recent study conducted—perhaps unsurprisingly—at Penn State Medical Center in Hershey, Pennsylvania, found that even self-professed milk chocolate lovers enjoy dark chocolate, once they give it a chance.

The researchers enrolled 99 participants in the study. At the outset, about half the participants said they preferred sweeter, milk chocolate. And the other half said they preferred darker, "semi-sweet" chocolate.

The researchers randomly gave out five different chocolate samples. The samples contained 35 percent, 50 percent, 65 percent, 80 percent, or 100 percent natural cocoa powder. Then they recorded the participants' responses.

Overall, more women than men preferred darker chocolate. About 20 percent of the total group accepted the 100 percent cocoa powder. This makes sense, as this powder tastes the most bitter. In fact, it has no sweetness to it at all.

About 20 percent of group also accepted the 80 percent cocoa powder samples. But here's the interesting part…

It didn't make a difference whether they were self-professed milk chocolate lovers or dark chocolate lovers. About the same number of people who said they preferred milk chocolate as those who said they preferred dark chocolate accepted the highly bitter, 80 percent cocoa powder sample.

So therein lies the lesson.

Even if you think you're a milk chocolate lover, you can probably tolerate a more bitter chocolate...something with at least 65 to 80 percent cacao. If you already like the taste of dark chocolate, try some with 100 percent cacao and see what you think.

Chapter 35

Can cleanliness contribute to Alzheimer's?

Over the centuries, our lives and communities have become much more hygienic. And that's mostly a good thing. But according to scientists at the Biological Anthropology Laboratory at Cambridge University, UK, there's a startling downside to all this cleanliness. It seems to be correlated with an increased risk of Alzheimer's disease (AD).

By comparing data from 192 countries, the researchers discovered that the most industrialized, wealthiest countries with large urban areas and good sanitation have the highest rates of AD. The reason, the researchers believe, has to do with the "hygiene hypothesis." This is the idea that immune systems that are overly protected against exposure to germs are weaker and less able to ward off disease.

In well-off, highly sanitized countries, our immune systems are "protected" through the widespread use of antibiotics, chlorinated water, antibacterials, and artificial surfaces. All these factors can lead to insufficient development of white blood cells, including the T-lymphocytes, which attack invading microbes.

Previous research has noted deficiency of certain types of T-cells in the brains of people with AD. What's more, an underdeveloped immune system exposes the brain to the inflammation associated with AD.

This idea is not as new as it may sound. The immune system requires some exposure to microbes in order to develop properly. When exposed naturally to germs early in life, the body develops lifelong natural immunity.

Since the 19th century, many populations have had less and less exposure to "friendly" microbes in soils, animals and manure, which strengthen the immune system, and had always been present throughout earlier human history. But as our exposure to germs has decreased, so has our resilience.

For example, polio became a big problem in the late 19th to mid-20th centuries (before the vaccine was developed) when a large proportion of the population began practicing "better" hygiene. This new level of cleanliness kept people from being exposed to polio as babies, but it didn't do them any favors later in life. There is even evidence from ancient Egypt that the royal elites who were protected from germs had more problems with viruses such as polio later in life.

Polio is one of many viruses that travel through the environment—in this case infecting humans through contaminated water supplies. It is basically an intestinal virus.

But in a small minority of cases, the virus passes into the spinal cord and can cause temporary or permanent paralysis. The vast majority of babies infected in infancy simply experienced an acute viral infection. Paralysis or partial paralysis is very rare. (This may be due in part to the "passive immunity" that babies retain from their mothers—especially if they're also breastfed). That exposure in infancy confers lifelong immunity.

If, on the other hand, better hygiene staves off your exposure until you're an adolescent or young adult, you have a much greater chance of having it spread into your spinal cord and cause paralysis.

Each person infected with polio will on average pass the infection to several other people. So, we can see how the virus hitting a previously uninfected population of "baby boom" adolescents would have caused an epidemic during the 1950s…as it dramatically did.

But don't ditch the soap just yet…

No one is suggesting that we stop washing up. In fact, as I've explained in previous in the past handwashing is the best way to prevent the influenza virus from spreading.

But don't use antibacterial soap or hand sanitizer. And it's important to only use antibiotics when they're absolutely necessary.

If you want to further support brain function, nature provides a number of options, including berberine and carotenoids such as lutein and zeaxanthin. And dirt—if we believe the new study's hypothesis.

So, don't be afraid of getting a little dirty while working in the garden, enjoying nature, or visit a working farm. And let your children or grandchildren play out in the dirt too!

Chapter 36

Natural brain booster hiding in plain sight

In a large telephone survey conducted in 2013 by the Centers for Disease Control (CDC), one in eight men and women over 60 years reported experiencing memory lapses that have been "happening more often or getting worse" over the past 12 months. Plus, 35 percent of these men and women said their confusion or memory loss interfered with their work, social activities, or ability to do household chores.

Yet, astonishingly, just 19 percent of them reported ever discussing their memory loss concerns with a healthcare provider.

The fact is, mainstream medical practice has very little to offer when it comes to supporting cognitive health. And in terms of public health, two "decades of the brain" initiatives have still not been enough to get adequate attention or funding from the government. Let alone effective treatments. Instead, funding gets funneled to the never-ending "war on cancer" and misguided heart disease campaigns.

So older adults who want to stay mentally sharp must find their own solutions.

It's no wonder online "brain training" programs like "Lumosity" now have more than 60 million users. Games on these websites are designed to exercise cognitive abilities such as attention, flexibility, memory, processing, and problem solving. These games "exercise" the brain on a computer screen, so you "use it" and don't "lose it."

But there is much more you can do to support your brain besides playing computer games.

Three years ago, I recognized this gaping void in mainstream care and began to formulate some natural solutions to brain health. Of course, the "natural know-it-alls" are now climbing on the brain bandwagon too. They realize various nutrients are important for brain and nervous system health. In fact, the natural products industry now offers any number of gimmicky, catchy, "new" brain health products.

These products may sound "high tech," but they usually rely on some "magic bullet" approach that's been recycled from a "heart" miracle…or "anti-aging" answer…into a supposedly "revolutionary" brain solution.

Don't be fooled.

The real natural brain boosters are hiding in plain sight.

In fact, a recent scientific review evaluated the use of coffee (*Coffea arabica*) and caffeine to prevent or delay age-related cognitive decline and dementia. The study also evaluated the influence of coffee and caffeine on aging and age-related diseases.

Of course, previous research showed caffeine and caffeinated coffee can improve short-term alertness, attention and memory. But controlled clinical trials and longer-term studies that follow the impact of caffeine on the eventual development of *actual brain diseases* cost much more. And funding for this kind of serious, long-term research is scarce in the government's drug-addled world of grants.

Despite these funding limitations, the reviewers found a clear trend toward cognitive protection and positive effects of caffeine in dementia prevention.

In my experience, when researchers observe a clear trend—despite limitations in the research—it's usually a sign the effect is strong enough to be seen even without stronger research design and methods.

In other words, "where there's smoke, there's fire."

And when it comes to preventing and delaying dementia, a steaming cup of hot coffee may be just what you need.

Caffeine appears to have many positive influences on the body. For example, it positively affects blood circulation, vascular supply, inflammation, and glucose metabolism. All these factors play important roles in preventing cognitive diseases, as well as cardiovascular diseases and diabetes.

Of course, as with all natural approaches, dose is important. And it appears you need to get about 350 mg of caffeine—or about three cups of coffee—per day. We don't yet know how many years you have to drink three cups per day to gain these benefits. (Again, there is no funding for controlled long-term or "lifetime" studies.)

Of course, researchers know coffee contains many other beneficial constituents in addition to caffeine. For example, several polyphenols appear to have even greater neuroprotective effects than caffeine.

Bottom line?

Drinking three to four cups of caffeinated coffee per day has clear, short-term brain benefits. And probably long-term benefits as well.

Chapter 37

Why brain training games won't help you

Mainstream medicine has nothing to offer men and women who want to prevent or reverse dementia. So it's no wonder people turn to brain training games in an attempt to forestall the devastation of this disease. I have reported before about the proliferation of these brain training games on the internet. It's a rapidly growing, $2 billion annual industry.

But there isn't much evidence that playing brain games by yourself does any good. On the other hand, going to a community center and participating in a group program may offer some benefits. In my view, engaging in any kind of group activity—which involves social interaction—offers some benefits, regardless of how flawed or insubstantial the program itself may be. It's simply the social interaction itself that helps support healthy cognitive function as you get older.

Of course, the creators of brain training programs make many people believe their cognitive training will prevent or delay dementia. They often cite the theory of neuroplasticity, described as the brain's ability to form new connections to enhance or maintain cognitive function.

Yes—neuroplasticity is useful in rehabilitation from stroke and some other sudden onset brain diseases. But it's not relevant in the chronic, degenerative brain diseases most commonly causing dementia.

You see, cognitive function is complex. It involves auditory and visual attention, executive function, manual control tasks, memory, processing speed, reaction time, reasoning, and spatial ability. And the pattern of cognitive dementia always shows declines in multiple areas of these brain functions.

So even if there *is* a way to prevent decline in one area, it's unlikely to preserve or improve daily function because other areas of the brain are also compromised.

For example, just slowing memory loss (if possible) would still not delay dementia. Driving a car, for example, would still be impaired due to losses in other cognitive functions such as executive function, reaction time, and spatial relations. The same applies to cooking, working around the house, or using the internet. These activities require attention, motor skills, and processing abilities, in addition to adequate memory.

Study results don't live up to the marketing hype

Researchers have studied cognitive training in both younger and older people, and in those with and without normal cognitive function, or dementia. Studies show it can lead to some improvements in *targeted* areas of cognitive function limited to the specific function for which the training was offered. For example, "memory training" may improve performance on the same kinds of memory tests in the future. But it doesn't affect processing speed.

One excellent study directly demonstrated that cognitive training doesn't reduce dementia rates. The ACTIVE trial assigned 2,802 older adults to one of three cognitive training groups on memory, processing speed, or reasoning. The fourth group—a control group—received no cognitive training. After five years, the researchers found no significant difference in dementia rates between the cognitive training groups and the control group.

This large study began in 2002 and appeared in publication 10 years later. But it's only been cited in scientific literature five times in the three years since publication.

No wonder the public hears far more about the bogus "benefits" of brain training—thanks to some aggressive marketing—than they do about this solid, factual, scientific study which barely made it into print.

Thankfully, leading experts in the neurosciences strongly oppose these efforts to mislead the public. In fact, two experts described the fallacy of these approaches in the *Journal of the American Geriatric Society*. They say there's no reasonable "mechanism of action" nor any scientific evidence that such approaches could work.

Plus, in October 2014, the Max Planck Institute for Human Development in Berlin published a report called, "A Consensus on the Brain Training Industry." They concluded that "exaggerated and misleading claims exploit the anxiety of adults facing old age for commercial purposes. Perhaps the most pernicious claims, devoid of any scientifically credible evidence, is that brain games prevent or reverse Alzheimer's disease."

An active daily life is the best brain booster

As I mentioned earlier, cognitive training concentrates on just a single cognitive function—without cross-over to other abilities. Furthermore, the modest amount of time actually spent on cognitive training per week is insignificant compared to actual daily activities involved in working, playing, studying, reading, and thinking. So—even if these computer games *could* work to delay dementia, it's highly unlikely that a few hours, or even a few hundred hours, could help build cognitive capacity to any adequate degree.

It makes a lot more sense to sustain cognitive ability by continuing to perform daily life tasks. Join a book club. Spend some time out in Nature. Most of all, stay active and engaged every day in the world around you.

Chapter 38

Four simple steps for avoiding Alzheimer's disease

Here are a few natural approaches you can use to counteract those risk factors.

In the first-ever comprehensive analysis on AD risk factors, researchers found four dietary factors offer strong protection against AD: coffee, folate, vitamin C, and vitamin E. Let's go through them one at a time to review the main points:

1. Coffee

Many studies show drinking three to four cups of coffee per day benefits the brain. Coffee comes from a natural plant that contains many biologically active, beneficial constituents that may act by protecting and supporting brain cells directly. These constituents also support healthy blood circulation to the brain.

2. Folate

Folate is the key B vitamin that reduces homocysteine, the real risk factor behind cardiovascular and heart disease. Plus, high homocysteine is also a major culprit in AD. Unfortunately, many people still remain deficient in folate and all the B vitamins. So, as I always recommend, make sure to take a high-quality B complex vitamin daily.

3. Vitamin C

Vitamin C is one of nature's prime anti-oxidants. It's so important, all animals except humans and guinea pigs make their own. We must get vitamin C from foods and/or dietary supplements. Fortunately, many fruits and vegetables contain lots of vitamin C. But you should also supplement with this essential nutrient daily to help protect against AD.

4. Vitamin E

Thank goodness someone is finally waking up to the power of vitamin E for brain health. Especially when it comes to AD. In a study that compared vitamin E to a new AD drug in men and women with dementia, patients who took vitamin E demonstrated dramatic improvements. Patients who took only the drug showed no improvements. And the patients who took both vitamin E and drug experienced no improvements.

How do you explain that last outcome?

Well, it appears the AD drug actually canceled out the benefits of the vitamin.

Of course, that study followed men and women who already had dementia. Imagine what this potent vitamin can do for someone like you who just wants to prevent brain aging.

You also want to stay active and maintain a healthy weight to stave off dementia as you get older. Eating protein with every meal will also help maintain muscle mass, skeletal health and vitality, all of which are associated with longevity.

Plus, you should take dandelion extract and aspal, the South African herb, daily to help stay physically strong as well. You can find these ingredients in some of the higher quality dietary supplements. You can even find them in water-soluble powders that you can add to water or another beverage. Look for aspal and dandelion together in the same product(s) and make sure you get the right doses of both every day.

Big pharma runs around trying to develop new drugs based on flawed, failed theories about what causes AD. In the meantime, you can take your health into your own hands with these simple steps to prevent AD.

Chapter 39

The battle against brain disease

While the U.S. government-industrial-medical complex keeps coming up short, Nature offers a number of science-backed solutions

Despite the first Bush administration declaring that the 1990s was the "Decade of the Brain," mainstream medicine is no closer to discovering how to treat—let alone eradicate—deadly brain diseases than it was 25+ years ago. As a recent article in the medical journal *The Lancet* pointed out, compared to cancer, diabetes, and stroke, research on brain diseases is often neglected or ignored altogether.

One reason could be that worldwide, brain diseases still account for only about 4 percent of all deaths from non-communicable diseases, and about 5 percent of all disabilities. But as the global population grows older, those numbers are expected to increase dramatically. In fact, some researchers believe that by 2050, one in 85 people worldwide will be diagnosed with Alzheimer's.

But Alzheimer's isn't the only brain disease striking fear into Americans. Other neurological diseases—like Parkinson's, *amyotrophic lateral sclerosis* (ALS), and multiple sclerosis—are equally terrifying. And equally devastating. Particularly because, in most cases, there are no effective mainstream treatments.

Fortunately there *are* some simple, **natural** approaches you can use to boost your brain power and combat these four fearsome neurological diseases. And they are *scientifically proven to work*. I'll tell you all about them in a moment. But first, let's take a closer look at the different types of brain diseases.

Unknown causes, devastating effects

Dementia symptoms include loss of memory, mood changes, and problems with communication and reasoning. Alzheimer's disease is the most common form of dementia.

Although mainstream medicine remains baffled about the cause of this increasingly frequent disorder, some research shows that if you're exposed to a lot of herbicides, pesticides, aluminum, copper, lead, or zinc (in heavy metal form), you may be more likely to end up with dementia.

Parkinson's disease has multiple symptoms, including tremors, walking and balance problems, speech pathologies, and depression. Yet nearly 200 years after a British doctor first described "the shaking palsy," the cause remains unknown.

But a growing body of molecular research suggests that cell abnormalities might be a factor. Which would help explain why several metabolic poisons may increase the risk—including pesticides and wood preservatives. Excessive exposure to copper, iron, lead, and manganese may also be a factor.

Motor neuron diseases are characterized by progressive paralysis due to degeneration of neurons in the brain, brainstem, and spinal cord. The best known of these diseases is *amyotrophic lateral sclerosis* (ALS—also known as Lou Gehrig's disease).

Ironically, although the vast majority of motor neuron diseases are not genetic, most of the research over the years has been on genetic factors. There have been few studies on environmental causes.

But some research shows that people who work with electricity or agricultural chemicals may be more susceptible to motor neuron diseases. A history of head injury, including sports injuries, may also be a culprit.

Multiple sclerosis is a neuro-inflammatory disease that damages the protective coverings of nerve cells in the brain and spinal cord. Like Parkinson's, it has many symptoms, including fatigue, walking difficulties, vision problems, and cognition issues.

As with other brain diseases, MS remains a mystery to the mainstream—

although there is some evidence that exposure to chemical solvents increases the risk.

In fact, it's very likely that a significant proportion of all brain diseases are associated with environmental and occupational toxin exposures.

But, as I mentioned above, despite a "decade of the brain," we are still decades behind on basic studies on this topic.

Another little-known casualty of the "war on cancer"

Biologists and medical scientists have known for centuries that the brain is our most sensitive organ, taking up one-third of all the blood, oxygen, and glucose in our bodies. So you'd think that any disease affecting this vital organ would be a top research priority. But in its infinite wisdom, the U.S. government had chosen to focus (almost solely) on cancer instead in terms of statistical searches for "causes." Why? The answer goes back many years.

Epidemiology and biostatistics are the main methods used to study the causes of diseases in human populations, including brain disease (epidemiology comes from the Greek "*epi*," or upon, and "*demos*," the people). Initially, epidemiology was a very effective tool for studying infectious diseases. But by the late 1960s and early 1970s, health policymakers declared infectious diseases had been "conquered" by antibiotics and vaccines. Instead, attention—and funding—shifted to waging a "war on cancer."

Of course, the brief armistice on infection proved to be short-lived in the West (and there never was one in the third world) when AIDS hit the scene in the 1980s, followed by antibiotic-resistant bacteria. But in the meantime, epidemiologists shifted from studying acute, short-term infections to chronic, long-term diseases like cancer.

This shift required quite an adjustment, but was helped along by billions of dollars in new taxpayer funding. And of course, any time money is involved, statisticians follow.

By the time I got to the National Cancer Institute in 1983, the statisticians were calling the shots—rather than physicians or biologists. That's akin to putting accountants in charge of the troops in a real war. In fact, statisticians were in charge of two-thirds of the "war" on cancer—namely prevention and early detection.

And when it came to studying nutrition and cancer, these new careerists, calling themselves "nutritional epidemiologists," were designing the methods for and performing the studies on nutrition and cancer. Despite the fact that they knew almost nothing about human biology, nutrition, dietary behavior, or metabolism.

But while all of this cancer research was going on, there was another area of chronic illness that was being completely ignored by epidemiologists—neurological and brain diseases.

Even as early as 1977, when I starting on my master's degree in epidemiology and biostatistics at the University of Pennsylvania, program director Anita Bahn, Ph.D., was trying to get funding for training and research programs to study brain diseases, which were being left behind in the war-on-cancer feeding frenzy.

Sadly and ironically, Dr. Bahn died suddenly of a ruptured brain aneurysm. Instead of moving forward, the university decided to shut down her program altogether, transferring grad students to "nearby" Johns Hopkins in Baltimore or Columbia in New York.

(But because I was enrolled in the M.D./Ph.D. combined degree program, I was "stuck" at Penn in Philadelphia. Fortunately, I was soon approached by Nobel laureate Baruch Blumberg to enroll in his new biomedical anthropology program.)

The result of all this tunnel-vision research and funding is that the government has not kept track of brain diseases the way it has done for cancer for decades. And there have also been few long-term studies on human brain diseases.

So despite all the professed political concern in recent decades about brain health, the mainstream has little to offer when it comes to avoiding, preventing, or treating the modern epidemic of devastating brain diseases.

Fortunately, there is good evidence that some basic nutritional and mind-body approaches can be helpful. Let's take a look.

The science behind natural approaches for brain health

Doctors and researchers have long known that the eight different **B vitamins** are key for brain health. In fact, their effects on brain tissue are so well established that in Europe they're referred to as "neuro-vitamins."

New research shows that the B vitamins may be particularly effective against Alzheimer's disease—reducing the shrinkage that causes Alzheimer's by a whopping *90 percent.*

For optimum brain health, I recommend *at least* 50 mg per day of B1 (thiamine), 50 mg a day of B6, 400 micrograms of folate (B9), and 100 micrograms of B12.

You can get all of these amounts and more in a typical B vitamin complex supplement. But my recommendations are designed so you can take different supplement formulations that may contain some Bs as well.

Besides the Bs, there are a few other nutrients that are also critical for brain health.

Vitamin D. This essential vitamin is key for the brain and nervous system, and also helps combat mood disorders like depression. The latest research confirms that low vitamin D levels are associated with a substantially increased risk of Alzheimer's disease and dementia of all kinds. And there is growing research that a lack of vitamin D is a contributor to multiple sclerosis.

I recommend 5,000 IU of vitamin D per day, which, again, leaves room to take other supplements that may also include some D.

Vitamin E. Recent evidence suggests that high doses of vitamin E (2,000 IU per day) can help prevent Alzheimer's disease. This finding is so surprising and new—although very encouraging—that I would like to see more research. And the FDA still needs to sort out its own mistaken perspectives on vitamin E. For now, stay with 50—200 IU per day of E (as d-alpha tocopheryl acetate).

Lutein. I helped discover the role of the carotenoid **lutein** in human nutrition and metabolism back in the mid-1980s. Since then, research shows its ability to penetrate the blood-brain barrier and provide health benefits to both brain and eye tissue.

Even though you won't find any government recommended daily allowances for lutein, I recommend taking 12 mg per day.

Berberine. This herbal powerhouse is often overlooked by the natural-know-it-alls who are still talking about tired, old gingko. But there is increasing research showing that taking 500 mg per day of berberine results in impressive brain benefits.

Nicotine. Research shows nicotine lowers the risk of Parkinson's disease. You don't necessarily have to smoke cigarettes to get this effect, though. Nicotine gum, patches, or electronic cigarettes are all widely available. And a recent study showed that eating peppers, which naturally contain nicotine, can reduce your chances of getting Parkinson's by 19 percent.

L-Alpha glycerylphosphorylcholine (Alpha GPC). This compound occurs naturally in the brain. Alpha GPC is actually a precursor for a "memory chemical" in your brain, acetylcholine. This brain chemical is believed to be critical for memory, thinking, and learning, among many other critical nerve functions. I recommend 50 mg per day.

Healthy fats. Your brain tissue needs healthy fats and cholesterol from fish, lean meats, and/or high-quality fish oil supplements. Research shows that these fats may also help insulate nerves, lowering the risk of MS. I recommend taking at least 1 to 2 grams per day of omega-3 fatty acids from fish oil. There are many other health benefits as well.

Finally, there is a pair of lifestyle choices you can make that have demonstrable brain benefits.

Keep your weight in check. Many studies have concluded that obesity early in life is linked with dementia later in life. However, new research from Oxford University shows that this risk decreases as we age. Interestingly, researchers found that people in their 70s who were obese had no increased risk of dementia, and by age 80, obese people were actually 22 percent *less* likely to develop dementia.

So there's no need to "overdo" it with an overly restrictive diet or intense workout regimen. Following a healthy, balanced diet and getting moderate amounts of exercise will help keep your weight in check—and your brain healthy—through middle age and into your "golden years."

Meditation and yoga. Researchers at the University of Illinois recently studied 108 inactive people between the ages of 55 and 79. The study participants who did yoga three times per week for eight weeks had improved memory and mental skills. But the study did not find cognitive benefits for participants who only did stretching and toning exercises. So it appears that engaging the mind in a meditative practice like yoga provides more benefits than simple "mindless" exercise.

As the brain disease epidemic unfolds, hopefully there will be more research into the prevention and treatment of these devastating disorders. But in the meantime, as you've seen here, there is still much you can do to avoid devastating brain diseases and keep your mind sharp and healthy, no matter how old you are.

Chapter 40

Profits—not cures—for Alzheimer's disease

Over 20 years ago, I attended a big government event in Washington, D.C. where science bureaucrats announced the "Decade of the Brain." At the event, they claimed we would conquer brain and neurological diseases over the next 10 years. And they proudly proclaimed massive increases in spending on research for brain and nervous system illnesses.

But clearly, it was just a publicity stunt to get more new funding from the taxpayers for more of the same old research.

During that "Decade of the Brain," science made little—if any—real headway regarding treatments. Instead, we endured 10 years of disappointing clinical drug trials, with virtually no progress toward curing or preventing brain diseases.

In February of 2014, the Obama administration announced another "Decade of the Brain." But here again, it's just a publicity stunt to spend more of your tax dollars.

Of course, brain changes can occur 10 to 20 years before you experience any overt symptoms of AD. So, by the time doctors diagnose you with dementia, too much damage has already occurred.

So early prevention not only makes sense…it's critical.

But government health officials and mainstream medicine continue to ignore berberine and vitamin E as viable AD treatments. They also ignore the apparent risk of lowering cholesterol levels for the brain. And they certainly don't give credit to the role vitamin D and B complex play in protecting cognition and neurological function.

They simply want you to take "new" drugs to prevent a disease they can't treat.

So, what are some of the new drug approaches proposed to prevent dementia? And, do they present opportunities for *true* prevention?

One approach targets the formation of a protein called beta-amyloid. In AD patients, this protein clumps into plaques in the brain. It disrupts the flow of information across nerve synapses and causes nerve cell death. But—unlike vitamin E—these drugs fail to stop the progress of AD.

So now, they're trying the failed beta-amyloid drugs out as "preventative" drugs. They can then give these failed drugs to younger people, before they present with AD symptoms. Just look at what's happening in Yarumal, Columbia…

In this small town, men and women get AD in their late 40s—about 15 years ahead of the norm. Researchers discovered they carry a gene variant associated with early-onset dementia.

In a clinical trial that began in 2013, men and women in their 30s from this small town who carry the gene began taking a drug developed by Genentech. Researchers hope the drug will prevent AD by blocking or slowing the formation of beta-amyloid plaques in the brain.

Since people with this gene form beta-amyloid earlier in life, anti-amyloid drugs are supposed to help in this genetic form. I worry if the study shows even a glimmer of promise, doctors will one day begin doling out AD drugs to anyone like candy to "prevent" AD. Like they do now with statin drugs, with their claim to "prevent" cardiovascular disease.

And the consequences could be just as deadly.

Fortunately, with the information you've just read, you're armed with real, scientifically proven cures. Ones that can keep you and your loved ones from suffering the devastating effects of Alzheimer's and other forms of dementia.

And if you're interested in learning more, please consider my brand new Alzheimer's learning program… **Dr. Micozzi's Complete Alzheimer's Cure Protocol: An All-New, All Natural Protocol to Protect and Restore Brain Health and Reverse Memory Loss.**

PART 4

MASTER YOUR HEART HEALTH— NATURALLY

Chapter 41

Shocking results! Not all is as it seems

In 1976, I was among a small group of U.S. graduate students awarded a scholarship to study in Asia. The scholarship was awarded by the Henry Luce Foundation (Founder of *Time*, *Life*, and *Fortune* magazines—who had been born in China of U.S. missionaries). Though it was barely one year after the last of the Americans were evacuated by helicopter from the rooftop of the U.S. Embassy in Saigon, Vietnam, I decided to conduct my studies in Southeast Asia.

Unlike the other scholars who landed in large urban areas (what demographers call "primate" cities, like Taipei, Bangkok, Jakarta, Singapore, and Manila) I chose to go into the jungles of Mindanao, Philippines, bordering on the Spice Islands of storied history. There, I sought a more authentic encounter with indigenous cultures.

I went to an area called, *"Donde Non Hay Doctor,"* or "where there is no doctor." These tens of thousands of islands, as well as the Malayan Peninsula, of Southeast Asia make up a living archaeology of human settlements. The original peoples of the area were pushed into the deep interior of the jungle islands by the arrival thousands of years ago by the Malay peoples of today. During the ancient era, the expansion of Hindu culture, Chinese mercantile influences, and the expansion of Islam turned Southeast Asia into the perfect melting pot to observe traditional healing. Including shamans, herbalists, midwives, and other traditional healers. Pretty good for a place that claims to have no doctor…

My base in Davao represented a rapidly growing population. It was quickly moving from a rural to urban setting, resulting in conflicts among the many different cultures and languages of Southeast Asia. In this environment, school children were rigorously segregated according to their abilities in performance in school.

My goal was to establish standards for normal blood pressure in children. All we knew at that time is that blood pressure is low (and heart rate high) in younger children and blood pressure increases as children age, until reaching the "normal" blood pressure of adulthood, which we say is 120/80.

I gathered the data, class by class. And soon, a pattern became clear. The rate of "higher" blood pressure was much greater among the remedial students in each grade, in each age group. So the students who did poorly in school were the ones with higher blood pressure.

So I started to look for physiological causes for the high blood pressure. Something that might be making the children "sick," that might account for their poor performance in school. But I couldn't figure it out. I couldn't find any physiological reason for these children to have high blood pressure. Nor a connection to their poor performance.

When I returned to the U.S., I mentioned my conundrum to a friend of mine, a neighbor of my parents. He was the Chairman of Physiology at the University of California and an expert on environmental physiology and stress. He was running studies in the "space age" Human Centrifuge Laboratory where they exposed humans to high stress and measured the effects of stress on raising blood pressure. And he was quick to point out the error in my thinking. When I turned my analysis around, I realized that the increased stress of doing poorly in school, and being segregated and treated poorly by the teachers, was responsible for raising blood pressure in these poor students.

Now, it's important to note that back then, "modern" medicine gave very little credence to the role of stress in health (just as it ignored nutrition). So my theory was debated.

Some had suggested that the students with high blood pressure must be drinking water with more salt in it. But the body is normally able to remove excess salt unless there is a reason for it to hang on to excess fluid and electrolytes (like salt). This can happen in times of stress. And, in Southeast Asia, there were traditional fishing villages that had the highest intake of salt yet recorded…yet blood pressure was actually low in adults and the elderly. Only when those villages were disrupted and the fishing communities moved from rural to urban areas, did blood pressure levels rapidly increase in those displaced and stressed populations.

So I persisted in defending my conclusion that stress was actually the cause of the high blood pressure. And finally, I was able to publish my results, as a student, in the *American Journal of Public Health*.

Fortunately times have changed. And my research prevailed. Today, nearly everyone understands how important stress can be to blood pressure and cardiovascular disease. The problem now, however, is how overlooked—or perhaps I should say "overshadowed"—blood pressure is as a primary risk factor for heart disease.

Cholesterol is NOT the most important risk factor for heart disease

A lavish amount of attention, effort, and money has been spent on controlling cholesterol. And the great medical-pharmaceutical complex has worked relentlessly to continue to lower the recommended cholesterol level for heart health. Of course, the end result is that more and more people will be caught in the net of taking dangerous cholesterol-lowering drugs.

But the truth is…half of the people who die of heart disease have *normal* cholesterol levels. And lowering cholesterol by a few points may not have any effect at all. Cholesterol is NOT the most important risk factor it's set up to be.

Blood pressure, on the other hand, is a *much* different story. Above all else, controlling blood pressure has the most direct and essential connection to cutting heart disease. The importance of controlling blood pressure should not be overlooked, or taken for granted. While lowering cholesterol by a few points may or may not have any benefit, lowering blood pressure by even a few points is *always* worthwhile.

And when it comes to your heart's greatest threat, I have what might be a *surprising* recommendation…

Seven critical heart health markers more important than cholesterol

Doctors routinely measure fasting blood glucose and insulin levels as well as hemoglobin A1C in people with diabetes. The first two of these tests are well known, but you may not be as familiar with hemoglobin A1C. This test gives a good long-term measure of your average blood sugar numbers over time.

Unfortunately, many doctors still don't measure homocysteine levels and do not take them seriously. But they should. Your body uses homocysteine to make protein and to build and maintain tissue. However, too much of this substance may increase your risk of stroke, certain types of heart disease, and peripheral artery disease.

So, without further ado, here are the targets for these four critical heart disease markers.

- **Fasting blood glucose.** The ideal range is 65 to 99 mg/dL. However, if your hemoglobin A1C is at a healthy, lower level, your doctor will likely be less concerned if your blood glucose is over 99 in a single test.

- **Fasting insulin.** A normal level is below 5 uIU/mL, but ideally you'll want it below 3.

- **Hemoglobin A1C** should be between 4.4 and 6.5 percent.

- **Homocysteine.** The Mayo Clinic says a normal level is between 4.4 and 10.8 µmol/L.

To help get all of these numbers where you want them, focus on improving your diet. (See Part 5 of this book for more on diet and proper hydration)

But there are a few more important factors to consider in assessing your overall heart health. And, unfortunately, your doctor is even less likely to monitor these markers. Unless, of course, you insist on it.

Three more heart health markers you should keep close tabs on

Other important measurements you should consider are C-reactive protein (CRP) and fibrinogen. CRP is a marker of inflammation.

Research has linked CRP to increased risk of coronary artery disease. And fibrinogen is a protein involved in blood clotting. Elevated levels can lead to dangerous artery-blocking clots.

Combined with the other parameters I mentioned above, these tests can help your doctor assess your overall risk of heart disease.

Your CRP level should be less than 1 mg/L, and your fibrinogen level should be between 200 and 400 mg/dL. To achieve this, follow a healthy, balanced diet. High-quality fish oils are particularly helpful at reducing the chronic inflammation that can boost your CRP level.

And keep in mind that research is also showing that your vitamin D level may be just as important as other tests in determining your risk of heart disease. A blood level above 50 ng/ml is healthy, and a daily dose of 4,000 to 5,000 IU of vitamin D is safe and appropriate for everyone.

One final heart-healthy tip: Avoid excess iron. It can potentially accumulate in your heart muscle and other tissues, eventually leading to organ failure in some people. I've also conducted research with Nobel laureate Baruch Blumberg that showed that excess iron in the body increases the risk of cancer in both men and women. Never take a supplement containing iron unless you have been diagnosed by a doctor with an iron deficiency.

Chapter 42

The ONE prescription I will always recommend for high blood pressure

This powerful cause of heart disease requires a potent remedy.

Admittedly, one of the challenges of natural, alternative therapies is that, while effective, they are gentler and generally take effect over longer periods of time as compared to their highly-potent drug counterparts. And when it comes to lowering high blood pressure, you need to use something that is going to work fast.

Extremists who reject ALL drugs in favor of natural supplements have nothing to talk about here, because there aren't really any dietary supplements that can bring down high blood pressure quickly. While some "natural experts" may claim to have nutrients that work for supporting blood pressure...don't be fooled.

There are many that can support heart health <u>overall</u>, which I will show you in Chapter 30, but none will compare to the most effective, and necessary approach—taking a blood pressure medication.

So, while there are many natural medicine "experts" who won't—or can't—recommend a drug medication, <u>I can and will when it is the best medicine</u>.

While there *are* many effective "mind-body" therapies that can help manage your underlying stress there is no acceptable alternative treatment that can substitute for fast and effective drug therapy for this dangerous condition. And fortunately, modern medicine has developed many safe and effective drugs to control blood pressure over the decades.

If you have high blood pressure you should have your blood pressure monitored and treated by a physician using these effective drug therapies. However, you and your doctor need not run to the latest, most expensive blood pressure drug offered by the drug industry. It is important to choose wisely.

What to look for...

Safe and effective drugs for blood pressure have been around for several decades with an immense amount of clinical experience on their best uses. Many people don't realize that even after a new drug is "approved" for use by the FDA, something called "post-marketing surveillance" is required to continue for many years.

It is during this surveillance, when drugs are being used by millions of people over many years, that so many of the disastrous side effects of many drugs are discovered. This is why we are constantly hearing that new drugs "approved" by the FDA are found to have dangerous side effects and the FDA issues "warnings" and restrictions, or they are pulled off the market altogether.

So when it comes to choosing a blood pressure drug, the safest course of action is to work with your doctor to choose one that's been around for many years. This could also save you a lot of money, since you'll have more generic drugs to choose from, which are a fraction of the cost of new, still-patented drugs. The point is—newer is not always better—or safer. Especially when it comes to anti-hypertensive medications.

Talk to your physician about trying out these older, effective drugs for controlling blood pressure.

Remember, everyone is an individual and may react differently to different medications. It may take some trial and error, with very close monitoring, to find the right medication for you.

The older drugs for blood pressure fall under the following categories:

1. Drugs that act to lower blood pressure through their effect on the nervous system

>Clonidine   Propranolol
>Methyldopa   Reserpine

2. Drugs that lower blood pressure by their effect on nerve endings

>Guanethidine Reserpine
>Monoamine oxidase inhibitors

3. Drugs that lower blood pressure by dilating blood vessels

>Diazoxide   Nitroprusside
>Hydralazine   Prazosin
>Minoxidil   Thiazides

4. Drugs that lower blood pressure by blocking nerve receptors ("Beta" and "Alpha" Blockers)

>Metapropolol Phenoxybenzamine
>Nadolol   Prazosin
>Phentolamine Propranolol

5. Drugs that lower blood pressure by influencing blood-pressure regulating hormones produced by the kidney

>Captopril   Saralasin

These drugs are given by their generic names as they are all off patent. Check with your doctor to see what is available by prescription and if they are appropriate for you.

Survival guide to blood pressure medications

Believe it or not, 100 years ago, blood pressure medicines contained cyanide. Not surprisingly, they caused some thoroughly unpleasant side effects. So it was often hard to get patients to stay on these medications. Unlike most drugs that address the symptoms of a disease, patients felt better when they stopped the medications.

Luckily, in more recent decades better, safer, more effective drugs have become available. There are still a few potential side effects. But in most cases, they're easily managed.

Beta-Blockers (like Propranolol) block adrenalin, relax and open the blood vessels for easier flow, and can reduce the speed and force of the heartbeat. But because they block adrenalin, they also can cause side effects such as faintness, dizziness, and cold extremities. They can also narrow the air passages in the lungs, which may cause wheezing, cough, and shortness of breath. Alpha-blockers are somewhat similar but may also increase cholesterol and weight gain, as well as episodes of sudden drops in blood pressure.

If you suffer any of these side effects, see your doctor about adjusting the dose or the prescription. And remember to ask about drugs that are "off patent." They're less expensive and have stood the test of time in establishing their safety.

Diuretics (or "water pills") are designed to eliminate excess fluids, making it easier for the heart to pump. They increase urination, which may already be a problem in men with prostate problems. And it may also allow key nutrients to escape in the extra urine. Most physicians recognize the potential loss of potassium, but may not be aware of the loss of other nutrients.

If you're taking a diuretic, make sure you are well hydrated and have adequate intake of vitamins and minerals.

Vasodilators relax and open the blood vessels, which allows blood to flow more freely and reduces blood pressure. However, they may cause problems similar to the ones listed above for Beta-Blockers.

Some of these potential symptoms may have you raising your eyebrows. But rest assured, if there's one thing modern medicine is good at it is managing diseases with drugs. And also managing the well-known and accepted side effects of those drugs. And in the case of high blood pressure, the benefit of swiftly and efficiently lowering it with the use of drugs far outweighs the risks of the side effects of the drugs.

But, again, one of the easiest ways you can help control the costs and the side effects of blood pressure medications is to consult your doctor about using a "generic." These have been around long enough to go "off patent," which dramatically lowers the price. And they've been used long enough that the FDA has had a chance to discover any hidden problems that emerged after they "approved" the drug. Which means your doctor will be well-equipped to spot—and deal with—any potential side effects that may occur. Some of these older drugs include Diazoxide, Hydralazine, Minoxidil, Nitroprusside, Prazosin, and Thiazides.

And, of course, it's just as important with high blood pressure as it is with any chronic condition to adopt a healthy diet and exercise program, lose weight, and reduce or manage stress through any number of effective "mind-body" techniques.

Chapter 43

Starting NOW—heart healthy relaxation tactics from the "Inside"

Once you have your blood pressure under control through appropriate drug therapy and monitoring by a physician, it is time to address the underlying stress that contributes to high blood pressure, heart disease, and many if not most other chronic diseases.

A basic approach in all of natural medicine is that the mind and body work together and each continually influences the other. Thus, nearly any effective therapy is essentially a mind-body therapy. However, some therapies are specifically called "mind-body" because they appear to draw directly on the power of our thoughts, emotions, and feelings to influence the disease or healthy states of our normal body functions. Literally, "mind over matter." There are several that are safe, proven effective, and widely available.

Biofeedback. We all learn as adults to control our emotions and feelings and to project a calm and controlled image to the outside world. But under the rigid exterior of the body, our feelings have a torrent of effects on our internal workings. Biofeedback gives us back information about how blood pressure, heart rate, and other vital signs are responding to environmental stimuli and stresses—and teaches how to consciously control our reactions for a healthier, stress-free response to life.

Guided Imagery. Visualization is a powerful ability the mind. You can literally create images in your "mind's eye" and train yourself to see your body becoming healthier. You can visualize a picture of immune system cells destroying cancer cells, for example. Or you can imagine yourself in a calm, healing environment and literally take your body to that place physiologically, lowering your blood pressure along the way.

Hypnosis. Today, hypnosis is understood as using the "power of suggestion" to move mind-body connections in proper alignment for healthier outcomes.

Meditation & Yoga. There are different approaches to meditation. Transcendental Meditation (TM) came to the U.S. from India, but there are strong traditions of meditation, or "contemplative thought," in the early U.S., dating from our Founding Fathers, such as Adams and Jefferson, to men of American letters, such as Emerson and Thoreau. And today, it can be seen as a simple, practical "break" from our hectic day. We can think of this form as Mindfulness Meditation. Simply paying attention to what is happening in the moment and how you are feeling about it.

Likewise, yoga is used to enter meditative states. There are several approaches in India but the Hatha-Yoga tradition, emphasizing physical postures and breathing, has become most popular in the west (probably because of its emphasis on the physical vs. mental aspects of meditation). Either way, yoga and meditation are pathways to the mind-body connection whereby entering into a more peaceful, calm state has clear benefits in lowering blood pressure and improving health.

These are just a few of the prominent mind-body techniques that are available. Though keep in mind, not all of these techniques will work for everyone. To find out which will work best for you, take the "Find Your Boundary Type" quiz on my website, www.drmicozzi.com.

8 easy steps to soothe stress right now

In the meantime, you can get started now towards any mind-body approach to managing stress by following these eight easy steps...

1. Pick a word or short phrase that has personal meaning, such as "love" or "peace," or the Christian "Lord is my shepherd," or Jewish "shalom"
2. Sit quietly in a comfortable position
3. Close your eyes
4. Relax your muscles
5. Breathe slowly, naturally, repeating your word or phrase silently, as you exhale
6. Take a passive attitude, dismiss all distractions
7. Continue for 10 to 12 minutes; do not stand for another 1 or 2 minutes
8. Repeat twice per day

Chapter 44

Heal your heart with what you eat and how you eat it

As you can see, you can control blood pressure with appropriate drug medications and reduce stress with effective mind-body techniques. These are important steps to reducing heart disease and promoting heart health.

But preventing the development of heart disease is an area where diet and nutrition, alternative treatments, and dietary supplements also have an important role. The body is not static—it has the ability to heal itself. This is an important basis of all alternative and complementary remedies, whether they are dietary supplements and herbs, or mind-body techniques.

In fact, my colleague, Dr. Dean Ornish (who co-chaired my medical conference on Complementary & Alternative Medicine in 1999) has shown the right diet can not only prevent but actually reverse heart disease.

Dr. Ornish emphasizes the benefits of the low-fat, high-carbohydrate aspect of his diet. Unfortunately, I think some of his recommendations are downright wrong. I'll discuss those in just a moment. But first, there is one aspect to the Ornish plan that I do agree with. He recommends that participants ideally eat together, and even cook and shop for food together. This provides much-needed social support and positive interaction with other motivated people.

Human diet is a behavior. People eat foods not nutrients. And the way we eat may be just as important as what we eat. Chinese Medicine and Ayurveda stress the way we eat: They place emphasis on the time of day, food and beverage combinations, family and social and community circumstances, even the seasons of the year. These are all aspects that are completely ignored by mainstream medicine and the natural products industry alike.

Fifteen years ago, epidemiologists puzzled over the "French Paradox"—that is, the French eat the "wrong" things in their diet (like cheese, liver pate, and pastries), smoke more, and drink more wine, on average—but their rate of heart disease is half that in the U.S.!

The epidemiologists did not know to take into account the traditional French lifestyle of taking two hours for lunch (often adding a little nap time). They eat slowly and in social circumstances, insisting on fresh and deliciously prepared dishes. And they take six or eight weeks off for the summer, with frequent long, three- and four-day weekends and holidays in between. The epidemiologists also did not understand the stress-reducing benefits of moderate wine consumption.

We had our own example of the French paradox here in the U.S. in the little Italian-American community of Rosetto, Pennsylvania. Residents here ate too much of the wrong foods, drank more wine, and smoked more—but were healthier. It turns out they were happy, had strong families, loved their neighbors and cared about their community. A little bit of kindness and love goes a long way for the "heart."

Our bodies are not defenseless when it comes to metabolizing rich foods, alcohol, or even tobacco smoke. A positive mindset and healthy habits of how we eat are just as important as what we eat.

And in terms of what we eat, when it comes to heart health, no two foods have been vilified more than salt and fat.

But do they really deserve their bad reputations?

The great salt scam

One of the wonders of the great American west is the Great Salt Lake. But today's informed physicians and scientists are wondering about "The Great Salt Scam." Promulgated, of course, by none other than the federal government.

For years we've labored under bad science when it comes to salt and blood pressure.

We've been fed a steady diet of misinformation that salt raises blood pressure, causes hypertension, and can lead to premature death.

But the fact is, if you have healthy kidneys, your body should be able to get rid of any excess salt. Subject those kidneys to a huge amount of stress however, and you may have problems.

Although it should be a settled issue by now, the great "war" against salt continues to rage even today. (Probably because the war helps keep a lot of political scientists and science bureaucrats employed working in the "salt mines.")

One anti-salt apostle even claims, "salt is the new tobacco." But this is an unscientific opinion. And it's not even half-right.

As you know, the U.S. government has made salt a public enemy for one main reason… They claim it causes high blood pressure.

As I always say, *stress* is the No. 1 cause of high blood pressure in most people. And salt is only a primary problem for a small minority.

But the government treats us all the same. And it treats salt like a villain, with a "zero-tolerance" policy. They recommend you limit salt intake to no more than 2,300 mg per day.

But this limit is ridiculous. Fewer than one-one hundredth of one percent (0.01 percent) of the population can achieve the government guideline. Plus, it's unhealthy—and lacks a fundamental understanding of human biology.

You see, sodium is an essential mineral. Your body needs it for all cellular communications, hydration, and essential physiologic functions. We should all make sure to get enough fluid and electrolytes. And what is *the* major electrolyte in the body? Sodium.

So your real goal should be to achieve balance. Not a nearly zero salt intake.

In fact, the optimal range for salt intake falls between 3,000 mg and 6,000 mg per day. That's 3 to 6 grams. (In terms of the government's "war on salt," we can think of this range as the "demilitarized" zone.)

In fact, a new study confirms my view…

Researchers recently conducted a new analysis of the PURE Study (Prospective Urban-Rural Epidemiology). They looked at data for 101,945 participants and found that men and women who consumed 3,000 to 6,000 mg of sodium per day had the lowest risk of cardiovascular disease events and deaths. But when patients went outside that zone, they landed in a salt pile of trouble.

Researchers found that men and women with either high or low sodium intake increased their cardiovascular disease risk. And this connection held up among people with and without high blood pressure.

Of course, the low-salt warriors immediately attacked these findings. They say the study's findings challenge the American Heart Association's (AHA) recommendations. (How dare the facts challenge the dogma?)

Like the U.S. government, the AHA says everyone should keep their sodium intake below 2,300 mg of sodium per day. Plus, if you're over age 51 years and/or African-American, the AHA says you should limit yourself to 1,500 mg of sodium per day.

That's half the lower limit of the PURE study's "safety zone." And it puts millions of Americans at risk!

You see, in the PURE analysis, the average sodium intake was 4,900 mg per day. According to the AHA, with numbers like those, everyone in the study should be dropping like flies. But only 8 percent actually had cardiovascular disease!

Overall, about half of the participants consumed between 4,000 and 6,000 mg sodium daily. Only 10 percent of participants consumed less than 3,000 mg per day. And nobody consumed less than 2,300 mg (the government and the AHA's ridiculous "maximum" limit).

But those who consumed less than 3,000 mg per day actually had a 25 percent increased risk of cardiovascular events *and* all-cause mortality! So, clearly the AHA's guidelines place everyone at risk of higher death rates and cardiovascular events.

Of course, it's important to note that there is a safety zone. And there *may* be such a thing as too much salt.

At the very highest end, men and women who consumed more than 7,000 mg of sodium per day had a 15 percent increased risk of death and cardiovascular events. (But remember, the low-salt group's risk went up by 25 percent!)

Now—let's look at the numbers for men and women in the study who did not have high blood pressure…

The low-salt group with normal blood pressure had an increased risk of cardiovascular events and death. But the high-salt group with normal blood pressure had no increased risk at all. So this confirms that the real problem is high blood pressure, not high salt. Or, put another way, these findings show that unless you have high blood pressure, there is no reason to worry about salt.

These results may surprise you. But they shouldn't. The PURE study isn't a lone shot in the dark. This kind of data has been around for a long time.

Data from two other major studies—the ONTARGET and TRANSCEND studies—support the PURE study results. Together, these two other studies followed 28,880 men and women at higher risk of cardiovascular disease. In these studies, men and women who consumed less than 3,000 mg sodium per day had an increased risk of suffering a cardiovascular event, such as a heart attack or stroke.

So, once again, the U.S. government and the AHA have been giving us bad advice all along. But real science shows you don't need to worry about salt (especially if you have normal blood pressure) except to make sure you're getting enough.

And while we're on the topic of bad advice, let's talk about another food you've been told to cut back on in the name of heart health…

Three big fat myths still being mouthed by "experts"

"Fat and cholesterol are bad." How often have you heard that? Even though these innocent nutrients are so essential that we literally could not live without them, we're still barraged every day by old myths and misconceptions promulgated by fat phobics and cholesterol cholerics.

Even worse, these myths continue to come straight from the mouths of paid experts who really should know better by now.

It is astounding to me that decades-old, ill-informed comments and recommendations about fat and cholesterol are still being made today. Despite the lack of any real proof—and a bunch of evidence to the contrary.

Here's a look at three commonly repeated fat and cholesterol "facts" that are as mythical as the nine lives of a cat.

Myth 1:
You'll have a heart attack if you eat saturated fat

The idea that saturated fat raises the risk of heart disease was initially based on flawed studies that clueless politicians, abetted by political scientists, somehow made into public policy.

The saturated fat myth is based on a chain of misconceptions. We've since learned that consuming saturated fat does not really appear to raise LDL "bad" cholesterol by much[3,4] (Even assuming that cholesterol is the culprit behind heart disease in the first place—see Myth 6).

Saturated fat actually appears to change LDL from small, dense particles that can clog arteries to larger, lighter particles that are mostly benign. Further, saturated fat appears to raise HDL "good" cholesterol.

So, if anything, saturated fat seems to actually *improve* cholesterol profile in terms of supposed heart disease risk factors.

Still not convinced? Consider this: In 2010, researchers reviewed data from 21 studies involving 347,747 participants and found no evidence that saturated fat consumption increases the risk of heart disease.[6]

You can't get much more proof than that.

Myth 2:
Foods that contain cholesterol will kill you

Cholesterol in food is broken down during digestion and has no correlation to the cholesterol that circulates in the blood. Nor does dietary cholesterol intake correlate to heart disease.

I repeat: Cholesterol in food is not the same as the cholesterol we've all been taught (misguidedly) to fear.

This tragic lack of basic knowledge and understanding has led to excellent, healthy foods such as eggs, lobster, and shrimp being consigned to the "bad list" simply because they contain cholesterol. To this day, so-called experts still drone on about how many eggs or shellfish servings you can "get away with."

There is nothing wrong with eating shellfish if you enjoy it. And eggs are actually nature's perfect food, packed with minerals, vitamins, and other nutrients. But keep in mind these nutrients are found in the yolk, which is also the part of the egg that contains cholesterol. Advising people to throw out the yolks and only eat egg whites is just about the most ridiculous and wasteful advice in the sad history of diet and nutrition recommendations.

Myth 3:
LDL cholesterol is evil

Mainstream medicine is obsessed with lowering total and LDL "bad" cholesterol in the blood. But while cardiologists drop the LDL limit ever lower, endocrinology doctors who are experts in human metabolism are crying foul.

Studies have found that total and LDL cholesterol levels are poor indicators of heart disease compared with other risk markers.

I also recently reported on a study of 231,986 patients hospitalized for heart disease. Half of them had normal LDL cholesterol levels.

And in older people, there are studies that show that the higher the cholesterol, the *lower* the risk of heart disease.

My late colleague, Dr. Arthur Schatzkin of the National Cancer Institute, first showed that low cholesterol is a risk factor for cancer nearly 30 years ago. Recent studies have found low cholesterol is associated with higher mortality worldwide—not only from cancer, but also suicide.

Despite all the research showing that these myths are nothing more than fairy tales that haven't come true, I continue to see warnings from nutritional "experts" about the evils of fat and cholesterol.

But now you know better. Just say no to these outrageous misconceptions that have been promulgated upon the American people over the last four decades. Your body will thank you.

Chapter 45

The heart disease battle plan:
Nine proven secrets for gaining control

As I mentioned above, there are many nutritional supplements that can benefit overall heart health. Following are nine of my favorites. These nutrients have been shown to help lower cholesterol, support the heart muscle, and promote free-flowing blood to the heart and circulation.

1. Gugulipid. Gugulipid, or gum-guggul, is from the resin of one of the remarkable gum trees found in South Asia, Southeast Asia, and Australia. Centuries ago, gum tree resins were employed in the ancient Ayurvedic pharmacy. The knowledge of how and when to harvest the resins, how to prepare and store them, and how to administer them are critical to achieving its therapeutic benefits. There are accordingly questions about the supply, formulation, and potency of different preparations, so check with your qualified health practitioner about the sources and uses of this dietary supplement. But when used appropriately, this therapy has been shown to lower cholesterol.

2. Garlic. The clinical studies of garlic on heart health address three areas: (1) lipids, like cholesterol (2) blood pressure, and (3) atherosclerosis and thrombosis. Investigators have explored its use as a treatment for mild hypertension and high cholesterol. Heavy consumption may lead to slowed blood clotting, perioperative bleeding, and spontaneous hemorrhage. Numerous studies have long documented garlic's irreversible inhibitory effect on platelet aggregation and fibrinolytic activity in humans, which makes the blood "thinner."

To benefit from the heart health effects of garlic take one or two fresh cloves per day; or if using a garlic extract, take 200-400 mg, two to three times per day.

3. B Vitamin and Flavonoids. The levels of a chemical called homocysteine in the blood are strongly and consistently linked to the risk of heart disease. The leading researcher who has worked for decades to demonstrate this effect lives in my home town in New England. I brought him to speak to the College of Physicians in Philadelphia over 10 years ago to try to get the word out about this critically important finding. All these years later, your doctor may *still* not know to do anything about homocysteine. But lowering homocysteine to healthy levels is easily achieved by supplementing with folic acid, vitamin B6, and vitamin B12.

Try daily doses of 800 mcg of folic acid, 25-50 mg of vitamin B6, and 100-300 mcg of vitamin B12.

4. Selenium & Vitamin E. Since selenium comes from the soil in which foods are grown, and livestock are grazed, selenium levels in the body often correlate. I studied the role of selenium in preventing cancer in China during the 1980's. But selenium is also important for the heart. Deep in the interior of Mainland China lies the land with the lowest levels of selenium anywhere on earth. In this low-selenium area of China, we find high rates of "Ke-Shan" disease, a deadly cardiomyopathy wherein the heart muscle itself does not function. Besides contributing to the health of the heart muscle, selenium also helps activate the important antioxidant enzyme, glutathione peroxidase, which is also important to heart health.

Selenium is often thought to work in combination with vitamin E, especially as an antioxidant. On its own, vitamin E protects low-density lipoprotein cholesterol from being oxidized and reduces heart disease.

Take selenium 100 mcg per day, and vitamin E 50 IU per day.

5. Magnesium. Magnesium deficiency can develop if you already have heart disease and are being treated for heart disease, especially with the use of digitalis and certain diuretic drugs. Some researchers believe that magnesium supplementation helps prevent the occurrence of sudden death in people with heart disease and helps increase survival.

Take 300-400 mg of magnesium per day for six weeks to restore healthy magnesium levels.

6. Hawthorn. Hawthorn is a member of the rose family with sharp thorns and small white or pink flowers that develop a bright red fruit, found in woodlands. The constituents improve heart muscle function, heart output, and blood flow in the coronary arteries and to the heart muscle. It also reduces resistance to blood flow.

Try a commonly used extract from leaves and flowers standardized on total flavonoid or procyanidin content, 160-900 mg per day for 4 to 8 weeks. If using a traditional preparation of the berries or fruit, try 4-5 grams per day.

7. Terminalia arjuna. This Ayurvedic herb has been well known in India for its heart benefits since at least 500 BC. It contains a flavone called arjunolone, as well as arjunic acid, and arjunetin and arjunosides, which are glycosides (like the better-known digitalis). Arjuna seems similar to other heart-active medicinal plants like Lilly of the Valley (*Convallaria majalis*) that help survival with heart disease. As with gugulipid, check with your health practitioner about appropriate sources and uses of this dietary supplement.

8. Coenzyme Q10. This critical enzyme co-factor is an essential component of mitochondrial membranes which are not only the energy factories of the cells but also produce water for proper hydration at the cell level (see *The Insider's answer to healthy aging and vitality*). The more active a cell needs to be in the body, the more immediate and important are its effects. The muscles do a lot of physical work, and especially the heart muscle. That's why drugs and chemicals that poison the mitochondria are so toxic to the heart and muscles as well as the other tissues and organs of the body. Coenzyme Q10 is coming to be considered a key nutritional supplement.

Try 30-50 mg of coenzyme Q10 per day.

9. Red Yeast Rice. Despite the hype and scare tactics that have surrounded it in recent years, red yeast rice remains a safe and effective option for lowering cholesterol levels. When choosing a red yeast rice product, look for four important things:

- Choose organic.

- Choose a product that has been processed to remove a potential toxin called citrinin, a by-product of the red yeast rice fermentation process.

- Choose a supplement made in the USA that meets FDA Good Manufacturing Practices (GMPs) and the standards of US Pharmacopeia (USP).

- Make sure it contains 1,200 mg of pure red yeast rice. Anything less and you will not be taking a clinically effective dose.

Red yeast rice can be combined with complementary ingredients to boost its effectiveness. Of course, as you now know, lowering your cholesterol is not enough for heart health. A more comprehensive approach is the best long-term solution.

A combined approach represents the best of complementary medicine: safe and effective drugs to control blood pressure, dietary supplements for heart health, a sensible program of diet and exercise, achieving and maintaining a healthy weight, and using effective mind-body therapies that match your emotional type for stress management.

10. Vitamin D. A new study from Germany highlights the heart benefits of the critical nutrient Vitamin D, which has so many healthy properties. Researchers found that vitamin D (a critical nutrient, deficiency of which is reaching worldwide "epidemic" levels) is associated with lower death rates in patients with heart disease, and overall. These researchers measured actual levels of vitamin D in the blood, rather than looking at daily intake of vitamin D.

Taking 1,000-2,000 IU of vitamin D is appropriate for most people.

Prevent heart disease with this key vitamin

New research shows older men and women who have adequate blood levels of vitamin D have lower cardiovascular disease risk.

You probably know the visible effects of inflammation—pain, redness, heat, and swelling. And you've probably experienced it after twisting an ankle or straining your back. In these cases, the inflammatory process is the first step toward self-healing.

But not all inflammation is the same. Some inflammation occurs inside the body—and it does not lead to healing. It only leads to destruction. In fact, inflammation in your cardiovascular system can cause damage to your heart and blood vessels.

So, as I've mentioned, it's very important to ask your doctor for the C-reactive protein (CRP) test.

If your numbers are too high, it means you have a lot of harmful inflammation in your cardiovascular system. And, therefore, you have a much higher risk of developing heart disease.

In a new study, researchers explored the role of vitamin D in inflammation and chronic disease in 957 healthy, older adults. At the study's outset, the researchers measured the participants' vitamin D levels. They defined anything above 75 nmol/L as "sufficient" vitamin D. And anything below 25 nmol/L as "deficient."

They found that men and women *deficient* in vitamin D had higher levels of biomarkers linked with cardiovascular disease. In fact, they had significantly higher levels of C-reactive protein and interleukin-6 (another marker of inflammation tied to heart disease) compared to those who had sufficient vitamin D levels. The men and women were also more likely to have other inflammatory conditions, such as multiple sclerosis (MS) and rheumatoid arthritis.

In an interview, Dr. Clifford J. Rosen of Tufts University School of Medicine underscored the importance of this study. He said, "I think all of us now think that inflammation is a critical factor in a lot of disease… so there's some rationale for thinking about trying to reduce chronic inflammation with something as simple as vitamin D. And it may have a further effect on atherosclerotic risk of cardiovascular disease."

In other words, lowering your cardiovascular risk and protecting yourself from just about every other chronic disease may be as simple as getting more vitamin D.

Unfortunately, as much as 80 percent of the U.S. population is vitamin D deficient. And those statistics won't get any better any time soon as long as health "experts" in this country continue to push propaganda to avoid the sun completely.

The truth is, you can—and should—spend 20 minutes a day in the sun without sunscreen. This healthy exposure will help boost your vitamin D levels naturally.

Plus, ignore all the medical experts who continue to claim that taking vitamin D and measuring blood levels isn't important.

You should take a vitamin D supplement. Currently, the Institute of Medicine (IOM) recommends 600 international units (IU) of vitamin D daily for adults up to age 70. After age 71, the IOM recommends increasing intake to 800 IU. But these recommendations are based on findings regarding bone health.

Ongoing research proves you need much higher doses to achieve and maintain optimal vitamin D levels in the body. I recommend everyone take a daily, high-quality supplement that contains 5,000 IU of vitamin D. If you don't like taking too many pills or capsules, look for a vitamin D in liquid form. You can take it straight from the dropper or add it to any beverage you like.

Chapter 46

The common pain "cure" that can increase your risk of heart attack and sudden death

Over the past few years, highly significant research has emerged showing that knee replacements are ot the easy effective procedures that conventional medicine seems to think they are.

And now, a large new study shows that knee replacement surgery is actually much more dangerous than many people thought.

In fact, getting your knee or hip replaced can substantially increase your risk of having a post-surgery heart attack. And it can also make you more susceptible to potentially fatal blood clots for years after the procedure.

Let's take a closer look at this shocking new research. And then I'll tell you how you can improve your joint health without surgery.

Trauma to your joints can cause trauma to your heart

Researchers analyzed data from 27,698 people, age 50 or older, who had been diagnosed with knee or hip osteoarthritis between 2000 and 2013. Half of those people had knee or hip replacement surgery, and half didn't.

The researchers compared heart attack incidences in the two groups. They discovered that 306 of the people who had knee or hip replacements had a heart attack in the month following surgery. But only 286 of the nonsurgical group had heart attacks during the same time frame.

To put it another way, people who had knee or hip replacements had a 5% greater chance of having a heart attack than people who didn't have the surgery.

The heart attack risk in the surgical group lessened over time. But what didn't lessen was the likelihood of blood clots after surgery.

Specifically, the people who had knee or hip replacements had increased risk of blood clots forming in their legs. And this risk persisted for years after the procedure.

Now, you don't have to be medical a specialist to understand that for blood to properly circulate in your body, it must be able to flow freely through the veins back to the heart. If blood flow gets blocked or slowed in the veins it has a tendency to form clots—especially in the legs.

And here's the really frightening part. Blood clots in your legs can travel to your lungs. And that can create a pulmonary embolism—which can kill you. In fact, pulmonary embolism is a leading cause of sudden death.

So how do knee or hip replacements help create these blood clots? Well, first of all, they're major surgical procedures. I'm talking about cutting and displacing muscles, tendons, ligaments, and bones—using the surgical equivalent of saws, hammers, and chisels.

It's hardly surprising that this causes immense damage to leg tissues, including blood vessels. And when blood vessels have been pummeled like this, or even cut out or cut off, there are major problems with blood circulation and drainage.

Voilà—increased risk of blood clots and pulmonary embolism, persisting for *years*.

All risk, no reward

So, thanks to this new research, we now know that knee or hip replacements can substantially increase your risk of dying from a heart attack or a pulmonary embolism—not at all surprising.

And there's a good chance that undergoing this surgery won't even make your knees feel or work better at all.

Researchers found that only 44% of knee replacement surgeries are "appropriate." Twenty-two percent were "inconclusive." And a whopping 34% were considered "inappropriate" in the first place.

That means the patient didn't meet the proper medical criteria needed for a joint replacement—but got one anyway. Often, these people only had slight or moderate pain or loss of mobility in their knees, and were younger than 55. But an orthopedic surgeon went ahead and did surgery anyway.

As if that weren't bad enough, a major study of 3.3 million people found that 10% of all knee replacements simply don't work or wear out. Meaning those poor people had to have another dangerous surgery to repair the first botched surgery.

So basically, when it comes to knee replacements, you have about equal chances of having an inappropriate procedure, an ineffective procedure, or an effective procedure.

And betting on one out of three is not good odds when it comes to having major surgery. As this new study has taught us, you may be literally betting your life.

Supplement your way to healthier knees

Putting it all together, at least two-thirds of the people who are considering, or being encouraged to get, joint replacements should not rush to surgery.

Not only because these procedures may not work, but because they also increase the short-term risk of heart attacks and the long-term risks of blood clots and pulmonary embolisms—all of which can be fatal.

So if you have aching knees or loss of mobility, what should you do instead?

The first step in naturally rebuilding cartilage is to reduce joint inflammation, which glucosamine and chondroitin can't do.

Fortunately, there are supplements that can. I like to call them the

ABCs, or the "three wise men" of joint health.

I'm talking about ashwaganda, Boswellia, and curcumin.

Ahswaganda and Boswellia come from ancient South Asian trees, and both are important treatments in Ayurvedic medicine. Ashwaganda is derived from the winter cherry tree, while Boswellia is a tree gum resin that's better known as frankincense. And curcumin is the active ingredient in the well-known medicinal plant and common spice turmeric.

Research shows that each of these natural substances is effective at reducing inflammation and pain. And when you put them all together, they are a formidable trio for joint health.

Based upon scientific studies, the individual doses of my ABCs of joint health are 400 to 500 mg each of ashwaganda, Boswellia, and curcumin. But there is good evidence that all of these botanicals have synergistic effects with the others when taken in combination, beating even the most potent (and dangerous) drugs.

So be like the Wise Men who brought these gifts to the Messiah on Epiphany (January 6)—and don't be caught without an effective joint remedy this year.

Chapter 47

The pill-free "prescription" that can cut your risk of heart disease in as little as one hour

Greece may be one of the few places where scientists are still able to observe the effects of an afternoon nap. Until the later 20th century, there was a strong tradition throughout Mediterranean countries of taking a long break midday. Workers and schoolchildren would go home for a hearty lunch followed by a nap or rest. Then they'd go back to work or school until 7 p.m., return home, and eat a light evening meal. And, of course, there is also the siesta in Latin American and tropical countries.

But this tradition may be well worth reviving, if this new study is any indication of its potential.

"Power nap" your way to better blood pressure

The Greek researchers gathered 200 men and 186 women with an average age of 62 years. All of them had high blood pressure.

The researchers discovered that the study participants who slept midday had 5 percent lower average blood pressure than the non-nappers. And this effect persisted after taking into account hypertension risk factors like weight, smoking, alcohol consumption, and fitness levels.

The midday nappers also had lower readings in other key measurements, suggesting they may have less damage from high blood pressure in their arteries and heart.

You may be thinking that a 5 percent reduction in blood pressure isn't much. But the researchers pointed out that simply dropping your systolic blood pressure (the upper number in a blood pressure reading) by 2 mmHg (out of a total of 130 mm Hg or more) can reduce your risk of cardiovascular disease by as much as 10 percent.

And a 5 percent dip in blood pressure is comparable to the drop associated with stress-reduction lifestyle therapies such as biofeedback, guided imagery, meditation, relaxation therapy, and yoga.

So how much should you nap each day? The longer the better, according to the study. But when you're strapped for time, the blood pressure effects were seen in as little as an hour.

Bottom line: Don't be afraid to be caught midday giving a "nod" to "winken and blinken." It might raise the blood pressure of your co-workers, but it will surely lower your own—and your risk of cardiovascular disease.

Chapter 48

The surprising vegetable that can help you slam the breaks on heart disease

The next time you're at the grocery store or farmer's market, I encourage you to pick up some fresh beets.

Why? Because beets are highly nutritious and contain a number of unique, biologically active compounds. In fact, beets are loaded with the cellular powerhouse betaine, aptly named since it was first isolated from beets.

And when it comes healthy aging, it's hard to beat betaine.

Betaine, also known as TMG or trimethylglycine, is a type of amino acid made from choline—an essential nutrient that's often grouped with the B vitamins.

It has remarkable ability to help protect cells against oxidation—a culprit in all kinds of chronic diseases, including cancer, heart disease, dementia, Alzheimer's, and Parkinson's.

But perhaps most unique are betaine's effects on homocysteine.

The biology of betaine and homocysteine

Of course, the most well-known risks associated with elevated levels of homocysteine are heart attacks and strokes. But the dangers of excess homocysteine go far beyond your cardiovascular system.

You see, too much homocysteine can disrupt the body's methylation process.

This is key because methylation helps control many important functions throughout your body. You need methylation for energy production, immune response, repairing cells damaged by free radicals, fighting inflammation, genetic expression and repair of DNA, detoxification, and even lowering your stress levels.

In short, virtually everything that helps you feel young and healthy relies on methylation. Unfortunately, your body's methylation capability can erode as you grow older. At the same time, your homocysteine levels can begin to creep up.

Although no absolutely "safe" level of serum homocysteine has been determined, research suggests that levels should be less than 12 mcmol/L—especially if you have other cardiovascular disease risk factors.

Ideally, studies show that homocysteine levels should be kept under 8.5 mcmol/L. But here's the kicker: You probably have no idea if your homocysteine levels are too high because you generally won't have any symptoms.

That's why it's important to have blood tests for homocysteine. And it's also a good idea to get your vitamin levels tested, along with tests for genetic defects that could cause your body to produce excess homocysteine.

If your homocysteine levels are too high, getting the proper nutrients from your diet and supplements is the most effective way to reduce them.

And that's key for healthy aging—including protection against heart attack and stroke.

How to feel younger, longer

I recommend the following daily supplement regimen to keep your homocysteine levels in check (and for overall good health).

These nutrients have been shown to either help keep your body from producing too much homocysteine, or help it metabolize and reduce homocysteine.

- 250 mg of alpha-GPC
- 250 mg of alpha-lipoic acid with biotin
- 100 mg of CoQ10 (ubiquinol)
- 3 grams of fish oil

- 200-400 mcg of selenium
- 500 mg of vitamin C (in two divided doses of 250 mg each)
- 200 mg of vitamin E (gamma E tocopherol/tocotrienols)
- 30 mg of zinc

I also recommend a high-quality B vitamin complex that contains at least 200 mcg of folate, 50 mg of B6, 12 mcg of B12, 50 mg of B2, and 50 mg of choline. Curcumin (200-900 mg a day) is also a potent, healthy addition to any diet.

And, of course, make sure to incorporate plenty of beets in your diet. You can eat them raw in salads, or cooked with any main course. They're particularly healthy—and tasty—when cooked with garlic. If you're not a fan of beets (or garlic), you can supplement with 2-4 grams of betaine a day.

Other supplements that can help you regulate homocysteine include micronized creatine (2-4 grams daily), lecithin (1-2 tablespoons of pure granules per day), serine (3-6 grams daily), N-acetyl-cysteine (600- 1,200 mg daily), and cysteine (500-1,000 mg daily).

To help repair any tissues that are affected by high homocysteine levels, along with the CoQ10, fish oil, alpha-lipoic acid, selenium, curcumin and vitamin C and E doses I mentioned above, I also recommend any or all of these nutrients and herbs:

- Garlic: 500-1,000 mg daily
- L-arginine: 500 mg daily
- Policosanol: 10 mg daily with evening meal
- Ginkgo extract: 120 mg daily
- Grape seed extract: 300 mg daily
- Green tea extract: 2 grams daily
- Bromelain: 500 mg daily
- Ginger: 10 grams daily
- Chromium: 200-400 mcg, once or twice daily
- Niacin (B3): 80-160 mg daily
- Pantethine (B5): 30 mg three times daily

A healthier use for beets

Historically, in marginally nourished populations living in climates that are relatively poor for crop cultivation, a "beet and potato" (versus the proverbial "meat and potato") diet has been able to sustain people. For example, in Eastern Europe and Russia.

In the U.S., "beet and potato" agriculture is also important to the economy of certain states like Idaho.

Idaho has a relatively small, close-knit population, and I developed close contacts with many business and political leaders there 12 years ago.

Some of those people made huge fortunes from supplying potatoes to McDonald's for French fries (which are simply a vehicle for unhealthy oils and excess calories). Others became wealthy by supplying beet sugar to food companies. But some were looking toward the future.

I told Idaho growers, as well as government agencies involved in agricultural and economic development, about manufacturing betaine from beets, instead of sugar. After all, people need a lot less sugar and a lot more betaine. Plus, I calculated that, pound per pound, betaine is priced over 10,000 times higher than sugar.

Former Sen. Larry Craig (R-Idaho) and his staff showed strong interest. They understood that sugars and carbs represent the past, and that growing healthy plant constituents like betaine represents the future. But then the good senator got caught in an airport literally with his pants down (although I never really understood what that had to do with anything). And, as a result, nothing ever came of my betaine suggestion.

It's a shame, because as more and more public health experts come around to the realization that sugar and carbs are driving the obesity, diabetes, and heart disease epidemics, the business of making sugar and French fried potatoes is starting to dry up.

And betaine could have been a real "rainmaker" to keep Idaho growers in the green.

Chapter 49

Eating right to control mild hypertension

I always advise doing everything possible to keep your blood pressure under control. That's because hypertension is the strongest risk factor for cardiovascular diseases and stroke. And it's just too big of a problem to tackle on your own. Plus, about half of people who have high blood pressure don't even know it. Or they aren't being treated for it.

And even when you *do* know your numbers, the treatment options just got more complicated. As I recently told you, some experts now question whether drug therapy is really appropriate for someone with "mild" elevation in blood pressure between 120/80 and 140/90.

If you fall into this category, you may consider trying yoga or another mind-body therapy. These can help you modestly lower "mild" high blood pressure. And help you avoid taking drugs.

So, what *else* can you do to help control mild high blood pressure?

The first thing most people now think of is to cut out salt. In fact, The National Heart, Lung, and Blood Institute created the DASH dietary plan to help people cut out salt. (DASH stands for Dietary Approaches to Stop Hypertension.) And it suggests you limit daily salt intake to no more than 2,300 mg. Or, ideally, no more than 1,500 mg.

But, as you know, the "great salt scam" is not based on real science when it comes to blood pressure control.

Fortunately, DASH also emphasizes eating more fruits, vegetables, whole grains, and low-fat dairy. It also tells us to eat less meat, fish, poultry, and sugars. So, DASH isn't just about cutting salt.

In fact, experts at the Boston Medical Center believe the DASH plan works because it combines lean protein with a high intake of fruits and vegetables. Yes, DASH encourages you to restrict salt. But it also encourages you add in fiber, protein, vitamins, and minerals. And together, these elements help to control your blood pressure as well as chronic diseases.

Plus, it turns out that the DASH plan is the only diet that actually has scientific data to support it. And it makes sense that DASH works. Especially when you consider that many experts have long questioned the role of salt as the lone cause of high blood pressure. And it also helps explain why simply restricting salt doesn't "cure" hypertension.

So how about other diets? Can they help lower your blood pressure?

As a matter of fact, there are some popular diets that can help lower blood pressure. Unfortunately, they're not all created equal when it comes to providing you with optimal nutrition. But let's start with one that does—the Mediterranean Diet.

Experts have long recognized the Mediterranean Diet for reducing heart disease and many cancers.

Traditionally, the Mediterranean diet includes healthy amounts of fruits, vegetables, whole grains, nuts, fish, and some red meat. They also use relatively large amounts of olive oil.

It is not a "low-fat" diet, per se, as it contains plenty of monosaturated fat from the olive oil. But this is a healthy fat, rather than an unhealthy fat. And, of course, the diet includes moderate wine consumption.

There is not a lot of science that the Mediterranean diet directly reduces blood pressure. But we do know that men and women who follow the diet reduce their risk of heart and cardio-vascular diseases, which are caused by high blood pressure. And that is the bigger issue at stake.

The Ornish Diet is another popular regimen that has been shown to prevent and even reverse heart disease. It is an extremely low-fat, vegetarian diet. Less than 10 percent of the calories come from fat. Instead, it's heavy on the carbs, fiber and vegetables.

Essentially, the Ornish Diet is a "high-carb" diet.

And that concerns me. In terms of basic human biology, I question the value of restricting natural fats to extremely low levels. And keeping carbohydrate levels high can cause metabolic problems.

Also, fiber is a complex issue. It is not simply a question of eating a "high" fiber diet. You have to be careful about the types of fiber you eat. For example, eating a cereal bar with added fiber doesn't improve your metabolism and disease risks like eating fruit will.

Furthermore, humans simply cannot obtain healthy levels of all nutrients from vegetarian diets alone. And any diet that eliminates entire food groups found in nature reduces the universally healthy effects of dietary diversity. This also makes the diet difficult to follow.

So how does the Ornish program get such good results, when it comes to heart disease?

I have a theory that is supported by lots of other research…

One key feature of the Ornish program is that participants shop together. Prepare food together. Eat together. And participate in other group activities. I always believed this social support helped Ornish followers to lower their stress and improve their mental health. According to much research, those effects also help participants lower their blood pressure.

Here's another major problem with the Ornish plan…when people try this at home, on their own, it doesn't work well. I gleaned this from my own observations and from my late colleague, Lee Lipsenthal, who worked with Dr. Ornish for many years.

The one positive thing about the Ornish program is that when followed properly, it *does* reverse heart disease. Yet for decades, mainstream doctors claimed heart disease could *never* be reversed. Only treated and "managed." The Ornish program proves otherwise.

In my view, it is not the Ornish diet alone that does it. But it may well be the social support and the blood pressure reduction that comes with it.

Another popular diet out there is the South Beach Diet.

This diet is unnecessarily complicated. And based on some "gimmicks" and "myths" that in my view do not fit well with human biology. Plus, it is difficult to follow. Especially long-term. It may have some heart health benefits, but like the Ornish diet, the quality of the nutrition is questionable.

In the end, I recommend you make eating more fruits and vegetables your top priority if you have mild hypertension. Start there. It makes sense for many reasons.

Next, limit consumption of processed foods. Basically, when you go food shopping, stay mainly on the outside aisles of the grocery store.

However, keep in mind that if your hypertension is beyond "mild," even a "heart-healthy" diet is probably not enough. The stress that most people face in modern life may simply be too difficult to overcome with natural approaches alone. That's why I always recommend working closely with your doctor to make a personalized plan. One that may include the use of safe, proven blood pressure medications.

But no matter what your blood pressure is, you have many healthy options for getting it—and keeping it—right where it needs to be.

Chapter 50

The "controversial" pennies-per-day heart cure every cardiologist in the country should be recommending

The *New York Times* recently published some very interesting statistics. Over the last half-century, from 1958 to 2010, the annual U.S. death rate from heart disease declined by a monumental 68 percent. And, during that same time period, the death rate from strokes fell even more—79 percent.

So, looking at it a different way, back in 1958, 56 out of every 10,000 Americans died from heart disease. In 2010, that number plummeted to just 18 people.

And in 1958, 18 out of every 10,000 Americans died from strokes— compared to only 4 out of 10,000 in 2010.

Why the dramatic reduction?

Well, in 1978, 20 years into this trend, a nationwide conference of experts was convened by the National Institutes of Health to answer that very question.

The experts noted that the decline in deaths from heart disease and stroke was evident before the government's misguided dietary recommendations and major anti-tobacco campaigns and lawsuits went into effect, and long before any drugs were available to address the myth of "killer cholesterol."

So, faulty dietary advice, smoking cessation and prevention, and anti-cholesterol drugs could not be responsible for this early decline.

The experts looked at other potential factors. In 1978, there had already been some favorable trends in physical activity. Plus, more intensive and effective hospital management and treatment of heart disease and stroke would have been expected to help reduce mortality.

But at the same time, Americans were eating more fat and meat, and gaining more weight.

So the experts were flummoxed. They couldn't identify a probable cause for why so many fewer people were dying of heart disease and stroke.

Nonetheless, the government-industrial-medical complex embarked on its faulty campaign to reduce consumption of meat, saturated fats, and salts, and to push cholesterol-lowering drugs. None of which had anything to do with the actual decline of heart disease and stroke that had already occurred.

But I and my colleague, Dr. Kilmer McCully, think we have the answer. And it's a simple one.

We believe the reduction in heart disease and stroke is because Americans are consuming more of three simple nutrients: vitamins B6 (pyridoxal), B12, and folate/folic acid (B9).

What B can do for you?

These B vitamins are required for normal metabolism of an amino acid called homocysteine. And high levels of homocysteine in the blood can result in cardiovascular disease.

Dr. McCully is a pioneer in B vitamin/homocysteine/heart disease research. He also introduced the "homocysteine hypothesis" way back in 1969. At the heart of this hypothesis is the belief that introduction of highly processed foods during the early 20th century caused lower B vitamin intakes and higher heart disease rates during the 1940s to 1960s.

Food processing involves heating, chemical treatment, extraction of purified carbohydrates and oils, and milling of grains—all of which strip foods of their naturally occurring B vitamins.

In fact, in the rice-dependent populations of Asia, it has been observed that removing the B vitamin-rich bran layer to convert brown rice to white rice leads to beriberi, a vitamin B (thiamine)-deficiency disease.

Along with unprocessed foods, B vitamins are also found in meat, eggs, dairy products, and whole grains. That's why vegans and vegetarians can have difficulty getting enough Bs to keep them—and their hearts—healthy.

For example, in the country of Chad in Sub-Saharan Africa, the population subsists on beans, cassava, ground nuts, millet, and sweet potatoes. The semi-arid climate and poor soil results in poorly nourished livestock, with fewer dairy foods and rare consumption of meat.

Dr. McCully and a colleague conducted a study in which they found that even though people in Chad eat very little saturated fat and have low cholesterol levels, they have high homocysteine levels. And even more tellingly, they have *more* cardiovascular disease than people in other African countries who get more protein and B vitamins in their diets.[2]

Need more convincing? In the U.S., the famous Framingham Heart Study found that the participants who were between the ages of 67 and 96 had major nutritional deficiencies during the 1950s, which led to them having low vitamin B status for years. Consumption of vitamin B6 rose from 0.23 mg a day in 1955 to 3.5 mg a day in the 1970s.

Likewise, folic acid intakes increased beginning in the 1960s, and in 1998, the FDA mandated fortification of processed grains with folic acid. The Framingham Heart Study demonstrated that folate blood levels doubled after this fortification began. And homocysteine levels decreased by 15 percent.

In addition to this compelling research, several large-scale studies conducted in the 1990s and 2000s evaluated whether supplementing with vitamins B6, B12, and folate could prevent heart attacks or strokes.

In the HOPE 2 trial, people who supplemented with B vitamins had a notably significant 27 percent reduction in strokes. And in the VISP trial, people who had the highest blood levels of vitamin B12 had a 21 percent reduction in heart disease, stroke, or death.

Why mainstream medicine is B-fuddled about heart disease

You'd think this research would convince doctors that low B vitamin intake and high homocysteine levels are the real risk factors for heart disease. So why is the medical profession and the general public so uninformed about this key finding?

One answer has to do with what happened to Dr. McCully after his pioneering B vitamin/homocysteine/heart disease studies.

Since then, over 17,500 scientific studies have shown that high homocysteine levels can also lead to blood clots, cancer, dementia, kidney disease, low thyroid levels, osteoporosis, retinal degeneration of the eyes, and mental illness.

But while some of these studies were underway, the mainstream was marginalizing Dr. McCully's research linking homocysteine levels with heart disease.

He says there was a "violent" reaction against his findings on homocysteine from the "cholesterol cartel," and he consequently was denied promotions and tenure and was blackballed within the research community and industry.

In fact, after a decade of groundbreaking research on this subject at Harvard Medical School and Massachusetts General Hospital, Dr. McCully was exiled to try to continue his work at the VA Medical Center in Providence, Rhode Island.

Dr. McCully believes his findings were not a threat to the multibillion-dollar food or pharma industries. But many of his colleagues disagreed. In fact, in the late 1990s I received funding from a private, non-medical foundation to bring Dr. McCully to speak at the College of Physicians of Philadelphia, a bastion of traditional biomedicine. But I was quickly reminded about the Biblical story of trying to "bring pearls before swine."

Dr. McCully's expulsion from Harvard came just at the time that big pharma was getting ready to launch its new "blockbuster" cholesterol drugs. And therein lies the conflict. If you can prevent heart disease by taking a simple B vitamin supplement, why bother with the dangerous and expensive new drugs?

The fact is, this simple, inexpensive, safe, natural approach should be the very first recommendation made by every cardiologist and general physician to any patient at risk of heart attack or stroke.

For optimum heart health and overall good health, I recommend taking a high-quality vitamin B complex that contains at least the following dosages: 50 mg each of thiamine, riboflavin (B2), niacin/niacinamide, B6, and pantothenic acid, plus 400 micrograms of folic acid/folate, 12 mcg of B12, and 100 mcg of biotin.

But beware—you must get started with B supplementation early. Once you have well-established cardiovascular disease, B6, B12, and folic acid supplementation may not be enough alone to reverse the disease.

Chapter 51

How to avoid heart disease when you have Type II diabetes

Contrary to popular belief, having Type II diabetes isn't an automatic, mandatory sentence for getting heart disease too. Many patients remain completely free of heart disease even after they have diabetes for many years. In fact, according to a new case-control study, two key factors keep patients safe from developing coronary artery heart disease more than 10 years after developing Type II diabetes.

For this study, the researchers recruited 76 patients with Type II diabetes. The patients had been treated for more than 10 years and were undergoing angiograms to detect possible coronary artery disease.

The researchers also took the patients' clinical history, recorded their anthropometric body measurements, analyzed biochemical parameters, and assessed insulin resistance. They also performed multiple analyses to determine the factors most strongly associated with the absence of heart disease.

Two factors linked to heart disease in diabetics

Turns out, the Type II diabetes patients who remained free from heart disease possessed two key characteristics...

First, their insulin resistance (IR) factor was less than 2.5.

Second, their level of albumin in the urine (microalbuminuria) was less than 20 mg/l. Albumin (protein) in the urine is a sign of diabetic kidney damage. So by that measure, absence of kidney damage meant absence of heart disease.

By contrast, blood lipids (cholesterol) had **zero** effect on the development of heart disease. So—this study presents further evidence that, contrary to popular myth, cholesterol isn't the main culprit for heart disease, even in diabetics.

Furthermore, the researchers learned that BMI, waist size, hip size, and waist-to-hip ratios did not affect the patients' risk of developing heart disease.

Of course, as I told you in the past, research shows that BMI is a flawed measure of excess weight or health anyway. Furthermore, extra body weight is not the universal and inevitable cause of chronic diseases that some experts make it out to be.

Perhaps the most surprising finding from this study is that the differences in fasting blood sugar and hemoglobin A1C were _not_ significant in predicting heart disease. Of course, these patients were already being treated for Type II diabetes for at least 10 years. So common sense tells us these patients didn't have **uncontrolled** diabetes. Rather, they probably kept their blood sugar levels down through medical intervention. And the study shows, below that controlled level, there was no difference in the development of heart disease.

Finally, women tended to develop less heart disease than men in the study. And we have known gender plays a role in the development of heart disease for many years from many other studies.

You can't do much about changing your sex (with apologies to Bruce/ Caitlyn Jenner). But you can make sure to keep your blood sugar levels under control by cutting out sugars, cutting back on carbs, and engaging in regular moderate physical activity.

The one and only Type II diabetes drug I recommend

When it comes to drugs for blood sugar control, I recommend metformin. It's a safe, effective and affordable prescription drug to lower blood sugar and hemoglobin A1C, the long-term measure of blood sugar.

Metformin also lowers the risks of other chronic diseases—including the difficult-to-treat pancreatic cancer. It's also the only drug treatment for Type II diabetes that also reduces the long-term complications of the disease in the eyes, heart, kidneys, and peripheral nerves. None of this information about metformin surprises me as it derives from an ancient European folk remedy called French lilac.

If you have Type II diabetes, your doctor should also monitor your insulin resistance, kidney function, and albumin with regular urine and blood tests.

With some careful monitoring and close control of your condition, you *can* stay completely free of heart disease, even after many years of living with Type II diabetes.

Chapter 52

10 real risk factors for heart disease

For decades, the government has been promoting politically correct, pet theories about the causes of heart disease. They tried to blame cholesterol, eggs, meat, saturated fats, salt, alcohol…you name it. But, one by one, real science has shot down each of these theories.

Unfortunately, many primary care doctors aren't aware of the current research. And they continue to use all the wrong numbers and ask all the wrong questions.

Plus, last year, the American College of Cardiologists and the American Heart Association muddied the water even further. They developed a new, mysterious mathematical formula for assessing your heart disease risk. And if you have more than a 7.5 percent risk for suffering a stroke or heart attack over the next 10 years, they recommend you take a statin drug. This misguided advice would put 70 percent more of the population on statin drugs.

The truth is, there are 10 very clear risk factors for heart disease:

Risk factor No. 1: High blood pressure

High blood pressure is the No. 1 cause of heart disease.

Higher pressure in the arteries places more stress and wear and tear on the linings of the blood vessels, which contributes to the development of atherosclerotic arterial disease. And atherosclerotic arterial disease is the cause of heart disease, stroke, and peripheral vascular disease. This factor is particularly apparent when blood pressure hits 180 or higher—a level where treatment is mandated, and may even represent a medical emergency.

Of course, on the other end of the scale, low blood pressure can also pose serious risks, including weakness, dizziness, and fainting. Extremely low blood pressure can deprive your organs of oxygen-rich blood, which can lead to heart, kidney and/or brain damage

So it is important to keep your blood pressure "just right." High enough to maintain adequate blood pressure in order to provide enough blood, oxygen, and glucose to the brain, heart, and other organs. But low enough to keep arteries and blood vessels smooth— and stop cardiovascular diseases from taking hold.

Risk factor No. 2: Age

Heart disease risk goes up for all of us as we get older. For men, it starts creeping up after age 45. For women, it's after they hit 55.

Risk factor No. 3: Pre-existing conditions

Men and women who already have coronary artery disease or another chronic condition like diabetes have a 20 percent greater risk of experiencing an actual heart event over the next 10 years. (Coronary artery disease is narrowing of the arteries that supply the heart muscle.)

Risk factor No. 4: Smoking

Of course, cigarette smoking is also a risk factor for heart disease. But only for men and women who smoke more than one or two packs per day. This behavior also increases lung disease and lung cancer risk. But smoking isn't the only factor contributing to these risks for most people.

And remember, several important, large studies looked specifically at the effects of *light* cigarette smoking or cigar-/pipe-only smoking. (Most studies lump all smokers together.)

These studies found light cigarette smokers and cigar-/pipe-only smokers do *not* have higher heart disease risk. In fact, their overall chronic disease risk was the same as nonsmokers. Plus, these light smokers even had a healthier weight.

So, if you smoke and you want to lower your heart disease risk, it's important to cut back to less than half-a-pack per day. (Less than 10 cigarettes per day.)

Risk factor No. 5: Family history

If you have a close male relative who had heart disease before age 55 years or a female relative who got it before 65 years, you run a higher risk of developing it too.

Risk factors No. 6 thru 10: Specific blood markers

You and your doctor should also pay very close attention to these four important numbers: homocysteine, blood sugar, hemoglobin A1C, and C-Reactive Protein (CRP). You can learn more about these critical numbers in the article "Seven critical heart health markers more important than cholesterol" that appeared in the May 2014 issue of *Insiders' Cures*.

Obviously, some of these risk factors are ones you can't control (like getting older and family history). But there are steps you can take to lower your overall risk of heart disease.

First of all, keep your blood pressure under control. As I mentioned earlier, it's the No. 1 thing you can do to prevent heart disease.

Second, manage your stress. It's easier said than done, for sure. But many mind-body techniques can help. Including biofeedback, meditation and yoga. They all help lower stress. And they help lower blood pressure as well.

But not everyone responds in the same way to these techniques. For example, some people respond very well to meditation. And others, may not at all.

Third, you should also follow a heart healthy diet. But don't let the government's food edicts confuse you. You don't need to avoid natural foods that contain cholesterol—such as eggs, shellfish and healthy meats. These foods are actually very nutritious and good for your health—and your heart. Plus, you shouldn't cut out all saturated fats. Or even cut out all salt.

And if you take a statin drug (which I hope you don't), be extra careful about your diet. In "The Statin Gluttony" study, it was found that men and women who take statins tend to loosen their lifestyle habits. Eventually, they gain weight and increase their blood sugar—which are real problems!

Also it is important to make sure to get some healthy exercise too. The biggest improvements come when you stop being a sedentary "couch potato" and start some light, regular exercise—like yard work, housework, walking, or swimming—every other day. Adding more exercise adds some marginal benefits. But don't overdo it. Extreme exercise harms your joints and your heart muscle.

Last, make sure to keep your vitamin D levels optimal. Research shows adequate vitamin D levels may also help lower your risk of heart disease (not to mention other chronic diseases). A blood level above 50 ng/ml is healthy.

Chapter 53

Getting off the sodium obsession

I mentioned this briefly above, but it's worth repeating: The government's long campaign against salt is NOT based on scientific evidence.

For years we've labored under bad science when it comes to salt and blood pressure. We've been fed a steady diet of misinformation that salt raises blood pressure, causes hypertension, and can lead to premature death.

But the fact is, if you have healthy kidneys, your body should be able to get rid of any excess salt. Subject those kidneys to a huge amount of stress however, and you may have problems.

In fact, if you lower your salt intake to the levels the government recommends, you may actually be doing more harm than good! Fortunately, from this standpoint the number of people who can actually achieve these salt restrictions is ludicrously small in reality.

Now, some experts are advising the government to finally take a more sensible, "holistic" approach to the prevention of high blood pressure and heart disease. And recommending that appropriate emphasis be placed on lifestyle.

Finally, another voice of reason taking a stab at something I've been advocating for decades.

The lifelong connection between lifestyle and high blood pressure is something I've understood since I did my own research on blood pressure back in the 1970's for which I was awarded an undergraduate research prize from the American Heart Association. Research that uncovered a clear link between stress and high blood pressure starting in childhood.

The evidence shows that lifestyle approaches simply lead to better results. And <u>that</u> is what government guidelines should be all about—evidence and results.

But these are the two most relevant and critical factors that, over and over again, are missing in action (or inaction, as the case may be) from bureaucratic fumblings and mumblings. And the concept of actual results when it comes to government health programs?

So, after all the waste of taxpayer money and precious time ignoring the evidence…what has another new "panel of experts" just come up with? The exact same lifestyle approaches we have known and recommended for decades for maintaining all-around good health and longevity:

- Manage weight
- Eat fresh fruit and vegetables
- Engage in moderate physical activity
  AND
- Moderate alcohol intake

And of course, if you have high blood pressure, I recommend immediate action with the right blood-pressure medication in addition to all of the above.

Salt is simply NOT the issue for most people.

The experts were convened by the International Food Information Council Foundation (IFICF) which is supported primarily by the broad-based food, beverage, and agricultural industries.

But regardless of the source, the facts are the facts. And we should be happy that someone else is pointing out the actual evidence when it comes to preventing and managing high blood pressure and heart disease.

Chapter 54

Can slightly elevated blood pressure actually be good for your health?

As you know, stress is the silent killer when it comes to cardiovascular diseases, metabolic diseases, and other chronic illnesses—in part because it can cause your blood pressure to spike.

But it turns out that not all boosts in blood pressure are bad for you. In fact, surprising research indicates that moderate increases in blood pressure as you get older may actually be good for your health.

That's right: Studies show that blood pressure levels that are slightly higher than the currently accepted "gold standard" of 120/80 *may not harm* your cardiovascular or cognitive health.

The research is so compelling that a government committee of medical experts recently increased the "safe" blood pressure levels for people over age 60. The committee recommended that treatments to reduce blood pressure for this age group should not begin until BP levels are over 150/90.

Other medical professionals are a bit more conservative. Discussions in both the *British Medical Journal* and the *Journal of the American Medical Association* recommended raising the level at which drug treatment should begin. (The BMJ article suggested 160/100 as the threshold, and JAMA suggested 140/90).

So how did these eyebrow-raising developments come about? After all, for decades, the most common blood pressure adage has been "the lower, the better." And as I've often noted, managing blood pressure is the single most important step you can take to reduce your risk of cardiovascular disease.

But the practice of medicine is both an art and a science, and it is continually evolving. New, expanding research on different age groups of adults is revealing that my frequent admonition—"moderation in all things"—also appears to be applicable to the concept of healthy blood pressure.

One thought is that blood pressures slightly above "normal" may actually assist older people in maintaining adequate blood circulation to the heart muscle and brain—thus helping to stave off heart attacks and strokes. And slightly higher blood pressure may also help pump more oxygen and glucose to sensitive tissues like the brain, preserving memory and cognition.

Let's take a closer look at this new research, along with steps you can take to manage your blood pressure in light of these new findings.

Moderately high blood pressure may *not* lead to heart attacks or strokes

A blood pressure reading between 120/80 and 140/90 is considered mild, or early, hypertension. Traditionally, many doctors prescribe blood-pressure lowering drugs to people in this range.

But new research is showing that this practice may actually be dangerous for your health.

Although earlier studies indicated that the risk of heart disease progressively increases as blood pressure rises above 115/75, a 2014 study showed that lowering systolic blood pressure *below* 120 in adults with hypertension *did not* reduce the rate of heart disease or stroke.

In this study, 4,480 people were followed for 21 years. At the start of the study, nearly three-quarters of the participants were taking a blood pressure drug, almost one-fifth had diabetes, two-thirds smoked or drank alcohol, and about one-quarter had "high" cholesterol (as defined at that time).

At the end of the study, the researchers found that people whose blood pressure was lowered to a level below 120 didn't have any less risk of cardiovascular disease than the people who remained at the 120 to 139 level.

What's more, the researchers concluded that using drugs to reduce blood pressure below 120 may lead to dizziness, fainting, and other side effects—which can actually increase health care problems and costs over the long run.

An even more recent study found that overly aggressive lowering of blood pressure actually made people's health *worse*.

This study reviewed data on 398,419 people taking blood pressure medications for three to five years. The researchers found that lowering blood pressure below standard levels resulted in greater risk of end-stage kidney disease, kidney failure, and even death.

The lowest risk was associated with a blood pressure reading of precisely 137/71. In people with diabetes (who are at greater risk for kidney disease), the lowest risk was at 131/69. For people age 70 or older, the ideal level was 140/70.

Of course, today's new drugs for treating blood pressure may be riskier than staying with the old generic standbys that have already been proven effective over decades for millions of people. My colleague Donald Light, MD, recently published a review of all of the drugs approved by the FDA in the past 30 years. He found that only 10 percent of the new drugs were more effective than the old drugs they were meant to replace. But fully 50 percent of the new drugs were less safe than their older counterparts.

In light of this evidence, I bet that researchers would find that treating blood pressure under 140/90 is less risky if doctors considered using only the older, safer drugs. Unfortunately, that's not likely to happen anytime soon.

Taking pressure off the brain

Of course, blood pressure doesn't just affect the heart. It's also a key component in brain function, including cognitive decline.

Thirty years ago, doctors like me were taught that a "normal" systolic blood pressure was 100 plus your age. So an 80-year-old with blood pressure of 180 was nothing to worry about. Over the years, that thinking changed, and doctors began using more drugs in more patients with elevated blood pressure levels. But interestingly, new research is showing that—at least in relation to the brain—my early medical school teachings may have been right all along.

And a recent study from Johns Hopkins University found that people who developed hypertension only after age 68 didn't have any more cognitive decline than people with normal blood pressure.

But there is a caveat: The researchers also found that high blood pressure during middle-age was linked to steeper cognitive decline as they grew older.

Lower your blood pressure without drugs

The good news in all of these recent findings is that it looks like we can afford to begin relaxing blood pressure control somewhat—especially as we grow older. And once again we can look to the golden rule of moderation as our guide.

But if you do have blood pressure above the now-recommended treatment levels of 140/90 or 150/90, you should check with your doctor about starting a treatment program (just be sure to insist on older, proven, safer drug treatments).

But there are also non-drug treatments that can help you manage your blood pressure. In fact, there are many proven, effective, and widely available mind-body techniques that can help reduce blood pressure.

One final note of caution: If you monitor your BP at home and find a reading over 180/110, check it again. If it persists, you should seek urgent care to lower it. And be sure to check both arms!

Chapter 55

Eat more butter to lower your heart disease risk

I don't want to keep beating a dead horse—or cow. But I just have to keep coming back to the government's admission that their decades-long advice to cut dietary fat and cholesterol was completely wrong. The implications for your health are huge.

For example, after all the government's twisting, turning, and churning, it turns out butter is one of the healthiest fats on the planet. And butter from grass-fed cows is even better. In fact, a recent study found that men and women who eat the *most* butter from grass-fed cows have a dramatically *lower* risk of developing heart disease.

It's a wonder to behold how cattle can convert cellulose from grasses—which is indigestible to humans—into meat, milk, essential fats, and vitamins. Cellulose is a long chain of sugars linked together, and it gives wood and plants their incredible strength. It appears in plant cells, which have double-sided walls vs. the single membranes of animal cells. So it provides tremendous strength and durability.

Cows break down this tough substance with specialized teeth, and multiple stomachs and specialized digestive tracts. They also have special bacteria that help break down and metabolize cellulose in their stomachs.

Clearly, cows make for natural vegetarians by design. They can easily get these nutrients, which are indigestible to humans, out of plants. But the human digestive system isn't equipped the same way. So we need meat and dairy for optimal nutrition.

Now, back to butter...

In the 1960s and 1970s, government health experts portrayed butter as a disaster-on-a-plate. Feeding off the flawed dietary guidelines, they called margarine a "healthy" alternative to real butter.

But as you know, margarine is essentially an industrial waste chemical for which manufacturers had to find a way, and an excuse, to dump on an unsuspecting public. Marketeers based their misleading margarine ads on zero real science. These ads were breathtaking in their stupidity, even for the lame stream media.

In fact, studies now show men and women who followed this faulty advice and substituted margarine for butter ended up suffering double the rates of cardiovascular diseases.

Butter is basically just milk fat, also known as butter fat. It contains all the healthy essential fats and 400 different fatty acids.

And, as I mentioned earlier, butter from grass-fed cattle is your best choice.

It has five times more conjugated linoleic acid (CLA) than butter from grain-fed cattle. It also contains many more omega-3 fatty acids, which benefit the heart, brain, and immune system. It's also higher in vitamin K2, which you should always obtain from food sources rather than dicey dietary supplements.

Of course, all butter contains saturated fats, which government health "experts" swore would cause heart disease.

But now we know the government's decades-long stance on saturated fat was complete bunk. The government itself now admits it was wrong about fat. Plus, three huge review studies in 2010 and 2014, which followed hundreds of thousands of people, showed zero association between saturated fats and heart disease.

Now, when it comes to *preventing* heart disease, the health benefits of butter seem to vary depending upon the country in which a study is done. In countries where cows are grass-fed, people who eat the most butter have a dramatically reduced risk of heart disease.

In a recent study done in Costa Rica, researchers looked at CLA levels in the fat tissue of 1,813 heart attack patients. (CLA is a direct marker of grass-fed, full-fat dairy consumption.) They compared those levels to 1,813 healthy people who hadn't suffered heart attacks.

Turns out, men and women who had the most CLA were 50 percent less likely to have a heart attack. Plus, researchers found a dose-response effect between eating more grass-fed butter and having a lower risk of heart attack. In other words, the more grass-fed butter they ate, the lower their heart attack risk.

In another study from Australia, people who ate the most full-fat diary had a 69 percent lower risk of heart disease.

Of course, real butter also contains critical fat-soluble vitamins like D and E. And vitamin D plays a huge role in preventing just about every chronic disease known to man.

But chances are, you haven't heard as much about vitamin E. Mainstream medicine often neglects this essential nutrient for a variety of reasons. First of all, it's difficult to measure the amount of E that's actually circulating in your body. So the government is basically clueless about how much of the vitamin humans really need for optimal health.

But vitamin E is definitely not something to be taken for granted. Research shows this nutrient is crucial for every stage of life—from helping fetuses develop normally to staving off Alzheimer's disease. It's also important for your heart, eyes, and immune system. And it's vital for brain health. Unfortunately, a shocking 93 percent of people aren't getting enough of this essential nutrient. (Consequently, I recommend taking 50 mg of vitamin E per day in supplement form, in addition to incorporating vitamin-E rich food into your diet.)

So keep spreading a little butter from grass-fed beef on your toast. Feel free to sauté your vegetables and grass-fed steak in it too. It will give you plenty of essential fats and so many vital nutrients hard to get anywhere else.

Chapter 56

The lifesaving "winter weather advisory" you won't get on the evening news

Part of medical lore is that there are more heart attacks during winter. It was presumed that these heart attacks occurred because men who don't (typically) exercise regularly are suddenly out in the cold, strenuously and furiously shoveling tons of snow to clear their driveways so they can get to work (or to that NFL playoff game).

The classic causes of having an acute heart attack are exercise, emotions, and eating. Franticly hurling snow meets two out of three of those criteria, combined with the potential effects of metabolic stress caused by the cold air. (Of course, it wasn't always like that when it comes to shoveling snow. In fact, before the automobile became the "go-to" mode of transportation over the last century, snow and ice actually made it *easier* for farmers and other workers to get around outdoors by working with nature. They had sleds and sleighs to smoothly ride over the snowpack, and ice made it possible to ride over the frozen, flat, smooth surfaces of ponds, lakes and some rivers, instead of having to go all the way around them on bumpy roads. Thus, Robert Frost could write a poem about stopping by the woods in the snow, with his horse-drawn sleigh, on the darkest evening of the year—the winter solstice, December 21- 22.)

There's also speculation that blood may have a greater tendency to clot during cold weather. And of course, clots in the blood vessels that supply the heart and brain can cause heart attacks and strokes.

But while these theories make sense logically, there hasn't been scientific research to prove them. Until now, that is.

In fact, three different teams of researchers recently decided to see if this winter-weather lore is really true. Their findings were striking—and offer some important insights that could very well save your life this winter.

When the temperature drops, heart attacks and strokes rise

Taiwanese researchers examined data from nearly 290,000 people with atrial fibrillation, a condition in which the atrium chamber of the heart doesn't contract effectively. And that can cause blood to pool in the heart, potentially forming blood clots that can travel to the brain and boost your risk of stroke.

The researchers found that over a three-year period, about 35,000 of the study participants had a stroke. And stroke risk was 19 percent higher in winter than summer. It didn't even have to be a particularly cold winter. The researchers found that the chances of people with atrial fibrillation having a stroke were significantly higher when the average lower temperature was even rather mild (anything below 68 degrees)

But colder weather also comes with some significant risks. According to another new study, freezing temperatures increase heart attack risk.

Researchers checked databases in Winnipeg, Canada—one of the coldest large cities in the world—and discovered there were 1,816 severe heart attacks over a six-year period.

And when the mercury plummeted, heart attacks soared. In fact, there were 16 percent more of the severest form of heart attacks (ST-elevation myocardial infarction, or STEMI) in Winnipeg residents when the temperature went below 32 degrees (freezing).

Finally, another new study found that the weather (and air pollution) may affect how long it will take to recuperate—and even your chances of survival—if you do have a heart attack.

In heavily industrial Silesia, Poland, researchers collected data on 2,388 people who had heart attacks between 2006 and 2012. They discovered that within the first month after a heart attack, people were more likely to die on days when it was cold, sunny, and less windy.

Why? No one knows for sure, but the researchers suggested that wind blows away outdoor pollutants that may irritate the lungs and heart. And cold temperatures result in more home heating and combustion products, which generate more indoor pollutants.

How to keep your heart healthy
when the snow falls

You can dramatically decrease your risk of a heart attack or stroke year round with some simple measures.

My accountant in Florida gave me the most convincing and lengthy argument I have ever heard as to why moving to Florida is going to result in slower aging and greater longevity. As you know, I have always found accountants and actuaries to have some of the best information on mortality and longevity because, after all, that's where the money is. And biostatisticians can't manipulate mortality data the way they do clinical outcomes on drugs, for example.

Also, knowing about the amazing benefits of sunshine and vitamin D for health, I am tempted to consider that possibility as well to help account for the health benefits of warmer climates and more sunshine.

As I have written in the past, people with low levels of vitamin D in their blood have a *27 percent* higher risk of having a heart attack or stroke. And a whopping 62 percent more chance of dying.

So no matter where you are over the holidays and this winter, make sure to take 10,000 IU vitamin D daily.

CONQUERING EVERYDAY HEALTH PROBLEMS

Chapter 57

Natural ways to soothe common digestive issues

Your digestive system is one of the most active parts of your body. But it's an often-ignored area of health. That is, until something goes wrong. And you get constipated. Or the opposite.

Maybe you've tried upping your fiber. You've tried a probiotic. Perhaps you've even given up dairy. But still no improvement. It could mean that your digestive system is missing three key nutrients.

Which ones?

Well, remember, the human body in an engineering marvel. So, let's think about this for a moment…

Your body must get certain essential vitamins from foods you eat. It can't make these vitamins on its own. So, when you eat food, what part of your body breaks down and begins to absorb these essential vitamins?

You got it—your digestive tract.

And these three key vitamins are *exactly* the ones that your digestive system needs. Unfortunately, very few of us get enough of these three essential vitamins from diet alone. So, what should work like a charm can turn into a vicious cycle when you don't get enough of these vitamins.

So, let's look at three main vitamins you need for a healthy digestive system:

1. **The B vitamins.** There are actually 8 B vitamins. And they are all essential for digestive health. But since they are water-soluble vitamins, you can't store them in fat cells or tissues. Therefore, you must get a regular supply from the foods you eat. Or from a dietary supplement.

How do B vitamins aid digestion?

In general, they help move energy obtained from food into the tissue cells, where it is needed. In particular, vitamin **B1** (thiamine) helps convert carbs in the diet into energy. This fuels your cellular metabolism and helps regulate your appetite.

Vitamin B2 (riboflavin) helps keep the mucosal lining of your digestive tract in good shape. It also helps to break down proteins, fats and carbohydrates in the foods you eat. Without vitamin B2, you may have trouble digesting food. And converting the nutrients into energy. Low B2 can also cause tongue and mouth sores and swelling. Clearly, this uncomfortable situation will also interfere with normal eating and digestion.

Vitamin B3 (niacin) plays an important role in the breakdown of carbs, fats and *alcohol*. Lack of niacin causes pellagra, with severe vomiting and diarrhea. Obviously, this too will interfere with digestion and absorption of nutrients. And it can lead to dehydration.

Vitamin B6 (pyridoxine) helps the body process proteins in the diet.

Biotin helps produce healthy cholesterol. And remember, every cell in your body needs cholesterol. Biotin also processes proteins, carbs and fatty acids. And it helps eliminate the waste your body produces when it breaks down protein.

Folic acid is the final B vitamin related to healthy digestion. Research links higher levels of this vitamin with a lower risk of colon cancer. In addition, we know that low folic acid in women can result in birth defects. This is why many foods today, such as cereal and bread, are now fortified with folic acid.

You can find B vitamins in meat, dairy, eggs, green leafy vegetables, beans, seafood, and whole grains. However, studies show that many people don't get enough B vitamins from their diet. So, I recommend everyone take a high-quality B supplement.

2. **Vitamin C.** All the connective tissues in your digestive tract contain collagen. This protein helps hold your tissues together. Your body

regularly replenishes this collagen to keep your tissues strong. And to heal damaged tissues in your digestive tract.

But you need vitamin C to make this all happen.

In fact, vitamin C helps your body produce enough collagen to keep the tissues of your digestive tract healthy. So, if you suffer from a bout of irritable bowels once in a while, make sure to take plenty of vitamin C to help your tissues recover.

Vitamin C is also important for healthy teeth and gums, a key to proper eating and digestion. Vitamin C also helps with healthy iron balance. (Most people do *not* require iron supplements. Getting plenty of vitamin C will help you get all the iron you need without supplements or fortified foods.)

Good natural dietary sources of vitamin C include berries, broccoli, citrus fruits, peppers, and tomatoes.

3. Vitamin D. Of course, many studies link low levels of the "sunshine" vitamin with a higher risk of colon cancer.[1] Indeed low vitamin D seems to increase your risk of many types of cancer. Deficiency also increases overall mortality.

But researchers are now beginning to look more closely at the importance of vitamin D in the colon, specifically. In fact, we now know that men and women who live farther away from the equator, in latitudes where the sun is weaker, get Irritable Bowel Diseases (IBD) much more commonly. Researchers think IBD, like multiple sclerosis, might have something to do with low vitamin D levels. Indeed, we already know that vitamin D plays a role in taming inflammation. And regulating the immune system. So it makes sense that Crohn's disease and ulcerative colitis, both inflammatory problems, might respond to vitamin D.

You find vitamin D naturally in foods like eggs, liver, and oily fish such as salmon and tuna. But about 1 billion men and women worldwide have a frank vitamin D deficiency. Including millions in the U.S. And up to 75 million having inadequate levels. So, I believe most people in the U.S. would benefit from a high-quality vitamin D supplement.

Of course, these three vitamins have many health benefits beyond keeping the digestive tract healthy. But as I said earlier, few of us can get to adequate levels from diet alone. So, I recommend finding high-quality supplements.

Drinking plenty of water is also essential when it comes to healthy digestion. Or better yet, drink **red bush** in your water. For 12 years I've focused a large part of my own research on a plant called red bush, or **rooibos**, native to South Africa. One of the most impressive effects of red bush is that it improves hydration all the way down to a cellular level. But I can also tell you about another benefit I've always heard about—both from doctors and South Africans who drink red bush: It also works wonders on digestion. Specifically, it helps digestive complaints such as indigestion and constipation. And red bush is safe. In fact, it's so safe mothers in South Africa give red bush tea to their infants because it helps with colic. From my experience, red bush is actually safe to drink instead of plain water—all day, every day.

These steps will help lay the foundation for overall healthy digestion. But you may need some additional support if you're suffering from a specific gastrointestinal disorder. Luckily, there are natural approaches that can help.

The drug-free way to put an end to irritable bowel

Inflammatory bowel disease (IBD) is becoming more commonly known each day. Which is good, because it can be a debilitating problem. So the more people know about it and talk about it, the more comfortable sufferers will be to seek help.

However, it's critical to choose the right kind of help. And it's not just people with diagnosed IBD (a.k.a. Crohn's disease and colitis) who need to be concerned about it. Irritable bowel syndrome (IBS), with related symptoms that afflict up to 15% of the U.S. population, may be a warning sign that IBD is coming for those who don't make a change.

IBS is a prime example of how the mind and body are connected. It's no surprise that the people who experience it and the chronic gastrointestinal pain or discomfort it involves often have a history of childhood trauma such as physical or sexual abuse, parental divorce, major illness or accident, or death of a loved one. It's the body's expression of the mind's suffering.

IBS also runs in families, so biomedical scientists are quick to claim some kind of genetic basis—but lifestyle factors run in families just as much as genes do.

How thin are your boundaries?

Tufts University professor Ernest Hartmann developed a "boundary concept" to explain differences in personality type. He found that people have differing levels of boundaries, ranging from thick to thin. Thin-boundary people tend to be more artistic, more connected with their dreams, and more likely to see themselves "merge" in their relationships with others. Thick- boundary people see clear divides between themselves and others and tend to see the world in black-and-white.

My colleague Michael A. Jawer and I suspected that this boundary concept could explain some mysteries of physical health, and we were right. In our book *Your Emotional Type*, we demonstrate that people with thin boundaries are more susceptible to a dozen illnesses with mind-body components—including IBS.

A common denominator among these ailments? Low serotonin levels. Serotonin is a key neurotransmitter found in the brain—but 95 percent is found in the neuroendocrine tissue of the gut. (Ever wonder why we have "gut feelings," and feel like we've been "punched in the gut" when we get bad news? It's likely related to these neurochemicals—chemicals that relate to thoughts and feelings—that are actually present in the gut.)

The level of serotonin in IBS patients (and, for that matter, fibromyalgia sufferers) is low compared with individuals experiencing the thick boundary condition of chronic fatigue syndrome. And while serotonin is far from the sole actor, the difference points toward a meaningful distinction in boundary type among these conditions.

Sufferers are often described as "overly anxious" and even "driven." It also often co-occurs with seasonal allergies and allergic eczema. And people with IBS are more likely to suffer from fibromyalgia and migraine. All thin boundary conditions.

A mind-body solution for a mind-body problem

If you have IBS, chances are you are a thin boundary type. (Find out your boundary type at www.drmicozzi. com.) Since the mind is clearly a critical part of what happens in this syndrome, your best bet for treating it is using a mind-body therapy that is most effective for your type.

Hypnosis is perfectly suited for people with thin boundaries. Biofeedback is another safe and effective technique for thin-boundary types. And acupuncture can be a powerhouse across the board—even for many people who have had no luck with other therapies.

When the syndrome becomes a disease

If IBS progress to an inflammatory bowel disease like Crohn's, treatment is a lifelong process. For many sufferers, conventional treatments offer little relief. Experts recommend complementary and alternative medicine (CAM) approaches, even beyond the mind-body disorder of IBS, as a powerful treatment for IBD.

My colleague, Joyce Frye, DO, who has contributed several chapters to my medical textbooks over the years and was previously with the Center for Integrative Medicine at the University of Maryland School of Medicine, was recently interviewed on this topic. "It's not a question of if you should use these alternative and complementary therapies," she emphasizes. "It's a question of using them correctly."

Another reason I urge you to find the CAM therapies that are proven to work for *you*—based on your individual type.

According to Dr. Frye, "The first goal is to treat the underlying imbalance that has caused a problem, so we can allow the body to heal itself. The second goal is to provide symptom relief in the meantime."

One of the best things about CAM therapies is that they are safe and unlikely to interfere with your conventional medical treatment. What's more, they can actually help you to replace essential vitamins and minerals your body is losing because of the disease.

Here's a closer look at some of the most effective mind-body remedies for bowel disorders.

Acupuncture

A recent review of studies on acupuncture and gastrointestinal diseases found acupuncture treatments to be helpful. One study in particular found that quality of life for Crohn's patients improved significantly after acupuncture treatments.

Mind/body techniques

Meditation, guided relaxation, yoga, and tai chi do not treat Crohn's disease directly, but they *do* reduce stress—and stress is known to trigger flare-ups and worsen symptoms. (If you choose the technique best suited to your emotional type, you may have even better luck.)

Hypnosis

According to a review by the University of Maryland Medical Center in Baltimore, hypnosis may help the functioning of the body's immune system and also give you the expected relaxation benefits of other mind/body practices, such as **easing stress and anxiety**.

Massage

Although it has no clear effect on Crohn's disease, massage is a popular stress reducer. If you experience the relaxation that comes from massage, ask your doctor for specific guidelines based on your medical condition, including whether the massage therapist should completely avoid your abdomen and how light or deep the massage should be.

Ginger, as well as verbena and linden teas may also help with digestion. In fact, I have some personal experience with the digestive benefits of these teas. They've been used in my family for at least five generations. But watch out for green and black teas which contain caffeine, tannins and oxalic acid—and can disrupt digestion.

Beware of this common peptic ulcer "cure"

Like other digestive disorders, peptic ulcers have frustrated mainstream doctors for decades. Their favorite 20th century approaches to medical problems—drugs and surgery—could not treat them. Much less cure them. In fact, you may have heard the old joke:

Q: *Who decides how to treat a peptic ulcer?*

A: *The doorman at the medical office building. If he points you to the internist's office, you get a drug. And if he points you to the surgeon's office, you get surgery.*

Truthfully, neither surgery nor drugs are good options for curing peptic ulcers. Both disrupt digestion, nutrition, and metabolism. And the drugs especially disrupt the absorption of critical B vitamins.

But about 20 years ago, many physicians thought we'd finally discovered the cause of peptic ulcers—a simple bacterium called *Heliobacter pylori* (H. pylori). They claimed we could "cure" the ulcer by killing the bacteria with antibiotics.

Proponents hailed this discovery as some great miracle. In fact, I knew a few of the simple-minded believers at the College of Physicians in Philadelphia, which I directed during the late 1990s.

A particularly delusional pair of doctors at the College had no patience for anyone who suggested that perhaps H. pylori was a normal part of the stomach's "microbiome." And they would never acknowledge that something else, such as stress, caused ulcers.

Instead, they could not wait to indoctrinate every physician with the new gospel. And they were disappointed when our program committee did not devote the entire year's continuing medical education program to this great discovery.

Well, somehow over the past two decades, they got someone to buy into this nonsense. In fact, they got a lot of people to buy into it. Today, many doctors give patients antibiotics in an attempt to eradicate H. pylori infections "causing" the ulcers. To add insult to injury, they give these patients proton pump inhibitors (PPIs) to reduce stomach acid while the stomach ulcer "heals."

But the healing never happens. Plus, you've wiped out normal H. pylori in the gut. And you've artificially lowered stomach acid with a drug. So now, when the patient goes off the PPI, the stomach acid comes back with a vengeance.

Plus, in a new study, Australian researchers found a strong connection between the eradication of H. pylori infections and rising obesity rates in the western world.

In their new analysis, the researchers looked at 49 studies with data from 10 European nations, Japan, the United States, and Australia. They found the higher the obesity rate in a population, the lower the rate of H. pylori infections. For example, research shows less than 50 percent of U.S. adults have the H. pylori bacteria in their gut. And we have one of the highest obesity rates in the world. Plus, in previous controlled trials, patients experienced significant weight gain after they eradicated their *H. pylori* infections with antibiotics.

These insights really aren't new.

We warned about it 20 years ago in Philadelphia. And Martin J. Blaser, M.D., Director of the Human Microbiome Program at New York University knew about it too.

In an interview, Dr. Blaser said, "In 1998, I predicted that doctors of the future will be giving H. pylori back to children. We should not be so fast in eradicating H. pylori."

It's just not nice to fool around with Mother Nature's plans, especially with antibiotics. These "magic bullets" are really "friendly fire." They cause more and more medical disorders and diseases.

Thankfully, more and more scientists like Dr. Blaser are now starting to realize the gut contains H. pylori for a reason. In fact, most people have H. pylori in their stomach. And most of them never get peptic ulcers!

In fact, we now know there's much more to the peptic ulcer story...

Peptic ulcers actually have a very strong mind-body connection. In fact, certain personality types (or emotional types) are more likely to develop them. And stress plays a major role.

Of course, my colleagues in Philadelphia never had any patience for the role of emotions in medicine. Except when it came to inflicting their own toxic brew of negative emotions on their colleagues and people like me whom they thought worked exclusively for them.

If you have a peptic ulcer, you should investigate ways to decrease your stress. Many mind-body approaches can help. You just need to figure out which approach works best for your personality type. For example, some people respond quite well to meditation. Others, not at all. Refer back to the techniques I outlined above for some additional suggestions.

Of course, a good diet supports good digestion. And good digestion nourishes the body. So do yourself a favor and start there. I'll tell you how in the next chapter.

Chapter 58

The top of the food chain cure for obesity

There's a remarkable thing about nature: In all the various environments, or ecological niches, animals sort themselves out in a kind of "pyramid scheme"...with the biggest animal species at the top of the food chain.

In the ocean, the big fish eat the little fish, and the little fish eat the littler fish, and the littler fish eat...the plankton. But keep in mind that the biggest fish (actually a mammal returned to sea, probably related to the hippopotamus), the whale, actually feeds on plankton by straining tons of water through baleen (or whalebone) instead of teeth. How can tiny plankton cells feed the largest creature on the planet? The secret is volume and continuous feeding.

On land, the "top dogs," or the biggest animals at the top of the food chain pyramid, are fierce creatures like bears in North America and Europe, or lions in Africa, or tigers in India and Malaya.

One thing the bear knows...it's lonely at the top (of the food chain).

These animals, because of their large size, tend to eat alone and over relatively large areas... it takes a lot of food sources over a lot of territory to feed them. They are omnivores (eating everything) or carnivores (eating meat—the most concentrated source of food with plenty of essential fatty acids, bioavailable minerals and nutrients, calories and total nutrient density).

The exceptions to the solitary rule for animals at the top of the food chain are wolves and humans, who like to hunt and eat in groups (and there are some significant health benefits associated with this dietary "pack mentality.") However, while humans are like canines in eating together, we are like bears in eating everything, omnivorously.

A bit like the whale in the ocean, the bear feeds by taking in lots of little things—pounds and pounds of nuts, berries and other foods, including fish and meat when available in season. When some bears want to get their feet wet, they go jump in the river (in season) and are able to feed on salmon making their return runs to spawn—thereby getting plenty of meat, fats, and essential fatty acids (the omega-threes). But normally, the only way to get enough nuts, berries, and other foods to feed a bear is to cover a lot of territory and keep other bears and predators away.

And herein lies the secret…

Eating like a bear

After trying various fad diets that most young women fall victim to these days…my daughter Alicia decided to stop and take a cue from Nature. After taking a few advanced courses in biology she came to follow what she calls simply "The Bear Diet."

It was the healthiest and most effective diet she had ever tried for losing weight. And since it is also one of the most nutritionally sound diets I have ever come across, I endorse it wholeheartedly.

The Bear Diet includes plenty of nuts, berries, vegetables, fruits, and some meat when available. In addition to the high nutritional value of fruits, nuts, and vegetables, eating the bear diet requires "frequent, small feedings throughout the day"—like a bear. This provides plenty of bioavailable nutrients and essential fatty acids, leaving the you satisfied but thinner.

This diet also avoids health-sapping processed sugars and fats, and provides basically the same approach that works in controlling diabetes, heart disease, arthritis, and other chronic health concerns.

The proof is in the past— our hunter-gatherer history

If you consider our prehistoric past, you'll find this approach makes perfect sense. Just don't get hung up on the misleading traditional picture of "Stone Age" humans that we've all been taught: "Man the Hunter." For the reality is actually closer to "Woman the Gatherer."

In fact, we have had the fortunate opportunity in modern times to observe actual human populations today that are essentially living in the "Stone Age" (*Neolithic*) in terms of the stone tools they use. Populations like the Tasaday of Mindanao, Philippines, the Bushmen of the Kalahari Desert, or even the traditional Inuit of the sub-Arctic. And in these "Stone Age" cultures, we observe that, mostly, it is the women who *gather* a lot of plants, nuts, berries, and small animals. And while the men may go away "hunting" large game, they mostly end up fooling around and getting into trouble.

A remarkable thing about wild game hunted and gathered is that the meat has only about 5% fat content—as opposed to the up to 50% fat content of artificially manipulated modern livestock raised for food. The USDA actually still considers that higher fat, "grade A" meat to be the better grades. But up until 100 years ago, cattle grazed on the western plains were still relatively lean—they had to be driven by cowboys (the original long-distance truckers) hundreds of miles to railheads for transport on trains to the stockyards in Chicago and elsewhere. Like the cowboys themselves, the cattle arrived pretty lean.

So while eating meat can be part of a healthy diet—watch out for what kind of meat. Natural, free-range livestock and wild game have the healthiest nutrient composition and are full of bioavailable minerals, vitamins, and other nutrients that are easy to digest and readily available to our metabolism. These lean, fresh meats will be free of the processed sugars and fats that are deadly causes of most modern ills.

And by the way, if anyone tries to tell you that humans should not eat meat…take a look at our teeth—do they look the teeth of a cow or horse?

On the vast American plains during the 19th century, Native Americans often suffered from what they called "rabbit hunger." During the depths of winter they could not hunt the declining populations of bison and other large game, instead, they had to rely on small game, like rabbits, which have very little body fat—and are very low in essential fatty acids. Contrary to some popular belief, not only is a little fat good for you, it is literally "essential" to health and life (that's why they are called *essential* fatty acids). Native Americans with "rabbit hunger" were starving from lack of essential fatty acids; when given just a spoonful of lard (rendered animal fat) they would return to normal health overnight.

In effect, getting the right amount of fat in the diet has always been a problem for people. Before the 20th century it was getting enough essential fatty acids, since they are rare in Nature, especially in plants. Today, we struggle from getting too much fat—and too many calories.

The Bear Diet provides just the proper balance. Plenty of bioavailable nutrients and essential fatty acids, which will leave you more satisfied… and thinner, too.

What to eat on the Bear Diet

Note that you do not have to count, measure, weigh, or otherwise obsess over what you eat down to the gram. This is a critical error that many of today's diet "gurus" and physicians make. Obsessive behavior around an activity of daily living, like eating, is not healthy and can be just another source of stress, which is counter-productive. When you follow the Bear Diet, how much you eat won't matter. And what and when you eat will easily become second nature.

1. **Eat all you want (like the bear), of the following vegetables. (Eat them raw or cooked, without butter, fat, or salad dressing.*)**

- Artichoke
- Asparagus
- Bean sprouts
- Beet greens
- Broccoli
- Cabbage (and pickled cabbage, or sauerkraut)
- Cauliflower
- Celery
- Chinese cabbage (bok choy)
- Cucumbers (and pickled cucumbers, sour or dill, not sweet)
- Eggplant
- Endive
- Escarole
- Fennel (fenocchi)
- Fiddle-head fern (in season)
- Green beans
- Kale
- Lettuce
- Mushrooms
- Mustard greens
- Onions
- Parsley
- Peppers (red, green, yellow; hot or sweet)

- Radishes
- Scallions
- String beans
- Turnips
- Watercress
- Rhubarb
- Spinach
- Squash (green and yellow; zucchini)
- Tomatoes

2. Eat no more than 3 servings of fresh fruits each day.

- Apple
- Apricot
- Berries (any kind; one-half cup = one fruit serving)
- Cantaloupe (one-half medium-sized = one fruit serving)
- Grapefruit (one-half medium-sized = one fruit serving)
- Honeydew melon (two-inch wedge = one fruit serving)
- Orange
- Peach
- Pear
- Plum
- Pineapple (one-half medium-sized = one fruit serving)
- Tangerine or tangelo

3. Spices and seasonings (all you want)
- Bouillon
- Horseradish, red or white
- Lemon, lime
- Mustard
- Tomato juice or paste (in cooking)
- Vinegar
- Herbs, including:

Basil	Chili	Dill
Garlic	Rosemary	Sage
Paprika	Pepper	Tarragon
Thyme	Cinnamon	Cloves
Ginger	Mint	Nutmeg

4. Eat several handfuls of mixed nuts (unsalted, not honey roasted). Especially almonds, pecans, and walnuts.

You can mix them with small amounts of dried fruits (careful, these can be high in sugar). You can have handfuls from a zip-lock bag throughout the day. This will definitely keep you from feeling hunger between meals. (Protein bars and "meal replacement" bars are not a substitute for anything. You will never need them and they should not form part of a healthy, weight loss diet.)

5. **Once per day: Eat 4 to 6 ounces (about the size of the palm of your hand) of fresh grilled salmon or other fish, shellfish or seafood, squid (calamari; cuttlefish), or octopus (wild caught)**

Grill fish with dill, natural yogurt, other fresh herbs, lemon-lime, cilantro, or onions to taste. Shellfish, while high in cholesterol, are low in fats. Eat mussels, clams, shrimp, lobster, or scallops cooked in their own broth, or sautéed in garlic and olive oil.

HOW to eat on the Bear Diet

Start by completely eliminating carbohydrates from the diet for the first 2 to 3 weeks. No sugars, breads, starches; no corn, no potatoes, avoid "pulses" like beans (except green beans) and peas. This will help get your metabolism back on track and also provide some relatively rapid weight loss, which will be a source of motivation important to the psychology of dieting.

Start the day like a "hungry bear" coming out of hibernation. Try to start with the largest meal in the morning, since your metabolism will have all day to burn. However, if you are someone who just can't eat in the morning, then go with what your body is telling you. Don't eat when you aren't hungry.

On this diet, there is nothing magical about breakfast, lunch, or dinner. The cultural tradition of "three meals per day" is not a metabolic reality. You can actually "snack" throughout the day, like the bear, with frequent, small feedings.

You can eat the recommended foods in any order at any time. If you could not finish dinner (stop eating when you no longer feel hungry— it takes the brain a few minutes to catch up with the "satiety" of the stomach) have the left-overs the next morning.

After 2 to 3 weeks, and observing some real weight loss, slowly add back some carbohydrates in the morning, like a slice of whole grain bread, or a cup of steel-cut oats (not rolled oats), or even a bowl of Cheerio's (no- or low-sugar).

After another 2 to 3 weeks, as an occasional "treat," instead of snacking on the nuts and berries, you can have a small bag of pretzels, or other salty snacks, once in a while, but NOT sugary treats. You will find that nuts and berries take the place of all these sugary snacks and desserts.

Helpful Hint: Take a few minutes to prepare zip-lock bags and small containers the night before so you can accommodate your schedule during the day. By measuring out your snacks the night before, you will avoid "overdosing" on snacks.

Mix it up

A diverse diet is also important to gain a balance of different nutrients. Poor diets, and fad diets, that rely heavily on only one or few foods are inherently unhealthy and may lead to malnourishment. Europeans had a hard time achieving dietary diversity before their "discovery" of the Americas. There were only 16 different cultigens (plants cultivated for foods) in Europe from ancient Rome until the introduction of foods from the Americans in the 1600's. Tomato sauce did not appear on an Italian menu until late in the 1700's.

Of course, the bear may not typically eat all of these foods (like eggs and olive oil), but you can—and you will be very well nourished, keep your metabolism going, and experience healthy weight loss. When you achieve your desired weight there are many other foods and food preparations you can add back to your diet to maintain your health and your weight.

Chapter 59

What B can do for you

We are constantly learning more about the health benefits of B vitamins. And now, research shows that the B vitamin folic acid may be a natural, inexpensive way to help you keep your cool in the summer heat. *And* help reduce your risk of heart attack and stroke to boot.

How can a simple vitamin serve as an internal air conditioner? Well, it all has to do with our blood vessels.

B vitamins have been shown in studies to help prevent blood vessel damage. Which may stop atherosclerosis and reduce your risk of cardiovascular disease. In fact, raising your B vitamin levels and managing your blood pressure are two of the most important steps you can take to dramatically reduce your risk of having a heart attack or stroke.

Bs also have other effects on blood vessels. For instance, you probably know about the flushing that can occur in your chest and neck when you take the B vitamin niacin. This flushing is completely harmless, but doctors use it as an excuse to give patients dangerous statin drugs instead of natural niacin. Even though niacin has been shown in study after study to reduce cholesterol.

Overall, B vitamins help our blood vessels stay healthy. And, of course, we need healthy vessels to keep our blood flowing smoothly.

The heat buster that's just as good as pricey pharmaceuticals

One way our bodies help cool themselves is to shift blood closer to the skin, where the heat can be released more easily. We do this cooling by dilating the blood vessels through the production of nitric oxide. (That's why nitroglycerin—a form of nitric oxide—has been a standby for nearly two centuries for dilating the coronary arteries and increasing blood flow to the heart).

But older adults have a harder time producing nitric oxide. Which gives us a greater chance of suffering heart attacks and strokes when the temperature rises.

The researchers behind this new study had previously discovered that a substance called tetrahydrobiopterin, or BH4, helps our bodies produce nitric oxide.

Folic acid helps produce BH4, so the researchers decided to find out if giving people extra folic acid would improve their blood flow and help them fight heat-related strokes and heart attacks.

They did two tests on 11 people with an average age of 71, and 11 people with an average age of 22. First, they put folic acid or placebo patches on the participants' skin. Then, they took the patches off and put the people in a type of wetsuit to control their skin temperatures. And they gave them either a placebo or 5 mg of folic acid a day for six weeks.

The researchers discovered that both of the tests increased the blood vessel dilation of the older participants, but not the younger ones. And the folic acid supplements were just as effective as the patches. Plus, the researchers found that folic acid showed the *same effect* on nitric oxide production as an expensive pharmaceutical drug.

Which just goes to show that after trying everything else, we can almost always count on coming back to natural approaches like B vitamin supplementation for safe, simple, and affordable solutions to staying healthy.

That's why I suggest you help beat the heat of the "dog days" of summer by taking a high-quality B vitamin supplement. One that contains at least 400 micrograms of folic acid.

And don't stop when the temperature drops. A lifelong regimen of B supplementation can do wonders for your circulation, heart, and blood vessels.

Chapter 60

Nine big fat myths still being mouthed by "experts"

"Fat and cholesterol are bad." How often have you heard that? Even though these innocent nutrients are so essential that we literally could not live without them, we're still barraged every day by old myths and misconceptions promulgated by fat phobics and cholesterol cholerics.

Even worse, these myths continue to come straight from the mouths of paid experts who really should know better by now.

It is astounding to me that decades-old, ill-informed comments and recommendations about fat and cholesterol are still being made today. Despite the lack of any real proof—and a bunch of evidence to the contrary.

Here's a look at nine commonly repeated fat and cholesterol "facts" that are as mythical as the nine lives of a cat.

Myth 1: Fat will make you fat and unhealthy

Yes, fat does have more calories than carbohydrates or protein. But this caloric density actually makes fat more nutritious. It's the only food source of vitamins A, D, and E, for example. And we all know how important these vitamins, especially D, are to good health—and how deficient most people are today.

Fat also tends to be very filling and satisfying, so there is less of a tendency to overeat. Which leads me to Myth 2…

Myth 2: Low-fat is the optimal weight-loss diet

During the 1960s and '70s, some influential scientists came to believe that saturated fat was the main cause of heart disease and some cancers. Although there was not a single study in humans that proved this misguided notion, politicians jumped on board. And the low-fat diet was recommended to all Americans beginning in 1977.

It became the largest uncontrolled experiment ever foisted on the American people.

But the low-fat diet has now been thoroughly studied. And it should have been put to rest following the largest controlled clinical trial in nutritional history—the Women's Health Initiative, which I originally helped to put together.

One Women's Health Initiative analysis of nearly 50,000 postmenopausal women showed that participants who followed a low-fat diet only weighed one pound less after eight years compared to the women who ate a normal, well-balanced diet. Plus, the low-fat group didn't have any lower rates of heart disease or cancer.

In other studies, a low-fat diet was actually associated with lowering HDL "good" cholesterol and reducing the size of LDL "bad" cholesterol. And while it seems counterintuitive, smaller, denser LDL cholesterol molecules are actually more likely to build up in arteries than larger, "lighter" particles.

So not only will you not lose weight on a low-fat diet, but it can potentially kill you. Talk about a big fat myth.

Myth 3: Processed, low-fat foods are healthy alternatives

When the low-fat craze took hold in the '70s and '80s, food manufacturers figured out how to remove fat from their products and make a bundle selling these higher-priced "healthy" alternatives. The problem was, without fat, the foods tasted terrible. So to combat this problem, manufacturers simply loaded low-fat foods with sugar, corn syrup, and tasty artificial chemicals instead.

But sugar—not fat—is the real culprit behind obesity and obesity-related diseases like type 2 diabetes and heart disease.

Nevertheless, sales of low-fat, high-sugar foods have skyrocketed as consumers attempt to follow faulty nutritional advice without having to give up their favorite foods.

In fact, according to a new study published in the *American Journal of Clinical Nutrition*, processed foods account for 75 percent of the added sugar in the average American's diet.

Of course, the best course is to avoid food that requires processing to make it low fat, low carb, or low anything. The purpose of eating is not to consume "low" foods with empty calories, but to eat highly nutritious foods.

Myth 4: You'll have a heart attack if you eat saturated fat

The idea that saturated fat raises the risk of heart disease was initially based on flawed studies that clueless politicians, abetted by political scientists, somehow made into public policy.

The saturated fat myth is based on a chain of misconceptions. We've since learned that consuming saturated fat does not really appear to raise LDL "bad" cholesterol by much[5,6] (Even assuming that cholesterol is the culprit behind heart disease in the first place—see Myth 6).

Saturated fat actually appears to change LDL from small, dense particles that can clog arteries to larger, lighter particles that are mostly benign.[7] Furthermore, saturated fat appears to raise HDL "good" cholesterol.

So, if anything, saturated fat seems to actually *improve* cholesterol profile in terms of supposed heart disease risk factors.

Still not convinced? Consider this: In 2010, researchers reviewed data from 21 studies involving 347,747 participants and found no evidence that saturated fat consumption increases the risk of heart disease.[8]

You can't get much more proof than that.

Myth 5: Saturated fats are the same as trans fats

Trans fats are also known as partially hydrogenated fats. They do not occur in nature, but instead are manufactured in a highly artificial— and toxic—process that makes liquid fats solid and thus easier to cook with. Trans fats extend the shelf life of processed foods, which is why you'll find them in everything from cakes to chips.

Trans fats pack a double health whammy: They raise bad cholesterol and lower good cholesterol, increasing your risk of heart disease, stroke, and diabetes. Even the FDA recognizes trans fats' harm and has belatedly banned them.

Many experts and organizations lump trans fats and saturated fats together and label them all as "bad fats." But as we learned above, saturated fats are safe. It's the artificial trans fats that are totally toxic and have no place in any diet.

Myth 6: Foods that contain cholesterol will kill you

Cholesterol in food is broken down during digestion and has no correlation to the cholesterol that circulates in the blood. Nor does dietary cholesterol intake correlate to heart disease.

I repeat: Cholesterol in food is not the same as the cholesterol we've all been taught (misguidedly) to fear.

This tragic lack of basic knowledge and understanding has led to excellent, healthy foods such as eggs, lobster, and shrimp being consigned to the "bad list" simply because they contain cholesterol. To this day, so-called experts still drone on about how many eggs or shellfish servings you can "get away with."

There is nothing wrong with eating shellfish if you enjoy it. And eggs are actually nature's perfect food, packed with minerals, vitamins, and other nutrients. But keep in mind these nutrients are found in the yolk, which is also the part of the egg that contains cholesterol. Advising people to throw out the yolks and only eat egg whites is just about the most ridiculous and wasteful advice in the sad history of diet and nutrition recommendations.

Myth 7: LDL cholesterol is evil

Mainstream medicine is obsessed with lowering total and LDL "bad" cholesterol in the blood. But while cardiologists drop the LDL limit ever lower, endocrinology doctors who are experts in human metabolism are crying foul.

Studies have found that total and LDL cholesterol levels are poor indicators of heart disease compared with other risk markers.

In the past, I have also reported on a study of 231,986 patients hospitalized for heart disease. Half of them had normal LDL cholesterol levels.

And in older people, there are studies that show that the higher the cholesterol, the *lower* the risk of heart disease.

My late colleague, Dr. Arthur Schatzkin of the National Cancer Institute, first showed that low cholesterol is a risk factor for cancer nearly 30 years ago. Recent studies have found low cholesterol is associated with higher mortality worldwide—not only from cancer, but also suicide.

Myth 8: Margarine is better than butter

As the U.S. government made the saturated fat myth official in 1977, margarine manufacturers and their ad agencies stepped up the opportunity to sell their unpalatable, slick chemical sticks as "healthy" substitutes for real butter.

But the truth is, most margarines contain large amounts of unhealthy processed vegetable oils and added trans fats. In fact, the well-respected Framingham Massachusetts Heart Study shows that eating margarine substantially increases the risk of heart disease, while butter has no effect.

And an Australian study of 458 men who had recently had a cardiac event found that those who increased their margarine and vegetable oil consumption were a whopping 70 percent more likely to die of heart disease than their butter-eating peers.

"Margarine, the toxic toast topper." Now that's an ad I'd like to see.

Myth 9: Corn and soy oils are heart healthy

I'll finish with a myth that seemingly came out of nowhere: The corn and soy oils sold in grocery stores are somehow healthy.

Vegetable oils contain unsaturated fats, and thus are touted as a healthy substitute for saturated fats like butter. But, the practice of irradiating corn seeds over many decades has created a genetically modified food and oil that is now virtually devoid of nutritional content.

Soybeans are even worse—93 percent of all soy planted in the United States in 2013 was genetically engineered.

And that's not all. Research shows corn and soybean oils are high in omega-6 fatty acids. Too many omega-6s can lead to inflammation— one of the chief markers for heart disease, type 2 diabetes, and other serious diseases. Furthermore, a study showed that soybean oils commonly sold in the U.S. can actually contain trans fats, which have been linked to heart disease.

Despite all the research showing that these nine myths are nothing more than fairy tales that haven't come true, I continue to see warnings from nutritional "experts" about the evils of fat and cholesterol.

But now you know better. Just say no to these outrageous misconceptions that have been promulgated upon the American people over the last four decades. Your body and your brain will thank you.

Chapter 61

The safe way to reduce belly fat and lower your risk of diabetes and heart disease— without eating less or exercising more

You may have heard how rosehips—which are popular in herbal teas, jams, and juices—are a potent natural source of vitamin C and other nutrients.

Maybe you've also heard how this fruit of the rose plant is traditionally used as a diuretic and laxative. And as a natural remedy for gout and rheumatism.

But rosehips have another health benefit that most people aren't aware of…

New research shows rosehips can actually help you lose that stubborn belly fat that's so dangerous for your health. *Without* cutting calories or exercising more.

And without the dangerous side effects of traditional stimulant weight-loss products that leave you jittery, make your heart race…and may even kill you

The natural way to lose abdominal fat

More than any other type of fat, abdominal fat has been linked to increased risk of metabolic syndrome, diabetes, and heart disease.

So how do rosehips help you shed this deadly fat? Well, as I mentioned above, along with vitamin C, these fragrant fruits contain an abundance of biologically active polyphenols.

Rosehips' most powerful polyphenol is called tiliroside. Studies have reported that tiliroside has antioxidant, anti-cancer, anti-inflammatory, and antiviral properties.

And, as it turns out, it also has anti-obesity capabilities. Let's take a closer look at the evidence.

How rosehips help you lose different kinds of fat... and why that's important

In one study, a rosehip extract prevented weight gain and body fat accumulation in non-obese mice—without any changes in their diets or the number of calories they consumed.

Other studies have shown that rosehips inhibit accumulation of lipids in fat cells. So in essence, rosehips can help prevent your fat cells from getting fatter.

Another study showed that rosehip juice also reduced blood lipids in obese people—*and* lowered their blood pressure as well.

The latest study involved 152 people who were divided into two groups. One group was given 100 mg of rosehip extract daily for 12 weeks, and the other group received a placebo.

All of the participants were asked to maintain their regular diet and lifestyle patterns.

Indeed, throughout the study, the researchers observed that both groups had almost identical food-intake rates.

But at the end of the study, the researchers observed that total abdominal fat, visceral fat (fat around the organs), body weight, and body mass index (BMI) all decreased significantly in the rosehip group.

Even though they ate just as much as the placebo group.

Another key thing to note about this study is the type of fat the people lost. Why does this matter? Because just looking at weight or BMI is a poor way of assessing body fat and composition in terms of health.

When I worked as a senior research investigator at the National Institutes of Health, I tried to get researchers to look beyond these simple, inaccurate measures of body fat when it came to their multimillion-dollar studies on health.

Measuring only body weight or BMI just doesn't tell doctors or patients what they really need to know about health status.

I didn't learn this truth in medical school—nor did I learn about diet and nutrition. Instead, I discovered it as part of my human biology training for my PhD in anthropology.

Sadly, medical doctors simply aren't taught in school what they really need to know about nutrition or assessment of the human body.

Why rosehips are safer than other weight-loss products

While rosehips stimulate the nervous system to burn fat, they're different than the typical "upper" type of weight-loss products.

These products hype up your adrenalin—which can make you jittery and increase your heart rate and blood sugar levels.

That's not only unpleasant (for you, and those around you), but dangerous for your health.

In fact, some of these products have even been associated with sudden deaths. In contrast, rosehips appear to accomplish fat burning *without* increasing adrenalin.

Researchers believe the tiliroside in rosehips helps us lose body fat through its effect on the autonomic nervous system—which controls basic body functions like breathing, heartbeat, and digestion.

Tiliroside is thought to stimulate the autonomic nervous system to increase fat burning both at rest and during exercise.

Even better, rosehips appear to target abdominal fat burning, rather than the subcutaneous fat that lies just under the skin throughout your body. This allows you to lose unhealthy belly fat without shrinking your skin and ending up with the gaunt look of someone hooked on stimulants.

Having some healthy subcutaneous fat also appears to actually *lower* the risk of many chronic diseases.

And it helps you maintain a more youthful appearance—in contrast to looking like emaciated old crows (feet and all).

You can find rosehips in some herbal teas. There are also rosehip supplements. Look for pills, extracts, or powders that contain at least 0.1% tilirosides. I recommend 100 mg of rosehips a day.

So now you are hip to the healthy body-fat benefits of rosehips. Lose some fat off those hips. Don't be fooled by other weight-loss supplements—a rosehip by another name is not the same.

Chapter 62

The surprising truth about Metformin

The "natural" blood-sugar remedy that had been sidelined for far too long

What I'm about to tell you may be shocking. And it's sure to ruffle the feathers of many of the "natural know-it-alls." But the science is clear, so I'm not afraid to say it:

If you have unmanaged Type II diabetes, you should consider the drug metformin as a first line of treatment.

And you won't get the full story anywhere else, since the natural health industry wouldn't be caught dead recommending a drug. So, please allow me to do the honors here…

Think of it as your emergency "get out of jail free card"

Diabetes is deadly. High blood sugar coursing through your body destroys your eyes, kidneys, heart, brain, and more. So the sooner you bring it down the better.

And the science is clear—the drug metformin has been proven safe and effective for most people. And since it's now a generic drug, it's highly cost effective, too.

Now don't get me wrong…I'm not saying diet and exercise isn't important. In fact, they're the best means for preventing and even reversing Type II diabetes entirely. Something metformin can't do. And there are certainly dietary supplements that can help with maintaining healthy blood sugar (like berberine).

But Type II diabetes doesn't develop overnight. And let's face it, changing the habits and consequences that got us there in the first place isn't an overnight task either. So if you need additional help, this is one rare instance where you shouldn't be afraid to look at a mainstream therapy.

And when an option this effective comes along to help kick-start your efforts safely (when taken properly), even if it *is* a drug...it's something you should consider seriously.

Indeed, it's rare to find such a safe and effective "drug" as the popular diabetes treatment metformin. In fact, this is one "wonder drug" that is steeped in natural history—like aspirin or digitalis—and was in "historic use" for centuries.

One of Nature's wonder remedies

Originally, metformin was known under the trade name Glucophage. But it's now been around long enough to go off patent and become generic. Which means it meets one of my primary requirements when it comes to taking a drug: Make sure it has undergone the seven-year post-marketing surveillance period required by the FDA. Which means it's been proven safe by the tens of millions of patients who have taken it over at least seven years, and now much longer.

As a drug, it was actually first synthesized in the 1920's. However, it was quickly overshadowed by the Nobel prize-winning discovery of the role of insulin in the treatment of diabetes. So metformin was swiftly set aside for a half-century.

However, its history goes back much further...where it was known throughout Europe as a traditional folk medicine for centuries. That's because this drug actually stems from a flowering plant called Galega officinalis, more commonly knowns as French lilac or goat's rue. The active ingredient is a chemical biguanide known as Galegine, after the botanical name of the plant.

As an herbal extract, Galegine was used traditionally to treat people with polyuria (excessive urination due to excess sugar in the urine) and sweet odor on the breath. Today, we recognize these as two leading symptoms of untreated diabetes.

References to this herbal treatment date as far back as ancient Egypt and it was in common use in Medieval Europe. It was even featured in an English medical treatise by Culpepper in the 17th century. And it was studied at the University of Edinburgh, a leading medical center of the 18th century from which the first medical school in America was established in 1765. It has also been used in Asia to treat influenza and is said to have antibiotic, antiviral, antimalarial, and antipyretic (fever) activities.

With such a long history as a potent herbal remedy, it's actually shocking that it took so long to be used for a major modern medical problem like diabetes!

So after languishing during the Great Depression and World War II, the French finally developed Galegine, or metformin, for clinical use in 1957. It was approved the following year in the United Kingdom, and made its way to Canada in 1972. But it was not approved by the FDA in the United States until 1994. And that was only after a U.S. drug company (Bristol Myers Squibb) acquired a French firm that manufactured the drug.

Getting to the root of the delay...

One reason for delayed approval in the U.S. was due to concern over a very rare side effect called lactic acidosis. This is a metabolic condition that results in a buildup of lactic acid in the muscles due to changes in levels of sugar and oxygen.

A poorly advised campaign was undertaken by the public advocacy group, Public Citizen, called "Do Not Use Glucophage". But when all the blowing smoke, and smoke-blowing, began to clear, a study found that the risk of this metabolic disorder was actually ten times higher with older diabetes drugs being used at the time (since discontinued). And eventually more studies observed no difference in risk between diabetics using the drug and those not using the drug—because the problem had actually been due to underlying medical conditions among diabetic patients, and not the drug itself.

So what's the final conclusion regarding the risk of lactic acidosis? If you have underlying kidney or liver conditions, then metformin is not for you.

Most side effects are minimal, and easily managed

The risk of lactic acidosis aside, the most common side effects associated with taking metformin are diarrhea and gastrointestinal upset.

But this is typically when first starting the drug, and rarely persists. And, because it lowers blood sugar (hence its use for diabetes) it may cause symptoms like tiredness or weakness, unless and until the dose is adjusted and/or the body adjusts on its own.

Relatively speaking, compared to most other drugs, these side effects are minimal for the benefits you may gain. And are easily managed by monitoring and adjusting dosage accordingly as with any medical management for diabetes.

At the same time, metformin is one of the few drugs that are safe for people with congestive heart failure.

Though it can interact with certain blood pressure medications, so be sure to check with your doctor.

All that said there are two concerns you need to know

1. You must supplement with vitamin B12.

Research has found that prolonged use of metformin can cause a deficiency in vitamin B12. Especially in those suffering from peripheral neuropathy. And unfortunately, the NIH and many doctors have yet to catch up to the research on this risk. So to be safe, you can supplement with a high-quality B vitamin daily for as long as you take metformin.

Look for a vitamin B complex that contains 100 mg each of vitamins B1 (as thiamine), B2 (as riboflavin), B3 (as niacinamide), B5 (as pantethene), and B6 (as pyridoxine) and 1,000 mcg of B12 (as cyanocobalamine).

And ask your doctor to check your vitamin B12 levels regularly. If you are unable to absorb sufficient B12, injections may be administered by your doctor. These doses may also help to enhance your immune system.

2. Beware of eating grapefruit.

As with other drugs, eating grapefruit may interfere with the effectiveness of metformin. So it's best to avoid grapefruit (which you should be doing now, to help reverse the disease in the first place).

Unexpected—and very promising—benefits

Metformin has ultimately gone on to be the most widely prescribed drug for diabetes in the world with over 120 million people taking it today. And with so many people taking the drug, some surprising beneficial "side effects" are now being observed.

In addition to controlling blood sugar, it has now been proven to prevent the common cardiovascular complications of diabetes, such as heart attacks and strokes. It also promotes healthy circulation to the limbs, kidneys, and eyes. And is the only diabetes drug that does not cause weight gain. (In fact, it's now being studied for use as a weight loss drug.)

It also helps reduce LDL cholesterol and triglyceride levels in the blood without the dangerous side effects of statin drugs. These are beneficial effects that are likely associated with metformin's effects on reducing blood sugar and helping to regulate normal metabolism.

But beyond these healthy effects, there is more...

Metformin is now the treatment of choice for the increasingly diagnosed condition of Polycystic Ovarian Syndrome in women of all ages. It also appears to be effective in the treatment of Multiple Sclerosis.

It is even being recommended as an "anti-aging" drug by some. This is likely due to the claims that it helps maintain healthy hormone levels such as estrogen in women and testosterone in men.

MD Anderson Hospital, the largest cancer center in the country, has observed that it lowers the risk of pancreatic cancer (notoriously difficult to treat) by <u>five times</u>. And it reduces overall cancer rates, including cancer of the breast, colon, lung, ovary, and prostate. Most of these cancers can be difficult or impossible to treat by conventional means.

Regarding the remarkable effects on lowering pancreatic cancer, I might speculate that by keeping blood sugar levels low, metformin reduces any effects to cause the pancreas to produce more insulin in Type II diabetes in order to counter high blood sugar or insulin resistance in the tissues. Thus, it doesn't promote the growth of pancreatic cells, some of which are responsible for producing insulin.

Several mechanisms are being investigated on the anti-cancer effects of metformin. Canada appears to continue to be ahead of the U.S. and is leading the way with clinical trials on using metformin to <u>actually treat</u> (not just prevent) breast, endometrial, pancreatic, and prostate cancers. The National Cancer Institute is playing catch up with trials on colon and other cancers.

And it seems metformin is particularly active against lung and oral cancers. Which adds even more proof that there is more to the story with these cancers than just tobacco.

And beyond all this, metformin has just been found to show promise for the most mysterious and alarming disease of our time—Alzheimer's dementia.

So here we have a safe, effective, inexpensive drug that actually treats the condition of diabetes, by lowering blood sugar (and not just "managing" symptoms). It also reduces all the major medical complications commonly associated with diabetes such as cardiovascular diseases. And the main long-term "side effects" are a list of additional health benefits such as reducing the risk of common cancers and probably helping to maintain healthy weight.

So the only mystery is why has it evaded comprehensive investigation of its multiple health benefits for so long?

Poisonous plant turned modern wonder "drug"

Ironically, the natural sources of G. officinalis are currently known in the U.S. as "Professor Weed" and the federal government lists it as a "Class A Noxious Weed" in their database of poisonous plants! This French lilac (also used for its fragrance) is just another weed to the U.S. government.

Perhaps the only answer to this modern government nonsense was provided by the 16th century Swiss physician, Philippus Aureolus Theophrastus Bombastus von Hohenheim (better known as Paracelsus), who would have known about the medicinal uses of this remarkable plant: "the right dose differentiates a poison from a useful medicine." Which could be said about many herbal remedies and almost all drugs as well.

Which is what makes the drug version of this herbal remedy—metformin—such a breakthrough. This modern "wonder" "drug" is actually little different from the ancient herbal remedy Galegine, widely known and used in Europe in the Middle Ages. It benefits from chemical simplicity and detailed clinical investigation. And endless drug vigilance has long settled concerns by the FDA and ill-informed public advocacy groups.

Of course, metformin will only get you so far...

It is possible to actually reverse diabetes through diet and weight loss alone. Researchers in the UK completely reversed diabetes in patients who were placed on 600-calorie-per-day diets under direct medical supervision. But the usual minimum caloric levels for healthy weight loss, working on your own, in women and smaller individuals are no less than 1,000 calories per day, and for men and larger individuals 1,200 calories.

These are guidelines you can achieve on your own following a healthy diet of caloric restriction. These are the caloric lower levels for weight loss, not weight maintenance. Healthy weight loss diets include lots of fresh fruits and vegetables and eliminate sugars and processed foods and fats. Lower body weight and body fat leads to lower blood sugar, cholesterol, and blood pressure.

Some dietary supplements may also help maintain healthy blood sugar levels.

- **Alpha Lipoic Acid (ALA):** 300 mg/day
- **Vitamin B6 (as pyridoxine):** 100 mg/day
- **Berberine:** 400-500 mg/day
- **Cinnamon:** 1 gram/day (food quantity)
- **Coenzyme Q10:** 150 mg/day

There are also some herbal remedies that are being investigated for their effects on maintaining healthy blood sugar. They include the traditional Chinese remedy bitter melon, cinnamon, blueberry leaf, dandelion leaf, as well as various traditional Ayurvedic herbs from India.

Finally, chromium, selenium, and vanadium are minerals and heavy metals that play important roles in managing blood sugar and healthy metabolism. As metals, they have potential toxicities, so check with your health practitioner.

Metformin for "Type III diabetes"?

New research has shown that metformin also stimulates neuron generation and memory, at least in laboratory animal models.[1] Of course, metformin is now being used for its metabolic effects, including healthy metabolism of glucose in diabetes.

One key to metformin's multifarious benefits appears to hinge on the enzyme called "atypical protein kinase." This enzyme is present throughout the body—and is responsible for metformin's primary metabolic effects in the liver. But protein kinase is also active in the brain for transforming stem cells into neurons.

The true miracle here is not necessarily the drug, but that the body uses the same enzyme efficiently and effectively for different critical functions among different tissues. Again, the key to all healing is stimulating the body to find ways to heal itself—as we often find in Nature.

Chapter 63

Skip these six "fad" diets

Not so long ago, having some "meat on your bones" was a sign of good health. It was widely considered healthy and desirable for thousands of years. In women, it was prized for bearing healthy children.

On the flip side, if you were underweight you were "sickly." This common sense approach lasted for centuries. And indeed, the research began to bear out this scenario decades ago. In fact, studies link being underweight with higher disease and death rates—versus the happy middle.

But today, it's "fashionable" to be "skinny." And somehow, these ridiculous fashion trends actually influence many medical practices (even medical specialties) and health approaches. They also bring about fad diets.

These diets come and go with the wind. But, unfortunately, many come back time and again. They're like *really* bad ideas that just keep bouncing back like bad pennies. In fact, these six fad diets are so ridiculous and off base in terms of science and human nutrition, it's hard to know where to begin. So we'll take them alphabetically.

1. The Alkaline Diet

This fad approach bars all meat, dairy, caffeine, and alcohol, as well as sweets and processed foods. It favors fresh fruits, veggies, nuts, and seeds. While the diet is half-right about foods, its goals of keeping healthy pH levels (acid-base balance) is ludicrous, unscientific, untested, and unproven.

The body must and does maintain proper pH in order to carry out basic metabolic functions. But the body maintains proper pH based upon a number of factors in addition to diet and digestion, including respiration, liver function, and renal function. In any case, there is scant scientific evidence that shows pH affects body weight.

2. The Blood-type Diet

I debunked this unproven, untested, unphysiologic diet before. It's based on pure myth and superstition that somehow different foods react chemically with different blood types. Blood types relate to blood cells as one of millions of different genetic variations that normally occur among different humans. But no evidence suggests that people with different blood types should eat different types of food. Or that blood type has any effect on metabolism, nutrition, weight loss, or maintenance.

3. The Five-bite Diet

For this diet, you must skip breakfast. Then, you can eat *anything* you like for lunch and dinner, provided you only take five bites. Lay's potato chips ("bet you can't eat just one") would not be a candidate for this diet. Again, the sensible advice of portion control is taken to a ridiculous, faddish extreme, which is neither sensible nor sustainable. This diet really bites.

4. The HCG Diet

I consider the HCG diet a near starvation diet. You consume just 500 calories per day while taking human chorionic gonadotropin (HCG), a powerful hormone that supposedly acts as an appetite suppressant. Of course, severe caloric restriction will guarantee rapid weight loss. And this kind of severe caloric restriction has been shown to reverse diabetes. But we don't have scientific evidence to back up its long-term safety. You should only attempt severe calorie restriction under doctor supervision on an in-patient basis. And, as with other hormone treatments, skip the HCG.

5. The Raw Food Diet

This diet starts with some good ideas. It emphasizes fruits and vegetables, and cuts out sugars and processed foods. But it takes things to extremes by banning all cooked foods. Proponents claim cooking destroys nutrients. But humans have been cooking food for about one million years. Research—including my own research with the USDA—shows that cooking does *not* reduce nutritional quality.

Any breakdown in some nutrients due to heat exposure is offset by making it easier to digest the tough, double-walled plant cells in fruits and vegetables that contain the nutrients. In some cases, cooking actually *increases* the bioavailable nutrients in vegetables. I discovered this fact while researching foods that contain lutein and lycopene.

(And don't forget about food-borne illnesses in uncooked foods.)

6. The Shake Diet

This diet requires you to drink specifically formulated shakes that provide very limited numbers of calories through the day. Then, you eat a "normal" dinner. Anyone can lose weight based on the caloric restriction alone, but it's certainly not a healthy approach. And it reverses the daily order of when calories should be consumed for optimal metabolism and health.

Overall, these six fad diets use unscientific, "half-baked" (literally in one case) approaches that ignore biology, nutrition, and science.

Diets that attempt to cut all fats and substitute with carbs deprive you of essential fats like those in meats, seafood, and nuts. Researchers have finally figured out that the real culprits in the nation's epidemic of obesity, diabetes, and cardiovascular diseases are sugars, high-carb foods, and highly processed foods. The "reduced fat" labels carried by many foods encouraged in some fads should be read as warnings.

There is no substitute for eating healthy foods, controlling portions, and getting some regular physical activity for healthy weight loss and maintenance. More sensible approaches include the "Paleolithic prescription" of our ancestors with animal proteins and essential fats, vegetables, fruits, and nuts. The Mediterranean diet of seafood, fruits, vegetables, and olive oil is another sensible diet. It's been widely studied for its many health benefits.

But everyone is an individual when it comes to nutrition and metabolism—not to mention tastes. You know you are following the right diet when you maintain a healthy weight. You should also feel mentally alert, happy, and energized.

Chapter 64

The only organic foods to buy

I've written about the barrage of organic foods flooding the marketplace in the past. And the truth is, many of the splashy, packaged "organic" foods lining supermarket shelves these days are a waste of your money.

But organic *produce* is a different story.

In fact, I often find myself opting to pay more for organic produce. I'll explain why in a moment. But first, let's talk a little bit about the incredible growth of the organic farming industry.

Since 1999, the area of farmland around the world certified as organic has increased 300 percent. And today, there are more than 91 million acres of farmland worldwide under organic cultivation. However, that amount still accounts for less than 1 percent of all agricultural lands. So, why does 99 percent of farming remain "non-organic"?

The organic farming sector faces three major challenges. First, there is a serious shortage of organic raw materials—such as grains, sugar and livestock feed. Without an adequate supply of these basic agricultural commodities, organic farmers cannot harvest sufficient products to make their businesses viable.

This shortage is partly why we pay a premium at the cash register for organic products. It's simply a matter of supply and demand. Demand is high. And growing higher by the year. Yet supply remains low.

The second challenge comes from food products marketed as "natural" or "locally grown." These savvy food producers capitalize on a consumer's desire to eat "clean" food. But they know many consumers don't understand the terminology.

So let's clear that up right now…"natural" and "locally grown" do NOT mean organic. When you read the word "natural" on packaged foods, it's an essentially meaningless term. Don't be fooled.

On the other hand, locally grown *is* an important concept. It supports local farming. It keeps food close to home. And it avoids the costs, pollution and preservation required for long-distance hauling.

Unfortunately, locally grown produce can carry a heavy synthetic pesticide load. (Although, even organic produce can contain "natural pesticides." And I'll explain more about that fact next week.)

Locally grown produce can also come from genetically modified seeds. So, the only way to guarantee you're not buying genetically modified produce is to buy organic. In fact, according to federal law, organic produce cannot be genetically modified.

The third—and largest—challenge faced by the organic farming industry is cost. Organic raw crop farming requires careful labor and management. So it costs far more up front to turn out an organic crop.

Conventional agri-business farmers use chemicals to reduce labor and increase raw productivity (although not nutritional value). However, in the long run, non-organic farming is just as expensive as sustainable farming. Or perhaps even more expensive than organic farming—at least in terms of indirect costs.

For example, non-organic farming takes a serious toll on the environment, wildlife, and human health with harmful, synthetic chemicals that contaminate the soil, water and air.

Of course, the Environmental Protection Agency (EPA) sets tight limits on permissible levels of synthetic pesticide residue allowed on organic and non-organic produce. And the Federal Drug Administration regulates these limits.

Even so, this fact may surprise you…

The pesticide residue found on produce in the U.S. falls below these limits more than 99 percent of the time. Even on non-organic produce.

So if pesticide residue isn't as big of a concern as some shoppers might think, why spend extra money to buy organic produce?

It all comes down to nutrition.

Simply put, organic produce contains more nutrients.

In fact, the actual nutrient content and quality of mass-produced, conventionally grown crops has significantly declined over the past 80 years. So, when you buy a conventionally grown apple, you ingest some unwanted, synthetic chemicals. But you only get a fraction of the nutrition compared to organic apples.

Several years ago, scientists compared the nutritional content of organic and conventionally grown produce. Over a two-year period, they purchased samples of both types of apples, potatoes, pears, wheat and sweet corn in the western suburbs of Chicago. They found that on a per-weight basis, the organic produce contained many more nutrients than conventionally grown produce. In fact, the organic produce averaged:

- 63 percent more calcium
- 78 percent more chromium
- 73 percent more iron
- 118 percent more magnesium
- 91 percent more phosphorus
- 125 percent more potassium
- 60 percent more zinc

Plus, the organic produce averaged 29 percent *less mercury* than the conventionally grown produce. The researchers published their findings in the respected *Journal of Applied Nutrition*. And that's just one study that focused solely on mineral content.

In 2008, a group of U.S. scientists reviewed 97 studies that compared the overall nutritional content of organic and conventionally grown produce. They found that organic produce provides about 25 percent higher nutritional content on average than conventionally grown produce.

So, if you want to achieve optimal nutrition from the foods you eat…and if you want to get the most bang for your buck, you may want to consider buying organic produce. But skip the "organic" and "natural" prepackaged foods on grocery store shelves. Just because that chocolate pudding is "organic" doesn't mean you should eat it!

Chapter 65

Remove these 5 dangerous items from your home today

Growing research suggests chemical toxins in everyday household products may increase the risk of autoimmune diseases, birth defects, cancers, and infertility. In fact, the Centers for Disease Control (CDC) now monitors 298 environmental chemicals found to accumulate in human tissues. Of course, the FDA is supposed to monitor the thousands of other drug chemicals put into the human body. And the Environmental Protection Agency (EPA) monitors thousands of chemicals put into the environment as well.

But we can't always count on the CDC, the EPA, or the FDA—so you have to take matters into your own hands. Here are some items around your home you may want to replace:

1. Food containers

Plastic food containers can break down over time, especially when exposed to heat in dishwashers or microwaves. Plastic can also release dangerous chemicals into the food, including phthalates, which act as endocrine-disrupters.

So avoid storing foods, or buying prepared foods, in plastic containers. And never heat your food in a plastic container.

Instead, look for glass storage containers. Then you don't have to worry whether ceramic containers or plates are "microwave safe." (You can't trust those labels from China anyway.) Glass is always microwave safe, as well as safe from chemical contamination.

2. Cooking pans

Many non-stick pans contain traces of perfluoro-octanoic acid (PFOA)—a fluoro-hydrocarbon like those found to be harmful to the Earth's ozone layer. The non-stick lining can scratch and scrape off right off into your food. So save the Teflon for politicians like Ronald Reagan and Donald Trump.

Instead, use olive oil and/or butter in stainless steel or cast iron cookware.

Remember, you don't need to (and shouldn't) scrub cast iron with soap and water. Just wipe out with oil to "cure" the cast iron.

If your stainless steel or cast iron cookware does get stained with burned contents, you will be amazed at what a little white vinegar placed in the pan and gently warmed will do.

3. Air fresheners

The incompetent EPA is killing our economy and destroying our freedoms to supposedly reduce *outdoor* air pollution. Yet research shows air pollution has been steadily improving since the 1960s.

But what about *indoor* air pollution? The EPA doesn't warn you about that serious problem at all! In fact, artificially scented candles and synthetic, plug-in scents often contain chemical phthalates. Eventually, these endocrine-disrupting chemicals can end up in your blood and tissues.

So don't allow artificial air fresheners into your living and working environments.

You can find candles made with essential plant oils, dried flowers, and spices. Or, even better, instead of covering up unwanted aromas around your home, use natural ingredients like baking soda and white vinegar to remove them.

4. Cleaning products

It amazes me how many harsh, chemical cleaning products I see on store shelves. But the government allows manufacturers to keep their chemical formulas a secret. So there's no way of knowing exactly "what's in there."

Here's a good rule of thumb: Don't use any product to clean your kitchen, bathroom, or any room in your home for that matter, if you feel like you should wear gloves to use it.

And skip the upholstery protection sprays. They often contain chemicals such as phthalates and surfactants. These stain blockers create a transparent plastic layer to "protect" upholstery. But when the plastic eventually wears off, it can release chemicals into the air.

So take a look under your kitchen and bathroom sinks. Throw out any harsh, chemical sprays you have hiding out under there. Instead, clean with natural products like baking soda, borax, hot water, vinegar, lemon, or soap powders. They work better and don't require covering your home with toxins and releasing them into the air you breathe.

5. Personal care products

Many antiperspirants, cosmetics, and perfumes pollute the air you (and others around you) breathe. So always use fragrance-free personal products.

Also, pay close attention to the ingredient list. Avoid deodorants made with aluminum-based compounds and other chemicals, such as parabens and "PEG-" numbered ingredients. You can absorb these chemicals through your sweat glands. And some research suggests possible concerns about cancer and dementia.

Cosmetics for personal care—from lipsticks to shampoos—can contain up to 126 different chemicals, according to the Environmental Working Group. The average American woman applies up to 12 such items to their skin and hair every day. Men are only half as bad; they use an average of six products daily. Although, I'm hard pressed to figure out what these men are using, since I manage with only soap, water, and toothpaste every day, and no spray anything.

So here are some tips for choosing personal care items...

Opt for ingredients labeled "organic." The word "natural" is essentially meaningless. Women should choose cosmetics with mineral-based pigments and moisturizers made with plant oils. Everyone should avoid soaps and shampoos that contain synthetic fragrances and chemicals such as triclosan.

You can look up just about any product on the market to learn how it rates on safety.

In the meantime, throw out all the chemical products found around your home. And go as pure as you can.

Chapter 66

Try these 4 tips for safe sun exposure

As I often report, you need regular exposure to the sun to maintain and achieve good health. In fact, healthy sun exposure activates the natural production of vitamin D in your skin.

So make sure to spend just 10 to 15 minutes outside in the sun without sunscreen every day between April and October. This will help keep your vitamin D at a healthy level. And if you want to spend more than 15 minutes in the sun, four simple tips can help you safely and naturally protect your skin, as I'll explain in a moment.

Of course, the cosmetics industry, some narrow-minded medical specialists, and clueless public health "experts" continue to generate ill-informed hysteria over sun exposure. But *real* scientific research links low sun exposure and/or *low* vitamin D levels with higher levels of the malignant skin cancer, against which all the photophobics try to protect us.

The fact is, only 9 percent of "skin cancers" are truly "malignant" melanomas that invade and metastasize. By contrast, 91 percent of what most mainstream dermatologists call "skin cancers" are really just skin "growths." These common skin growths almost never invade or metastasize like a real cancer. And doctors can easily detect and remove them before they ever cause problems.

Plus, science links *low* sun exposure and/or *low* vitamin D with virtually every common medical problem, such as other common cancers, dementia, Type II diabetes, heart disease, kidney disease, as well as mood disorders, anxiety, and depression.

Without a doubt, vitamin D is an essential nutrient.

But the Institute of Medicine (IOM) only recommends adult men and women up to age 70 take 600 IU of it daily. But researchers at University of California San Diego and Creighton University in

Nebraska discovered the IOM's ridiculous Recommended Daily Allowance (RDA) for vitamin D is too low by a factor of 10.

The science shows you need vitamin D. And an easy way to get more of it between April and October is to spend some time outside. But you want to avoid burning, which can harm your skin.

So how can you protect yourself from burning while getting the sun exposure you need?

Here are a few tips to try:

1. Sunscreen can wait

A lot of "experts" tell you to apply sunscreen before leaving the house. But as I mentioned earlier, you can spend the first 10 to 15 minutes outside without sunscreen. This will activate some vitamin D production in your skin. So take your sunscreen with you and apply it after you've given your skin some time to soak up some healthy rays.

2. Don't assume higher SPF is better

Many consumers believe they can spend more time in the sun if they use sunscreen with a higher sun protection factor (SPF). And they assume sunscreen with a sun protection factor (SPF) of 100 offers twice as much protection as sunscreen with SPF 50. In reality, the extra protection against ultraviolet rays is negligible. And using these higher SPF sunscreens gives sunbathers a false sense of protection, which leads to harmful burns. Plus, these higher SPF sunscreens may also contain additional toxic chemicals.

3. You only need SPF 20

Science shows that you only need sunscreen with an SPF of 20. It provides maximum blockage of ultraviolet sunlight. Anything beyond SPF 20 is a meaningless marketing gimmick.

4. Try products with plant oils

Many natural plant oils provide protection against the sun for reasonable amounts of time. Plus, they still allow sufficient sunlight to reach the skin so it can make vitamin D naturally. Furthermore, they improve the look and feel of your skin.

Carrot seed oil has a unique earthy, nutty aroma. Some people find it a little strong, but it naturally filters the sun's rays. In fact, it has all the sun protection of an SPF 20 sunscreen. Plus, it allows your skin to naturally build its own protection from melanin and imparts a natural light orange-tan color. Best of all, it contains plenty of alpha- and beta-carotenes.

Red raspberry oil is another option. It too has all the protection of a sunscreen. And it's high in vitamin E, which heals and protects the skin.

Wheat germ oil is right on the spot with an SPF factor estimated at 20. It's inexpensive and has no scent. Plus, it's lighter and less oily than carrot seed or red raspberry oil.

More natural oils with their SPF factors are: Almond (5), Avocado (4 — 10, up to 15), Coconut (2 — 8), Hemp seed (6), Jojoba (4), Macadamia (6), Olive (2 — 8), Sesame seed (4), Shea butter (3 — 6), Soybean/Non-GMO (10).

In the spring and summer, make sure to spend some quality time in the sun *without* sunscreen. And when you do cover up, choose carefully.

Chapter 67

9 ways to get a balanced diet on a balanced budget

Plenty of evidence shows that diet and nutrition is the single most important element for health promotion, disease prevention, and managing common medical disorders.

To some extent, you do have to pay more for better, healthier, tastier food—which is a sad comment on both "big food" and the modern agriculture industry, as well as our social values.

But the good news is that eating healthy does not have to break your budget. Just follow these 9 simple steps to cut out the waste. And as an added benefit, many of the same measures will help you cut back on your waist as well.

1. Forget fad foods

Slashing your grocery bill begins with avoiding food gimmicks, fads, and flaky diet ideas.

Some food manufacturers learned long ago that it costs far less for them to make hyped-up claims about supposed "new, improved" products than to make real innovations or provide better quality. I've often found the cheaper the ingredients, the bigger the breathless (and usually groundless) claims.

Unfortunately, the same rule tends to apply as much in the "natural" products world as it does with big food.

Goji berries are an example. These dried fruits from Asia look like red raisins, and certainly are an acquired taste. At $14 to $18 per pound you can get much better value when it comes to antioxidants from actual raisins—not to mention one of my favorite fruits, blueberries. And think of how many pounds of other healthy, organic fruits and berries you can buy for $18.

Another example is the ridiculous price of pomegranate juice—about $25 for 16 ounces of the most popular brand, POM Wonderful. A UCLA study found that pomegranate juice does have more antioxidants than other juices, but researchers also rated the much less expensive concord grape and cranberry juices high in antioxidants as well.

Of course, you do want to watch the sugar content of any fruit juice. Have you noticed the small size of a so-called juice glass? There's a reason. Juices from whole fruits without added sugars or artificial ingredients can be a healthy treat—but only in moderation.

Another healthy drink option is to add a little spice to your favorite beverage or cocktail with sauces made from different varieties of chili peppers. Like pomegranates, these fiery peppers are also high in antioxidants and vitamin C. But unlike pomegranates, a little bit of chili pepper goes a long way in terms of your budget.

2. Substitute some spice

Part of avoiding overpriced foods and beverages is making smart substitutions when it comes to recipes. For example, you can usually use plain yogurt (check the nutrients label to make sure it's low in sugar) instead of higher-fat, higher-cost ingredients like sour cream or heavy cream.

The same is true when it comes to spices. Some exotic Asian spices that require trips to specialty stores are priced as if sailing ships laden with them still had to travel thousands of miles to isolated locations—as was done by traders on the ancient spice routes.

Take pepper, for instance. There are all kinds of exotic, pricey types of pepper for sale today, but don't be fooled. They all come from the same plant. Different colors are often related to how the pepper is cultivated, harvested, and dried. But all pepper, no matter how colorful, has essentially the same beneficial ingredients and taste.

So instead of paying for exotic peppers in fancy packaging, invest in a good pepper mill and buy whole, black peppercorns. Grind only when ready to add to food on the stove or at the table.

Why? Well, with pre-ground pepper you can't really tell what you are getting. Plus, potency is rapidly lost when the natural shell or husk of the peppercorn is removed, cracked, or ground up.

When you buy whole peppercorns, and other herbs and spices in bulk (instead of pre-ground powders in packages), you also get better value. And you can buy more because most bulk spices stay fresh for one to two years. Powdered, ground spices typically last only six months.

3. Snack smart

When it comes to snacks, I'm appalled at how many people pay ridiculous prices to eat absolute junk—salt, sugar, and fats with artificial ingredients.

But that doesn't mean you have to give up between-meal treats altogether. For instance, many of the spices I mentioned above can also be used to add flavor to healthy, inexpensive snacks.

Popcorn for one. It's not only low-cal, but also a good source of fiber and the complex carbs your body needs to produce energy. You don't need to add butter (and certainly not oil) to this tasty snack for flavor when hot peppers, herbs, or a sprinkling of Parmesan cheese can do the same thing with a lot fewer calories.

One thing to keep in mind, though: Essentially all yellow corn grown in the U.S. is genetically modified, so look for organic, non-GMO popcorn kernels. Blue corn is a good choice.

Nuts are also a healthy snack. They can be expensive, but a little goes a long way. I've reported how study after study has found that just a handful of nuts a day can produce big benefits for your brain, blood sugar, and heart. Nuts are high in essential fatty acids and minerals, and they also help you feel full and satisfied —which can keep your weight down.

Also, while tree nuts (almonds, cashews, pistachios, walnuts) are relatively costly, the same health benefits have also been found for inexpensive whole peanuts. In fact, a new study reports that people who regularly ate peanuts were 21 percent less likely to die over a five-year period than people who didn't eat nuts.[3] And that was true even for the people who smoked, were obese, or had high blood pressure or diabetes.

One of the worst offenders when it comes to both your budget and your health are so-called "snack packs." Many candy bars, chips, and cookies are available in a 100-cal snack pack. But why waste 100 calories—not to mention several dollars—on absolute junk?

The same goes for most "granola" bars, energy bars, and other candy bars disguised in pseudo-healthy packaging. How much is 100 calories of this kind of junk? About one handful. Just say "nuts" to that.

Another terrible idea is "lunch snacks," or pre-packaged junk lunch meats with some crappy cheese product and crackers thrown in.

4. Know when to go organic

As I reported back in 2012, the U.S. government has turned the organic label into another quasi-government bureaucratic process—not to mention a procedure for essentially shaking down the little grower (check out "Deep into organic" and "Big food takes over the organic market" at drmicozzi.com). Since then, big food has found even more ways to infiltrate and pervert the organic labeling process.

But that doesn't mean the organic label is entirely unimportant for your health and nutrition. Every year, the nonprofit Environmental Working Group (EWG) publishes its "Dirty Dozen Plus" fruits and vegetables that are most contaminated by pesticides. These are the foods you should always eat organic.

This year, the list includes apples, peaches, nectarines, strawberries, grapes, celery, spinach, sweet bell peppers, cucumbers, cherry tomatoes, snap peas, potatoes, hot peppers, kale, and collard greens.

I also recommend that if you eat corn and soybeans, choose the organic ones. Most of the conventionally grown versions are genetically modified. And you'll avoid dangerous growth hormones and antibiotics if you choose organic meat and chicken.

But there are some foods for which you don't necessarily need to pay extra for organic versions. Foods with peels, for instance. If you completely remove a peel before eating, you're not likely to ingest any pesticides. Although there is still the environmental impact of using pesticides to grow that food.

Along with "peel foods" like avocadoes, onions, pineapples, kiwi, papaya, grapefruit, and cantaloupe, the EWG also put the following produce on its 2015 "Clean Fifteen" list for having the lowest concentrations of pesticides: sweet corn (although, as I said above, watch the GMOs), cabbage, frozen sweet peas, asparagus, mangoes, eggplant, cauliflower, and sweet potatoes.

If you want to save money, buy conventional rather than organic versions of these foods.

5. Bag the bagged lettuce and salad dressings

One of the most wasteful and dangerous (in terms of contamination) food products is prepackaged lettuce and salads. Why seal your salad in artificial plastic bags when you can buy lettuce and other greens out in the open—where they can breathe and are also watered regularly by the produce staff at your grocery store?

That's why I always buy salad and other greens by the head. They're not only fresher, but less expensive and safer than bagged salads.

As with flowers, you can carefully slice the ends off the heads of greens and place them in water to maintain a "fresh-picked" appearance and flavor for days. Just make sure to wash them so they'll be free of salmonella and other contaminants that can make their way into salads that are bagged—and stay there.

Bottom line: <u>bagged salads = bad idea</u>.

Bottled salad dressings are also a bad idea. These expensive concoctions are typically loaded with sugars, fats, preservatives, and artificial chemicals. They're also loaded with calories, which negates the weight-loss effect of the salads they douse.

All you really need to make your salad sing is a little red wine vinegar and olive oil (which is one of the healthiest foods on the planet). Don't like vinegar? Try lemon juice instead. Add a dash of mustard (3 calories) and virtually any and all spices for extra flavor.

To keep olive oil fresh, buy only as much as you will use within three months. Vinegar is already "aged" and can be kept almost indefinitely.

6. Get more bang for your beef buck

Beef is expensive. But judging by its nutritional content, it should be. Beef provides essential fats, B vitamins, and bioavailable minerals, as well as protein —which most people don't get enough of, especially as we get older.

The lost decades of government misdirection when it comes to beef (and also butter, cholesterol, eggs, and fats) are over—and the government finally admitted that its advice to avoid these foods was all wrong, all along. Now, we know it's important to include beef and other meat, as well as fish and seafood, in our diets at least twice per week.

Even if your grocery budget is tight, you can still afford beef. Stay away from the filet mignon and choose bottom round, shoulder, or tri-tip cuts instead. You'll get the same nutrition at a lower cost. These cuts can also be marinated in the same healthy spices, vinegars, and olive oil that add flavor to salads and other foods.

And, as I mentioned earlier, buy organic beef whenever you can. Also, research shows grass-fed beef is lower in unhealthy fats and higher in omega-3 fatty acids than conventional beef, which makes it good for your heart. It also has more cancer-fighting antioxidants than conventional beef.[6] So it's worth the splurge for this healthier meat.

7. Make sure you know beans about beans

You can supplement your beef consumption with another excellent source of protein—beans. They're also high in fiber and the B vitamin folate.

And dry beans can be bought for bargain-basement prices. Although they must be rehydrated and rinsed to eliminate natural anti-digestive toxins. Canned beans are more expensive, but still make it easily onto the budget list.

Slow cookers are a good way to make convenient bean casseroles and dishes. One of my favorites is beans, beef, and chili peppers—better known as chili con carne or simply chili. There are as many delicious chili varieties as there are chefs, and they make a good year-round meal.

8. Don't surrender in the battle of the beverages

You already know how important it is to avoid all bottled soda and soft drinks, whether they're made with sugar, high-fructose corn syrup, or artificial sweeteners. They're as harmful to your health and your waistline (even "zero-cal") as they are to your bottom line.

Stick with water. Or make your own fruit/vegetables juices with any or all of the healthy organic produce listed above. Investing in a restaurant-quality juicer will help ensure that you can juice just about anything.

9. Remember there's no downside to downsizing

In addition to choosing the right foods, controlling portion sizes is the single most important step to a healthy weight. Which, of course, helps promote a healthy life.

But portions of prepared foods at grocery stores and restaurants seem to keep growing and growing. I've found the best way to lessen the burden on your wallet and waistline is to share these supersized portions with another person—or yourself.

Cut your restaurant or grocery entrée in half and either share it with your dining partner or take it home. You will still get all the flavors, and you'll find yourself satisfied with less. Plus, you can sample more types of food (for those who have a hard time making up their minds with the menu).

Do the same thing with meals you cook at home. Combining leftovers has led to some of the great inventions in cooking. Pizza, for example. Leftover vegetables can also be made into soups, or vegetable broth or stocks. And stale bread makes excellent breadcrumbs and croutons.

Another benefit to portion control is that you won't waste food. Americans squander a whopping 30 to 40 percent of our food supply—the equivalent of *20 pounds* of food per person per month.

The mindless reading of expiration dates on perfectly good, unopened foods is another source of that waste. Don't throw out foods that still taste and smell all right. Your nose knows. On the other hand, choosing the later expiration dates on packages while still at the grocery store will postpone the point at which you even have to consider this issue.

Above all, be creative with cooking and leftovers. The kitchen is a place where virtually everyone can express themselves—which is healthy for body and mind.

PART 6

SECRETS TO STOP AGING IN ITS TRACKS

Chapter 68

New research reveals America's most-hated vegetable may hold the secret to a longer life

There is a great deal of hard science you never hear about from "natural-know-it-alls" or "Johnny-come-lately" experts in natural health.

I keep my eye on all of the important clinical-trial research (the kind the FDA has rigged up for drug studies). But I also understand how to read statistics and epidemiology-based research, as well as lab studies on animals, which can confound and confuse (sometimes on purpose) the typical doctor.

And that's what led me to an important new study—which should be of vital interest to everyone who wants to achieve healthy aging. Researchers have discovered that a compound found in one of the most hated vegetables in America—the "dreaded" lima bean—can help male fruit flies lower their glucose levels and improve their body composition. And that helped boost the flies' lifespan by a whopping *10%*.

Of course, most natural-know-it-alls have overlooked this study because it has to do with fruit flies, rather than people. But I'm going to share with you several key reasons why you shouldn't shoo away these findings. And why you really should eat more lima beans...

The simple insect that can teach you how to live longer

Anti-aging, healthy aging, or life extension (depending on which term you prefer) is of great concern to many people. But there aren't many good, clinical, human studies in this field. That's because these types of real scientific studies take a long time to do—literally a human's lifetime.

(Also, the vast majority of research funding is tied up in expensive clinical trials for drugs—because the crony-capitalist mainstream is far more interested in studying drugs than natural remedies.)

So when I look for good scientific data from valid, well-designed studies on prolonging lifespan (versus the hype you typically hear from the "anti-aging" gurus), I often turn to experimental biology research using animal models.

Particularly fruit flies. After all, scientists have been studying these insects for over a century, following their entire lifespans over multiple generations.

Much of the basic science of genetics was originally determined in inexpensive fruit fly experiments.

The lima bean study is a case in point. This research, which was conducted on fruit flies, is clear, simple…and compelling. Let's take a closer look.

The bean that could boost your lifespan by 10%

The study was published in February in the *FASEB (Federation of American Societies for Experimental Biology) Journal*. It revealed the life-prolonging properties of prunetin, a type of flavonoid found in plants—particularly lima beans, but also in other legumes and prunes.

Previous studies have detailed prunetin's anti-inflammatory properties. But this study was designed to go much further. Researchers wanted to determine whether prunetin can also affect lifespan, locomotion, body composition, metabolism, and gut health. What they discovered is impressive.

The researchers found that male fruit flies that consumed prunetin lived an average of three days longer than their counterparts that didn't receive prunetin. That's quite amazing when you consider the average lifespan of the fruit fly species the researchers studied is 30 days.

In essence, the prunetin fruit flies lived about 10% longer. Translated into human terms, that means prunetin could potentially increase a 70-year-old man's lifespan by *seven extra years*.

So how does prunetin do this? Well, the researchers found that the flies given prunetin had elevated activation of AMPK, an enzyme that helps cells (in both fruit flies and humans) produce energy. They believe the extra AMPK boosted the flies' fitness levels and improved their body composition.

Researchers found that the male fruit flies that consumed prunetin were able to climb up a test tube a whopping 54% faster than flies not given prunetin. And the prunetin flies had an impressive 36% reduction in glucose levels.

Interestingly, the researchers noted that the female fruit flies given prunetin didn't have the same longevity results as the males. They think that may be because female fruit flies already live longer than males, so prunetin may actually help the males catch up with the females.

The many reasons you should eat legumes and prunes

The editor of the FASEB Journal said, "This research shows the connection between diet and health is important for all living animals, no matter how complex or simple they are." He concluded: "It certainly doesn't hurt to add lima beans to more men's diets."

I also agree with the editor's qualification that "there is a lot of work that must be done before we would know if [prunetin] will be useful in humans." Which means, of course, that we need to keep the funding for experimental biology coming.

After all, previous studies have already shown us that lima beans and other legumes have plenty of lifesaving components.

Researchers have found that legumes are typically higher in protein than other plants (since they host nitrogen-fixing bacteria in their root nodules). And other studies show a link between lima beans and prostate health.

Legumes are also rich in biologically active plant alkaloids, flavonoids, and isoflavones—which have health benefits at the cellular level.

In fact, my favorite plant source for cellular hydration—aspal—comes from the South African legume that has been commonly known as rooibos or red bush.

There is, however, an important thing to keep in mind when it comes to choosing legumes. Soy is a legume, but it's also a common allergen. And, as I have warned before, almost all soy grown in the U.S. is genetically modified. You can avoid this by only choosing organic soy.

Along with legumes, prunes—or the more appetizing-sounding "dried plums"—are also packed with prunetin. Additionally, prunes are a very good source of vitamin C. And, of course, they're a well-known remedy for constipation and improved gut health.

The bottom line is that it's vital to increase the amount of research on plant compounds. That's because we typically find that if a plant compound is good for one aspect of your health, it's also good for other aspects of your health.

After all, that's the way Nature works. But sadly, most doctors don't know beans about that.

Chapter 69

Scientific secrets of successful aging

I often write that in addition to monitoring the amount of nutrients you get from foods and dietary supplements, you also need to know how many of those nutrients make it into your cells...and what happens once they get there.

This process is a major issue when it comes to so-called "antioxidants." Some of these compounds are inter-converted to oxidants and back to antioxidants depending on the environments they encounter in your stomach, intestines, blood, liver—and ultimately in the cells of your brain and every organ throughout your body.

Metabolites are an important aspect of this cellular nutrition process. Researchers are increasingly paying attention to these small molecules produced by the cells during metabolism. In fact, they're finding that metabolites can provide valuable information on how diet, lifestyles, and diseases can contribute to aging.

Which leads me to an interesting new study.

Japanese researchers analyzed the blood of younger and older people and found 14 metabolites that may be related to specific aspects of the aging process.

Basically, this means we may finally know some cellular reasons for why we lose strength and become more susceptible to chronic health problems as the calendar pages turn.

Help your cells age gracefully

So what can you do about these aging-related metabolites?

Well, the researchers simply said their findings demonstrate the importance of older adults consuming more antioxidants from foods and continuing to exercise their muscles.

This conclusion is consistent with the healthy aging advice I give you regularly. But based on other research I've reported, I would also add a few carefully selected supplements to your daily regimen as well.

Studies show older adults can almost always benefit from a high-quality B complex, 500 mg of vitamin C (divided into two daily doses), 100 mcg of selenium, and 200 IU of vitamin E.

Furthermore, older adults need to consume about twice the amount of meat and protein as currently recommended by clueless government dietary guidelines in order to maintain muscle mass—which helps to keep you strong and vibrant well into your "golden years."

Chapter 70

Fight the ravages of time at the cellular level— and add YEARS to your life...in just 6 weeks

In this chapter I will reveal my latest research on how you can slow down or even prevent age-related diseases in your body.

I've boiled the new studies down into three simple but effective steps. And they start with my favorite fruit.

Step 1: Eat blueberries, live longer — and better

News about the amazing health benefits of blueberries just keeps getting better.

As I discussed in the January issue of *Insiders' Cures,* there's compelling evidence that blueberries can help fight the oxidation that leads to age-related brain damage like dementia and Alzheimer's. They also help slow down aging in your body by lowering your risk of heart disease, diabetes, and obesity.

And now, a new study reveals that blueberries can improve functional mobility in older adults.

This discovery is a remarkable aging breakthrough. Research shows that maintaining mobility—including the ability to walk quickly and effectively—is the *single-best* predictor of longevity.

Blueberries have already been shown to improve motor function in animal models. And this new study demonstrates they can do the same for humans.

Boost your longevity in just 6 weeks

Researchers gathered men and women age 60 or older and divided them into two groups. One group ate two cups of frozen blueberries daily for six weeks, and the other group got a placebo.

At the end of the study, the researchers found that the blueberry group had noticeable improvement in grip strength, reaction time, and balance and foot placement while walking.

And they had improved walking speed…which equals improved longevity.

That's quite striking after just six weeks of eating blueberries.

Of course, eating two cups of blueberries every day might not be very realistic. Fortunately, you have other options. Look for powdered, water-soluble blueberry food extract, which you can add to any beverage. I recommend 400 mg a day of the water-soluble powdered ingredient to help slow down aging in both your body and brain.

Step 2: Fight aging at the genetic level

Until recently, the only way to really increase your chances of living longer was to have had parents who lived into old age.

But now, researchers have discovered that even if you didn't win the parental genetic lottery, you can still take steps to control aging at the cellular level.

In essence, you can actually *turn back* your biological clock.

How? Well, those who study longevity are focusing on telomeres, which are sequences of nucleic acids (thymine, adenine, and guanine, or TAG) that appear at both ends of all chromosomes in each gene. This "TAG" team helps keep chromosomes stable—similar to the way metal or plastic caps help protect the ends of shoelaces from fraying.

To understand how telomeres affect aging, you need to know that the cells in your body continually divide and replace themselves. So theoretically, you should always have "young" cells in your tissues, as long as they are properly nourished, energized, and hydrated.

But there is one catch. When new cells are formed in chromosomes, the telomeres don't duplicate. Instead, they get shorter with each new cell division. Eventually, they become so short that the stability of the chromosome is compromised, and cell division comes to a halt. No more new, young, healthy cells to replace the old.

That's why over a lifetime, cells can only undergo a finite number of divisions. Eventually, they enter a phase where they accumulate imperfections, lose their functions, and simply die. And that's a big factor in the aging process.

So it's no wonder that telomere shortening has been a focus of aging research at the genetic and cellular levels.

Gilgamesh was right—plants really can extend your lifespan

I think it's fascinating that much of this 21st century research was actually inspired by a king who ruled nearly 5,000 years ago. In the ancient Sumerian epic of Gilgamesh, the king of Uruk searches for a plant that can restore youth. This inspired Andrew Sokar, a child-prodigy-turned-doctor, to create the Gilgamesh Project to research how to prolong the human lifespan.

Dr. Sokar and other researchers have discovered that as cells age, genetic modifications accumulate and appear to affect our biological clocks.

We hear a lot about biological clocks in terms of pregnancy, but they also influence how we age. In my specialty of forensic medicine, for example, investigators might be able to determine the age of an unknown victim, or assailant, from blood or tissue samples at the scene.

Dr. Sokar and other researchers have actually discovered how to determine and detect "age accelerators," or factors that make our biological clocks go faster. They've also discovered which natural compounds help fight these age accelerators.

Interestingly, two of these compounds are found in plants, just as Gilgamesh suspected long ago. I'm talking about B vitamins and betaine—which comes from beets.

My colleagues at the NIH's cellular and molecular pathology lab tell me another important way to slow your biological clock is to nourish the mitochondria, which provide the energy and water that's critical for proper cell function and replication. You can do this by taking Co-Q10 every day, as well as aspal (rooibos, or red bush), dandelion, and blueberry.

Step 3: Don't stress about living longer

We're always hearing that "stress is aging us." But how, exactly?

Well, a new study on stress reduction and lifestyle modification provides great insight into this question. The study was done on African-Americans, who have long been recognized to suffer disproportionately from high blood pressure and heart disease.

When I was in medical training, researchers searched in vain for genetic causes for these differences in African-Americans. But after my research overseas in the late 1970s, I recognized stress was more of a factor for high blood pressure and heart disease among different population groups than genetics were. Of course, stress is now frequently cited as a contributing factor for many chronic diseases.

The new study looked at 48 African-American men and women with high blood pressure.

The participants were divided into two groups. One group followed a stress-reduction program that involved meditation and basic health education. The other group followed an extensive health program.

After 16 weeks, researchers measured both groups' blood pressure and their genetic expression associated with aging. Both groups showed improvements in each of these measurements.

Social support can outweigh diet and lifestyle factors

Based on this study, I am tempted to conclude that participating in *any* healthy group activity has longevity benefits. In particular, there are powerful stress-reduction benefits that come from having doctors and health professionals actually paying some attention to you and interacting in a healthful environment with other people.

In fact, as I noted in my special report *The Insider's Guide to a Heart-Healthy and Statin-Free Life*, research shows that over a lifetime, family and social support can outweigh the strongest dietary and lifestyle factors.

The Ornish diet program is a specific example of this phenomenon. People who participate in the diet program often report reduced blood pressure, which lowers their risk of heart disease. It seems the benefits of learning, eating, cooking, and even food shopping in a social group interaction can aid in weight loss, and improved heart health. But the Ornish diet itself isn't all that healthy—it's much too high in carbs and low in healthy fats.

How meditation can boost your lifespan

Beyond lowering the risk of heart disease, studies show that meditation can also help lower stress, anxiety, and depression in people with a chronic disease like cancer—and that can potentially help prolong life or even help reverse the disease.

And, as I have reported in the past, short periods of meditation can actually increase brain matter. Which, of course, can help fight diseases like Alzheimer's.

Mindfulness and stress reduction has also been shown to influence healthful gene expression (including the genetic expression associated with aging) in studies conducted by the "father" of relaxation therapy, Herb Benson, at Harvard University.

But you don't have to become a Buddhist monk to practice mindfulness meditation and gain its stress-reducing and anti-aging benefits. My book with Don McCown, *New World Mindfulness*, tells you how to practice mindfulness anytime, anywhere, in the middle of your busy life.

So, there you have it. The secret to living longer—and better—isn't flowing from some mythical fountain of youth. It's actually flowing within you.

And science shows that a common (but powerful) fruit, a few simple supplements, and meditation appear to be keys that will help you tap into it.

5 supplements scientifically proven to slow down aging

Here's my daily anti-aging "prescription" based on these breakthroughs in cellular and genetic research:

- A high-quality B vitamin complex that contains at least 200 mcg of folate, 50 mg of B6, 12 mcg of B12, 50 mg of B2, and 50 mg of choline

- 2-4 grams of betaine (or a serving of beets)

- 100 mg of CoQ10 (ubiquinol)

- 400 mg each of aspal and dandelion (you can find these combined in powders you can add to any beverage)

- 400 mg of blueberry powder (or a handful of fresh blueberries)

New research reveals this common drug can slow down aging—and add almost 5 years to your life

I've said before that dementia might as well be called "type 3 diabetes." After all, controlling diabetes markers like blood sugar and hemoglobin A1c are key parts of my upcoming Alzheimer's prevention and reversal cure. And, of course, preventing type 2 diabetes is vital for reducing your risk of serious disease and increasing your longevity.

Metformin is a proven, safe way to fight both type 2 and 3 diabetes. Even though it's a drug, it has ancient natural roots derived from the ancient herbal remedy French lilac.

And research shows there are also beneficial anti-aging "side effects" for metformin, including preventing lung and pancreatic cancer and helping you maintain a healthy weight.

But it turns out metformin can do even more. New research suggests it may even be able to *slow down* the aging process.

Scientists studied the effects of metformin on animals, and found that the drug can increase lifespan by nearly 6 percent. That doesn't sound that impressive until you translate it into human terms. An 80-year-old could live almost *five years longer,* thanks to metformin!

All the benefits of fasting without skipping a single meal

Researchers believe metformin mimics some of the benefits of calorie restriction—without actually having to cut calories. I find this effect particularly interesting because some of the strongest lab experiments for the past half-century show that increases in longevity come from either fasting or restricting calories. Cutting calories lowers blood sugar and substantially reduces your chance of developing metabolic syndrome and obesity—all of which are major risk factors for a variety of fatal diseases.

Apparently, this research has even impressed the government. I'm hearing that the FDA has approved human trials on metformin's effects on longevity. Although, considering how long the average person lives, we could be waiting a very lengthy time to get final results!

I'm not the only doctor who's excited by metformin's longevity potential. Dr. Jay Olshansky of the University of Illinois recently said: "This would be the most important medical intervention in the modern era—an ability to slow aging."

I met Dr. Olshansky when I gave a lecture to the medical residents at the University of Illinois medical campus in Chicago over 15 years ago. The new doctors-in-training were more interested in hearing about natural approaches to healing than were their faculty members—with the exception of Dr. Olshansky.

As old-line faculty challenged me, Jay spoke up in favor of my "new" healthcare ideas. I thought then that he would make a name for himself, and history has proven me right.

Chapter 71

The secret to feeling and acting younger that's been "hiding" on your kitchen counter all along

We have heard about the benefits of olive oil for years—both from researchers and generations of people who know their foods.

But lately, some Internet gurus have been trying to cast doubts about olive oil, claiming it has too many calories and too much fat to really be healthy. (Try telling that to Vito Corleone.)

The truth is, for decades, hundreds of scientific studies from around the world have demonstrated the benefits of olive oil for heart health, preventing strokes, and even lowering the risk of some cancers. And olive oil is a key part of the Mediterranean diet, which can help you maintain a healthy weight and live longer.

In addition to its benefits for the body, new research shows olive oil has cognitive benefits as well. A new study from Italy shows that consuming extra-virgin olive oil can significantly improve memory, anxiety levels, and coordination.

And even more amazingly, the researchers found that olive oil's polyphenols (antioxidant and anti-inflammatory compounds) appear to affect regulation of a gene linked to memory.

How olive oil can tackle brain aging and more

Researchers gave mice olive oil for six months. At the end of the study, the mice performed 74% better on motor coordination tests, and also had significant improvements in spatial memory and anxiety.

You may wonder why it's important to improve your spatial memory. Well, when that type of memory is combined with better coordination, it boosts your mobility—which helps you stay independent longer. And, as I have mentioned, functional mobility is the single-best predictor of longevity.

So it's no surprise that the aging mice that took olive oil started behaving like teenagers again.

There's another important takeaway from this study as well. The researchers observed that most of the genetic changes in the mice were in the cerebral cortex—the area of the brain involved in attention, awareness, memory, perception, and related functions.

This observation provides support for the idea that dementia is essentially brain aging. And that like physical aging, brain aging can be avoided or delayed with the right diet (including olive oil) and supplementation.

Furthermore, these "anti-aging" genes in the brain have an impressive range of functions, including helping to regulate bone and nerve health and glucose metabolism. Which once again shows how important the brain is for healthy aging.

In fact, these study results are so convincing, lead researcher Dr. Cristina Luceri stated that long-term treatment with olive oil could become part of a strategy for the prevention of brain aging and dementia.

So make sure your diet contains extra-virgin olive oil. A splash a day will do—either tossed over salad and vegetables, or as a healthy way to sauté meat or fish.

Chapter 72

Take out that hearing aid!
New research shows 5 safe, simple
nutrients can help reverse hearing loss

Our aging population and increasingly noisy environment means that hearing loss is all too common these days. In fact, hearing problems have become a major health issue, affecting about 48 million people—20 percent of all American adults.

And the statistics get even more dire the older you get. By the time you reach age 65, you have a one in three chance of becoming hard of hearing.

Shockingly, that ranks hearing loss as the third largest public health issue in the U.S.—just behind arthritis and heart disease.

And interestingly, scientists are discovering that our ears appear to be sensitive to environmental stresses such as oxidation and inflammation, and are also vulnerable to nutrient insufficiency.

So that means hearing loss may actually act as an early indicator of inadequate nutrition and a toxic environment—like the proverbial canary in a coal mine.

Hearing loss presents other serious health problems as well. A new study shows that people with hearing loss also have reduced cognition, which is associated with dementia. And another large study found that hearing loss can cause physical impairment, including a 31 percent increased risk of disability that could result in the need for nursing care.

But hearing problems don't have to be an inevitable part of growing old. In fact, new research shows that boosting your consumption of a few basic vitamins and minerals can dramatically improve your hearing.

The secret to a long, healthy life, deep inside your ears

The ear is a fascinating organ that is actually responsible for two important senses—hearing and balance. Loss of hearing results in deafness, and loss of balance results in vertigo.

Let's start with the balance aspects. The inner ear is important for maintaining proper orientation in space. It works with the eyes and the muscular-skeletal system to keep us oriented, upright, and walking correctly.

This is important as we age because maintaining balance and having a good gait are two of the strongest predictors of longevity—probably because they combine muscular-skeletal strength and abilities with central nervous system processing and coordination.

The other function of the ear—hearing—is also important, of course. This part of the ear is known as the cochlea (or shell—like a seashell, whose convolutions follow the natural ratio *phi*, also known as Fibonacci's number). Aside from listening to spoken words, music, and the sounds of nature, our ears' perception of sound waves is also a key component in the innovative healing fields of Acutonics, music therapy, and sound therapy.

Simple nutrients may help stave off—even reverse—hearing loss

The presence of free radical chemicals in the inner ear is a key factor in hearing loss, suggesting that antioxidants may play an important role in prevention and treatment.

And indeed, some animal experiments have shown that the antioxidant **vitamins A, C, and E** do have an effect on hearing.

Experimental studies have also shown that **magnesium** may be important in reducing hearing loss as well. It's thought that this versatile mineral helps restore blood flow to the hearing apparatus of the ear following damage by excessive noise.

Plus, we know that magnesium can help prevent headaches and migraines, probably because of its effects on blood flow in the brain. So it makes sense that it could also have a similar impact on our ears.

But despite these provocative findings, epidemiologists have been slow to study the effects of nutrients on human hearing.

That is, until —the *American Journal of Clinical Nutrition* published a new study on nutrients and hearing. The researchers found that higher intakes of vitamins A, C, and magnesium were associated with better hearing in nearly 2,600 participants, ages 20 to 69. This data came from the National Health and Nutrition Examination Survey— the single best source of data on nutrition and health in the U.S.

The beneficial effects of A, C, and magnesium were found at both normal speech ranges and high-frequency ranges of sound. Furthermore, the impact of all three nutrients acting together was stronger than the individual effects of each of the nutrients acting alone.

There is also experimental evidence that **vitamin B** supplementation can help prevent noise-induced hearing loss. And nicotinamide riboside (NR), a precursor to vitamin B3, appears to protect the nerves

Optimal nutrition, optimal hearing

Here is a quick recap of the nutrients your body needs for optimal hearing:

- Vitamin A
- Vitamin B complex—50 mg each of thiamine, riboflavin (B2), niacin/niacinamide, B6, and pantothenic acid, plus 400 micrograms of folic acid/folate, 12 mcg of B12, and 100 mcg of biotin.
- Vitamin C—500 mg twice per day
- Vitamin E—50 IU per day
- Magnesium—200 mg per day

that transmit sound input to the brain. Research shows that NR may be particularly effective for people regularly exposed to loud noises.

Of course, it's difficult to find NR on supplement shelves (it is, after all, a derivative of the "dreaded" nicotine). But you can protect your hearing with a good vitamin B complex that contains at least 50 mg of B3 (niacin).

Drugs don't sound like the answer

When it comes to drugs that help hearing, there are very limited treatment options. However, there are many drugs that can *cause* hearing loss, from antibiotics to popular pain relievers, including non-steroidal anti-inflammatory agents (NSAIDs) and acetaminophen (Tylenol).

Studies on these drugs using high-tech audiometric measurements are curiously lacking. But a new review of research involving more than 92,000 people does show that people who took NSAIDs had increased risk of self-reported hearing loss.

Specifically, those who regularly took ibuprofen had a 13 percent increased risk of hearing loss, and acetaminophen consumption was associated with a 21 percent larger risk.

So for good hearing, it's best to stay away from drugs and go back to the basic A, B, Cs of good nutrition. Think of the ear as nervous tissue. These nutrients benefit the brain and peripheral nerves, so it makes sense that they appear to help hearing as well.

Along with the vitamin B dose mentioned above, I recommend supplementing your diet with 500 mg of vitamin C twice per day, 50 IU of vitamin E daily, and 200 mg of magnesium. There's no good data on the optimal human dose of vitamin A, so I recommend getting the vitamin from dairy, fish, and meat. All of these foods contain essential fats, which is key because vitamin A is fat soluble.

You should also include lots of red-orange fruits and vegetables in your diet (for carotenoid vitamin A precursors), and green-leafy vegetables for other carotenoids such as lutein. Lutein has been shown to be important for brain and eye health, and I suspect it benefits hearing as well. You can now also get the carotenoid astaxanthin together with liquid vitamin A. I recommend 5,000 IU of vitamin A plus astaxanthin daily.

Follow this plan and it will help keep not only your ears, but your entire body, healthy and sound.

Chapter 73

Evidence shows statins speed up the aging process

The bad news about cholesterol-lowering statin drugs just keeps piling up.

It's not surprising when you understand the basic biology. Statin drugs are metabolic poisons. They interfere with normal cholesterol metabolism by design. But cholesterol is a key constituent of all your cells, brain tissue, nerve tissue, and hormones.

And in any case, the metabolic disruption appears to go far beyond cholesterol.

In a recent interview, one general practitioner said statins "just make many patients feel years older. Side effects mimic the aging process."

Now—I don't like to use the term "anti-aging." I prefer the term healthy aging. It seems to me if you're "anti-aging" it must mean you favor of the alternative—which is to <u>not</u> get older. But in the case of these drugs, it seems big pharma invented an "ANTI-anti-aging" pill. In fact, new research by scientists at Tulane University shows statins speed up the aging process by interfering with stem cell metabolism.

Stem cells help repair tissue damage, and replace brain and muscle cells. Plus, many experts now believe stem cells are the key to understanding cancer and other diseases. (Note: this important research comes from the use of adult stem cells, not fetal stem cells.)

For this study, scientists treated stem cells with statins under lab conditions. And they observed dramatic effects after just a few weeks.

Statins prevented stem cells from performing their main functions to reproduce and replicate other tissue cells to carry out repairs in the body. They also prevented stem cells from generating new bone and cartilage. These effects all add up to faster aging (not to mention a general disaster for your health).

Other known side effects of statins include cataracts, dementia, diabetes, fatigue, joint problems, and liver, muscle, and nerve dysfunctions.

In observing patients, researchers say statin drugs don't seem to outwardly affect a fortunate few. But for others, statins slow them down in more subtle ways. And for still many others, they experience serious side effects that help clinically confirm these disturbing toxicities from the drugs.

Dr. Malcolm Kendrick, a GP in the U.K., said, "This research reinforces what has long been suspected. The side effects of statins mimic the aging process."

As in the U.S., millions of men and women in the U.K. currently take statins to supposedly lower their heart attack risk. And a 10-year UK National Health Service Plan has already been introduced to prescribe these drugs to patients with only a 10 percent risk of heart attack over the following decade. They claim this step could save thousands of lives.

But critics contend much of the data has never been made public and the work needed to ensure that routine use is not harmful has not been done.

My suggestion?

Follow these six steps to keep your heart healthy:

1. Maintain a healthy diet filled with fruits, vegetables, fish and lean meat to get enough protein.

2. Cut sugars, carbs and "soft drinks."

3. Get some moderate exercise regularly.

4. Take a daily B vitamin complex to reduce homocysteine, which damages the heart and blood vessels far more than cholesterol.

5. Take 10,000 IU of vitamin D per day.

6. For healthy aging, the dynamic duo of *aspal* (South African red bush) and dandelion extract provide vitality to older men and women. Look for 400 mg of one or both ingredients in dietary supplements and water-soluble powder mixtures.

Chapter 74

Mother Nature's "secret weapon" for optimal health and longevity

One thing I learned early on about natural medicine is its ability to make the "impossible" possible. And there's no better example of that than adaptogens.

Their potential is so tremendous, I believe everyone should consider taking an adaptogen every day—right along with other essential nutrients like vitamin D and omega-3 fatty acids.

Adaptogens are individual herbs that have the unique ability to help your body adapt to changes, both internal and external. For example:

- If you're cold, they help you warm up

- If you're hot, they help cool you down

- If you're tired, they wake you up

- If you need rest, they help you sleep

And so on. In fact, they have more serious effects, too. They can help return abnormal cells to normal. They can help promote healthy, balanced blood sugar. And they can help keep nerve cells and synapses in the brain firing on all cylinders.

There is no single drug that can do all of that.

But the human body has many mechanisms to maintain homeostasis, a "constant" internal environment. And adaptogens work by activating all of those mechanisms.

Modern-day miracles steeped in tradition

While adaptogens are still a foreign concept in western medicine, they're well known—and commonly used—in Chinese and Indian medicine.

In China, the classic adaptogen is ginseng.

In Ayurvedic (traditional Indian) medicine, *Ashwaganda* is probably the best-known adaptogen. It is used for general longevity in Ayurveda (which itself means the "science of life, or "long life"), as well as for a number of specific indications.

But I've recently discovered another extremely powerful, yet little known adaptogen called *Sutherlandia frutescens*. Sutherlandia has been used in South Africa for centuries. And it is revered there for its tremendous potential.

In fact, in 1879, as part of its colonization of South Africa, the British army attacked an aging group of Zulu tribesmen. The aging tribesmen were armed only with short spears and crude cow hide shields. And the British army—regarded at the time as the strongest in the world—fully expected to overwhelm the Zulu in mere minutes and then move on easily to their conquest of South Africa.

But a mysterious thing happened…

Zulus stun the world with their energy and grit

After hours and hours of fighting, the Zulus never gave up, never retreated and never tired. They kept on fighting with the energy, strength and focus of men *half* their age, until eventually they overpowered the British forces in a stunning victory in the infamous Battle of Isandlwana.

The stunning defeat shocked the British—and, indeed, the world. But the Zulus weren't surprised in the least. Because they knew to rely on a coveted local herb to help boost their strength and vitality to newfound heights.

As time went by, that fierce battle reached almost mythical proportions in the history books. Yet the Zulu's legendary herb remained a puzzling medical mystery to the rest of the world.

But after countless hours of research with some of South Africa's brightest scientists and health professionals, I finally tracked down the answer to one of natural medicine's most legendary mysteries...

It turns out the Zulu tribesmen took *Sutherlandia* before the famous battle. And they also used it to calm their nerves and lighten their mood upon their return home. But as I discovered in my research that is really just the beginning of *Sutherlandia's* story.

As it turns out, this herb has a rich history around the globe... everywhere except the US, that is.

As usual, America is late to the party

During WWI Sutherlandia was widely used overseas to help support immune systems as well as boost energy to help people cope with the stresses of wartime.

And it turns out Sutherlandia and other adaptogens have been studied and researched outside of the country for decades.

They've been used by everyone from Olympic athletes, to soldiers, to astronauts because of their amazing ability to help protect and preserve your body's youthful vitality.

And Sutherlandia is known far and wide throughout South Africa. In fact, it's so popular it's being sought after like South African diamonds!

BBC news even reported that one health manufacturer bribed several local farmers to plant as many acres of the herb as possible for fear of over-harvesting.

Yet despite the overwhelming demand, it remains virtually unknown—and hard to find—here in the U.S.

But when I learned of its incredible potential, I knew this balancing herb was the "missing link" everyone in this fast-paced, "country of extremes" needed.

Of course, the centuries-old legend surrounding this herb is what first got my attention. But the science is what really "sealed the deal," so to speak.

Head aging off at the pass

While other "anti-aging" remedies claim to minimize the effects aging has *already* taken on your body, Sutherlandia helps head aging off at the pass by addressing subtle, stress-related changes that continually occur in your body on a <u>cellular level</u>.

As I often report, stress ages your body on multiple fronts.

Whether it's the physical wear and tear that takes its toll on your joints and skin, the psychological drain of a long day at work or the environmental toxins in the air you breathe, food you eat and water you drink.

When your body starts to sense these stressors, your cells shoot up tiny red flags—and that's where Sutherlandia goes to work.

It may help to calm your joints, replenish your energy, or support your immune system—just to name a few ways it helps bring your body back into balance. And science continues to point to the fact that balance is the key to optimal health and longevity.

Adaptogens, then, are like Mother Nature's "secret weapon" for achieving both.

Chapter 75

9 foods that cut your cataract risk

By age 80, more than half of Americans will develop cataracts, clouding of the eyes' normally clear lenses. Sunlight is one source of damage to the lenses. Which you may prevent by wearing protective sunglasses that filter out certain ultraviolet rays.

But increasing evidence shows poor nutrition and chronic inflammation in other parts of the body can damage the eyes too. Evidence also links cataracts with Type II diabetes and cardiovascular disease, probably for the same reasons.

Fortunately, research shows several foods help prevent cataracts and support eye health in general.

1. Avocados

Avocados are nutrient dense and contain high amounts of beta-carotene, lutein, vitamin B6, and vitamin E—all of which are important for preventing cataracts.

2. Blue-purple berries

Bilberries, blueberries, and blackberries all contain anthocyanins, which give the berries their deep blue-purple colors. These pigments also fight inflammation and keep the blood vessels clear that supply the retina and eyes.

In a lab model, bilberry extract completely prevented cataract formation in animals bred to have a 70 percent risk of developing them. I recommend a daily dose of 160 mg of bilberry or 400 mg of blueberry.

3. Broccoli

This cruciferous vegetable is rich in lutein and zeaxanthin, whose role in human metabolism and nutrition I helped discover in the mid-1980s working with a team of scientists at the National Cancer Institute and the USDA. These two nutrients fight inflammation and free radical formation, which can damage eyesight. Broccoli also contains sulforaphane, an antioxidant that protects eyes from the sun's ultraviolet radiation.

4. Yellow-orange vegetables

Your grandmother probably told you to eat your carrots to keep your eyes strong. And she was right! The alpha- and beta-carotene (the word comes from carrot) form vitamin A in the body, which is important for healthy eyes. But don't forget about the other yellow-orange vegetables— such as pumpkin, squash, and sweet potatoes. They also contain lutein, zeaxanthin, and other carotenoids. Again, these carotenoids help absorb harmful ultraviolet rays from sunlight, which can damage the eyes.

5. Eggs

Speaking of yellow and orange, egg yolks (not the whites) contain high amounts of lutein and zeaxanthin also. In addition, they contain the omega-3 fatty acid DHA (docosahexanoic acid), which is important for brain and nervous tissue, including the eyes.

6. Oranges

Oranges contain high amounts of vitamin C, of course. And studies show nerve cells in the eye need vitamin C. In fact, a study published in the *Journal of Nutrition* found high levels of vitamin C can reduce the risk of developing cataracts by 64 percent.

7. Salmon

Salmon is rich in astaxanthin, the marine carotenoid that gives this fish—as well as crabs, lobsters, and shrimp—their pink-reddish hues. Astaxanthin also protects the eyes from free-radical damage and helps prevent the formation of cataracts.

Salmon and other cold-water fish also contain high amounts of omega-3 fatty acids, which are powerhouses for your overall health.

Plus, a study found that women who ate fish three times per week reduced their risk of cataracts by 11 percent compared to those who ate fish only once per month.

Remember, only eat wild-caught salmon from the Pacific. Atlantic salmon is farm raised, which lacks nutrients by comparison.

Of course, you should also supplement with 1 to 2 grams of a high-quality fish oil every day. And you can also find astaxanthin in supplement form. Some formulas even combine this important carotenoid with vitamin D (another essential nutrient) in an easy-to-take liquid.

8. Tea (black and green)

In lab testing, researchers learned black and green tea reduced glucose levels in lab animals. It also reduced their risk of cataracts in half. Chinese researchers also found that catechins in tea protect the eyes from glaucoma (increased pressure in the eye chambers). A study published in the *Journal of Agricultural and Food Chemistry* by the American Chemical Society found the effects of catechins in a cup of tea last up to 20 hours.

9. Walnuts

Not only are walnuts a perfect snack or addition to side dishes, they also contain vitamin E and other antioxidants, as well as the essential fatty acids DHA and EPA, which are important for eyesight. These omega-3s also help reduce levels of C-reactive protein, a marker of chronic inflammation.

You should eat these nine foods regularly to maintain good eyesight. But there are also foods to avoid—mainly processed carbs and sugars. In fact, an Australian study found that people who ate the most carbs had three times the risk of developing cataracts compared to those who ate the least. I always recommend cutting out these foods for general health reasons. Plus, now we know they can contribute to cataracts.

PART 7

DRUG-FREE GUIDE TO DEFEATING YOUR DEPRESSION

Chapter 76

The tragic truth about antidepressants

If you're suffering from depression, the promise of relief in the form of a little pill can feel like a lifeline. So the fact that antidepressants have few—if any—real benefits is, well...*depressing.*

You're better off passing on the SSRIs—and using natural solutions instead.

That's the conclusion published last month in the British Medical Journal. And it's consistent with views I have presented before in Insiders' Cures. My practice in forensic medicine backs it up too. I've seen case after case of depressed patients committing suicide... *after they start taking "antidepressant" drugs.*

Making matters worse, it's not that antidepressants don't do anything—it's just that they do the wrong thing. The newer antidepressant drugs act as selective serotonin reuptake inhibitors (SSRIs). They artificially raise levels of serotonin in the brain by preventing its normal re-uptake into nerve cells after it's released into nerve pathways.

This is believed to help depression symptoms. And it does...but not the symptoms that need to be improved.

In my forensic medicine practice, I saw case after case of chronically depressed patients with suicidal thoughts. But they were too depressed to take action and do anything about it. *Until they got their dose of SSRIs, that is.* Once the drugs kicked in, the patients still had their suicidal thoughts, and now they had the energy to act on them. The results were tragic.

Even more tragic is that some mentally troubled, depressed patients have thoughts about harming others as well. Disturbing new analysis indicates many of the recent violent tragedies grabbing the headlines may be the result of antidepressants.

That's because depression has a built-in self-protection. It causes people to turn inward, close themselves off, and they lack the energy to carry out actions. Instead they just endlessly think these thoughts, many of them negative. Psychiatrists call this *thought substitution.* So even if people have thought of hurting themselves or others, they often don't have the energy or ability to do it.

Now give the depressed person Prozac. You haven't changed anything about the real causes of the depression. But, suddenly, the depressed person's brain is flooded with serotonin. And now they finally have the energy to act.

I'll leave it to statisticians to debate whether SSRIs cause suicide in depressed patients. But as a physician, the evidence in real cases of suffering human beings is all too obvious.

Still, serotonin is not just a loaded gun waiting to go off. And while I don't recommend artificially manipulating your serotonin levels as a treatment for any disease, I can tell you that there are natural approaches that really work. They help the body naturally restore its own proper levels of serotonin, acetylcholine, and other neurotransmitters. And that makes for a healthy mind and body.

I'll tell you more about these natural depression helpers in a minute. But first…

Antidepressants on the rise

Why are prescriptions for antidepressants going up and up, while the people taking them continue slipping down into their depression?

Some psychiatrists claim it's because of a small, but appropriate, increase in the length of treatment—not the number of patients being treated. That is, patients are being kept on the drug longer.

But why keep people on the same tired medication if it's not working?

The real issue is that too many people are being treated for something that's just a normal part of life—not a disease in need of a pharmaceutical cure. The current definition of clinical depression is two weeks of "low mood". I can think of a number of people whose moods were low for a couple weeks after the last election. But I wouldn't call it a disease—and I certainly wouldn't want to medicate it away!

A more serious mental illness is being so delusional that you can't recognize when bad and sad things are happening in reality—and that's much worse than two weeks of "low mood".

But some parties have reason to be in a good mood about the overuse of antidepressants. **Three-quarters of psychiatrists who write the definitions of depression used in the psychiatric manual have links to drug companies.1** So they have good motivation to put people on prescriptions and abandon more time-intensive—but effective—mental health treatments! (Think psychoanalysis, talk therapy, and even spiritual approaches.)

Depression may be the perfect condition for the drug industry: Incurable, common, long-term (even with these so-called "treatments"), and involving multiple medications. Some experts say contemporary psychiatry's relationship with the drug industry has created a pharmaceutical mindset to treat mental illness.

But the National Institute for Health and Clinical Excellence does not even support the use of antidepressants for mild depression. Instead it favors psychological talk-based therapies.

Of course, the government industrial-insurance complex doesn't want to pay health professionals for the time it takes to really help patients. Instead they push the quick treatment—the few seconds it takes to scribble on a prescription pad (often with the name of the drug also advertised at the top).

Perhaps *that's* why antidepressant prescriptions increased by almost 10 percent in 2011.

The upside of being down

Occasional "low mood" may simply be a fact of life. In fact, research shows that mildly depressed people are actually better at assessing and dealing with life's circumstances. Sometimes low mood is just our way of seeing that all is not well, and that we need to protect ourselves.

Shakespeare was no stranger to low mood when he wrote the character of Hamlet. When Hamlet perceives that "something is rotten in the state of Denmark," it leads to his famous soliloquy: "To be, or not to be—that is the question…whether to suffer the slings and arrows of outrageous fortune, or take arms against a sea of troubles, and by opposing them, end them."

Sounds like an appropriate response to a dangerous situation, doesn't it? To most of us anyway… But not to some ever-alert psychiatrists, who have used that soliloquy to diagnose Hamlet as depressed.

Nature's answer to depression

While antidepressant drugs may be worse than worthless for many or most people, many natural approaches can enhance brain, mind, and mood. And of course all of those work together, especially when talking about neurochemicals like serotonin. Here are just a few natural ways to get serotonin levels to their natural, optimal levels.

Omega 3s. Omega 3—rich foods (salmon, sardines, walnuts, flaxseeds, and olive oil for example) may help depression. And we already know they're powerhouses in other areas of health. Researchers think omega 3—rich foods affect structural fats in brain membranes, making it easier for nutrients to enter cells.

Folic acid (and other B vitamins). Low levels of folic acid and high levels of an amino acid—like chemical called homocysteine are associated with depression. Folic acid, as well as vitamins B2, B6, and B12, have all been shown to decrease levels of homocysteine and protect against heart disease, as we document in *The Insider's Secret to Conquering High Blood Pressure and Protecting Your Heart.* Find B vitamins in fruits, vegetables, nuts, whole grains, and legumes. If you're taking a supplement, look for 800 mcg folic acid, 2.5 mg thiamine, 5 mg B6, and 20 mcg B12.

Amino acids. Tryptophan is an amino acid needed to make serotonin. For many years higher tryptophan has been found to be associated with lower depression rates. Tryptophan is high in foods containing proteins (which are chains of amino acids), such as meat, fish, beans, and eggs.

Nucleic acids. Research at McLean Hospital in Belmont, MA, has shown foods high in uridine improves mood. Uridine is a nucleic acid found at high levels in beets and molasses. Beets are also a rich source of betaine, which is critical in maintaining proper antioxidant balance in cells.

Carbohydrates. Carbohydrates are broken down into sugar your brain needs to function properly. However, simple sugar or too much carbohydrate can cause or aggravate depression. Avoid this problem by eating a diet low in refined carbohydrates and sugar and high in fruits and vegetables.

St. John's wort. This European folk remedy has been used for centuries as natural treatment for depression and anxiety. In Germany, for example, St. John's wort has long been approved for its effectiveness in treating mild depression. General dosage is 300 mg three times per day (at 0.3% standardized hypericin extract).

Antioxidants. A new study in the *Journal of the American Academy of Nutrition and Dietetics* found that foods high in antioxidants (but not dietary supplements themselves) help stem depression in older adults. This is not surprising since foods contain a biological matrix that is important for proper absorption and metabolism. Plus most antioxidant supplements are of poor quality and not based on real science.

Proper hydration. What and how much you drink can influence mood as well. A small study of 25 women suggests dehydration can cause headaches, loss of focus, fatigue, and low mood. Now here's the really interesting thing. Even minor dehydration (about 1 percent lower than optimal) was enough to cause serious effects.

South African Red Bush (Rooibos). Of course, water alone is not enough to prevent dehydration. You need fluid and electrolytes—but not from so-called sports "hydration" beverages. Instead, I recommend the little-known South African Red Bush (rooibos). You've heard me sing this herb's praises before for all sorts of conditions. But it also packs a one-two punch for depression. It keeps you hydrated while also providing antidepressant effects and benefits for brain, mind, and mood. As a true adaptogen (helping the body adapt to stress), red bush will refresh you during the day and relax you at bedtime. I generally recommend replacing your 8-glasses-a day with 4-6 glasses of rooibos tea—hot or iced.

A truly depressing drink

Diet drinks are chock-full of nasty stuff. A new French study shows that diet drinks pose a higher diabetes risk than *even regular soda!* And now we're finding out they can affect your mood as well.

A just-off-the-press study links artificially sweetened beverages—especially diet drinks—with higher depression risk in adults. (Coffee, on the other hand, slightly lowered risk).2

Researchers studied 263,925 people for about 10 years. Those who drank more than four cans of soda per day were nearly one-third more likely to develop depression than those who drank no soda. The same amount of fruit punch caused an almost 40 percent increased risk. The same amount of coffee, on the other hand, came with a 10 percent risk reduction.

Think it's just the sugar? Think again. As with the French study on diabetes, this study showed an *even greater* risk for people who drank diet versions of these drinks.

So, do your mood a favor. Pass on the sweet drinks and go for a cup of Joe or rooibos tea instead.

Chapter 77

Feed your brain: What you should—and shouldn't—eat for better mental health

Want to improve your mental health? Start by improving your diet.

American psychiatrists are finally beginning to take note of what I've been telling you all along: Your brain needs nutrients just like your body does.

And what's the best way to get all those particular nutrients? From food.

In fact, a recent analysis of 17 different studies found that in nearly half of the studies, dietary changes significantly improved depression.

And during an annual meeting of the American Psychiatric Association, there was an entire session on the best foods to support mental health. Not surprisingly, those foods did not include processed junk, sugary foods, or white bread and pasta.

Let's take a look at what else you should—*and shouldn't*—be eating to fight depression and anxiety…and improve your overall mental health and mood.

5 foods you might not expect to boost your mood

Meat. We now know when it comes to eating meat, what we have been told by the government for decades is just flat-out wrong. We actually need to eat more—not less—of this food for both physical and mental health. In fact, the researchers who conducted the meta-analysis of 17 studies I mentioned above specifically recommended diets that <u>did not</u> reduce red meat or cholesterol intake.

Meat is a nutrient-dense source of minerals and vitamins A, B, and D. And of course, it's an excellent source of protein.

As I've reported before, B vitamins are so important to brain function, they're called "neurovitamins" in Europe. And there are scores of studies showing that vitamin D can help reduce depression and lower your risk of Alzheimer's disease.

Meat is also a good source of cholesterol and fat. The omega-3s in cholesterol and fat actually help build and support the structure of brain and nerve cell membranes (not to mention every other tissue cell in the body).

Bottom line: Every one of us needs cholesterol and fat for healthy brains and nerves. And one of the best sources of both of these nutrients is meat. While plants like chia and flax contain some omega-3s, they're not the same brain-building type that are found in meat.

There are, of course, many ethical problems with industrial meat production. Opt for organic, grass-fed beef instead of corn-fed (almost all corn grown in the U.S. is GMO now). These more natural agricultural practices are much less abusive to animals, and also result in much healthier foods.

Eggs. We have been ridiculously advised by the government to avoid this perfect food. But like meat, eggs are a good source of cholesterol and other nutrients, making them one of the best foods for the brain.

Making an omelet in the morning with some red peppers, for example, is a tasty and healthy brain treat. (The color of the pepper is a clue to its nutrient quality. The presence of bright red, orange, yellow, green, blue, and purple in natural foods is a sign that they're packed with vitamins, carotenoids, anthocyanins, flavonoids, and other valuable phytonutrients.)

As with meat, look for eggs from humanely raised animals. That means free-range and organic (which ensures the chickens aren't given antibiotics).

Oysters, clams, and other seafood. When it comes to nutritional value per ounce, few foods measure up to bivalves like oysters and clams. A half-dozen oysters on the half-shell provide 272 percent of the daily intake of vitamin B12, and 509 percent of daily zinc.

Zinc has been shown in a variety of studies to be critical for memory and cognition—especially as we age.

Bivalves and other seafood are also leading sources of vitamin D and omega-3s. And they're rich in chromium and iodine—two minerals important for brain function. The omega-3s in seafood also help support the production of a chemical called brain-derived neurotropic factor (BDNF). BDNF plays a role in the survival and growth of neurons. Research has also shown that, in patients suffering from depression, anxiety, and mood disorders, higher BDNF levels result in less severe symptoms.

Liver and organ meats. These foods also get a bad rap, but nothing is more nutritious. Predatory animals on the hunt always go for the organ meats first, since they are the densest sources of vitamins and minerals—literally storing them up for the rest of the body.

Not a fan of liver or other organs? You can disguise the taste and texture by adding them to delicious vegetable stews, or many different varieties of chili con carne.

Nuts. Like meat and eggs, nuts were also once "off limits" because they're considered high-fat treats. But that kind of thinking is "nuts," according to the science. A handful of tree nuts (almonds, cashews, pistachios, walnuts) can help ward off diabetes, heart disease, and obesity. And nuts improve brain health.

Nuts are full of bioavailable brain-boosting minerals like manganese and selenium. Not to mention protein, omega-3s, and vitamin E—which has tremendous brain benefits.

In fact, one study showed that adding nuts to a Mediterranean diet resulted in overall improvements in depression and mental health.

Until recently, researchers assumed that these benefits only came with relatively expensive tree nuts. But new research shows that peanuts (which grow in the ground) are just as healthy at much less cost. (Peanut butter did <u>not</u> have the same health benefits, probably due to the addition of sugars and other added ingredients.)

Finally, the information on the food labels for nuts is all wrong when it comes to calorie counts. One study showed that almonds actually have 25 percent *fewer* calories than thought. And there's speculation that calorie counts could be significantly lower for other nuts as well.

Sidestep these two mental-health minefields.

Vegetarian or vegan diets. Of course, we all know that plants have an important role in a balanced diet. But, as I have uncovered in the past, strictly plant-based diets are not healthier for body or brain.

B-vitamin deficiency is commonly associated with vegetarian diets and causes development delays in children and brain atrophy in adults. And some research shows a vegetarian diet is associated with increased anxiety and depression.

Plants just can't provide enough healthy fats, minerals, and vitamins that are crucial for good mental health. And, unlike meat and seafood, they also don't have the full range and variety of amino acids that are needed in proteins.

Gluten. Most of the health, metabolic, and weight problems associated with grains come from their high carbohydrate content. But the gluten protein found in wheat and other grains can also be a culprit.

We already know that gluten can cause allergic reactions, including celiac disease, in some people. And now there's evidence that it may be a factor in psychosis.

A large clinical trial demonstrated that people diagnosed with schizophrenia have significantly elevated anti-gliadin antibodies (gliadin is a component of gluten). The researchers found that over 23 percent of schizophrenic patients have high anti-gliadin antibodies, compared with only 3 percent of controls.

In one case, an underweight but otherwise healthy 37-year-old woman became paranoid and psychotic over a period of a year. She entered into the "downward spiral" of mental illness, losing her job, home, family, and friends. Numerous psychiatric drugs were useless.

But after only three months of a gluten-free diet, her mental condition became stable.

Later, she consumed just one gluten-heavy meal. She ended up back in the hospital. But when she went back to a gluten-free diet, she resumed normal mental health—without any drugs.

A growing amount of research also shows that gluten may influence the microbiome—the "good" bacteria in your gut. In addition to controlling digestion, the microbiome appears to be important for mental health.

Irritable bowel syndrome (IBS), is also influenced by the microbiome (and vice versa). And IBS is associated with anxiety and depression. That's because the digestive process may involve conversion of the amino acid tryptophan to serotonin—powerful neurotransmitter that influences depression and other moods.

Many of the bacteria of the microbiome actually make their own neurotransmitters, which communicate with the vagus nerve. The vagus nerve originates in the brain, as one of the twelve cranial nerves, and travels throughout the internal organs and gastrointestinal tract. Scientists don't yet know what the gut is saying to our vagus nerve, but they think the brain is listening.

If you do decide to try a gluten-free diet, remember that many non-grain-based foods are naturally gluten-free. There are also a growing number of delicious and nutritious gluten-free breads and baked goods. I have personally inspected, and highly recommend, Aleia's Gluten Free Foods. To find a store near you that sells these healthy goodies, or to buy them online, visit www.aleias.com.

In mental health, as in virtually all other aspects of health, diet is the best option we have for health promotion and disease prevention.

Chapter 78

Eat more of these foods to improve mental health

A good diet is a basic tenet of good physical health. And it's a basic tenet of good *mental* health as well. In fact, as I'll explain in a moment, you can improve your depression risk by up to 60 percent by making a few simple changes to your diet.

It seems American psychiatrists are *finally* starting to take note of the all the good research on nutrition and mental health. In fact, at an American Psychiatric Association's (APA) annual meeting, Dr. Drew Ramsey, assistant clinical professor of Psychiatry at Columbia University College of Physicians & Surgeons, led a session about the best foods to support mental health was included.

We all know a good diet supports body and brain function. And the body and mind are connected. So it makes perfect sense the foods that support good physical health would also support good mental health.

According to Dr. Ramsey, "Food is a very effective and underutilized intervention in mental health." He continued, "…patients have more resilient brains by using whole foods…by getting off processed foods, off white carbohydrates, and off certain vegetable oils."

Of course, you would never hear this advice from the mainstream. The only "solution" they offer patients struggling with depression is to take an antidepressant drug. But this "solution" does very little to actually help the patient—and all too often it causes more harm than good.

Plus, remember the infamous Harvard study on depression from 2002? In that study, researchers found neither SSRI drugs nor dietary supplements worked better than placebo for depression. But the "placebo" received by everyone in the study was 14 hours of counseling by a skilled mental health professional…and they *did* experience some improvements.

That Harvard study always reminds me that talking and listening to the patient is more effective than handing out any pill, whether drugs or supplements. And you don't have to conduct formal psychoanalysis either. Apparently just talking about anything important to the patient helps.

In fact, in another recent study, just *discussing diet* with a counselor for six hours over the course of two years decreased depression scores by 40 percent in elderly patients. Thankfully, many experts are beginning to recognize the psychiatry of food.

A paper published in the British journal *Lancet Psychiatry* attested: "Although the determinants of mental health are complex, the emerging and compelling evidence for nutrition as a crucial factor in the high prevalence and incidence of mental disorders suggests that diet is as important to psychiatry as it is to cardiology, endocrinology, and gastroenterology."

Plus, a 2014 meta-analysis of clinical trials showed dietary interventions improved depression comparable to antidepressant drugs in half the studies.

Now, back to the APA session…

Dr. Ramsey and his co-presenter took a stab at explaining human biology and evolutionary biology to support the importance of diet to mental health.

They made a good point about the importance of seafood to the human brain. They said the earliest human ancestors in the African Rift Valley lived close enough to the seacoast to have reliable access to seafood.

Of course, early modern humans emerged during the Ice Age on the northwest coast of Europe, where they clearly took advantage of seafood. In fact, as recently as 100 years ago, anthropologists observed healthy indigenous peoples on the northwest coast of North America who didn't farm at all. They gleaned most of their nutrition from marine foods such as fish and seafood.

Indeed, oysters, and other mollusks are very ancient marine creatures.

And they're very high in nutrients, including B vitamins, which are commonly deficient in vegan or vegetarian diets. The human brain needs vitamin B12 for neurotransmitter functions. It also supports healthy myelin, which insulates nerve endings.

Of course, oysters and other kinds of seafood also provide abundant natural cholesterol and omega-3 fatty acids for our brains, which are composed of 60 percent fats.

Humans only began cultivating and consuming agricultural products—such as grains, legumes (beans), and dairy—about 6,000 to 10,000 years ago. The history books call this an advancement of civilization. But I would disagree. Archaeologists found evidence that human health and nutritional status *declined* and growth became stunted among populations who adopted agricultural foods compared to hunter-gatherer ancestors.

Clearly, the government's advice to cut out cholesterol and fats from the diet was a disaster for our health—both physical and mental. And mainstream medicine still pushes the disastrous cholesterol-lowering drugs, which poison normal metabolism.

Plus, many Americans—when they tried to follow the government's advice to cut fats and cholesterol—ended up with a diets filled with processed grains and sugars, which lack nutritional value.

Also, many of the people who went to the extreme and tried to follow a vegan/vegetarian diet ended up following a high-carb diet—which usually amounts to a high-sugar diet and is unhealthy for all the same reasons. Indeed, pregnant women who follow vegetarian diets run the same risk of suffering from anxiety as those women who follow high-sugar diets.

I *do* respect ethical concerns about the treatment of animals. But it's hard to make the case for vegan/vegetarian diets based on that ethical argument alone. The human body simply needs the bioavailable nutrients found in meat and seafood.

A number of studies link the Mediterranean diet—high in fish, olive oil, nuts, and wine—with mental health benefits. In fact, recent studies show adults who follow the Mediterranean Diet most closely for four to five years had a 40 to 60 percent reduced risk of depression.

Of course, evidence shows the Mediterranean diet benefits the heart and circulatory system as well. And it improves mental focus, energy, and self-confidence. Indeed, a healthy diet is the first step in this virtuous cycle.

My colleague Don McCown is the Director of the Center for Contemplative Studies at West Chester University of Pennsylvania. He just visited with me in New England to work on our next book together. He shared a quip about what causes mental health and illness, "It's more about what's out there, than what's in here".

In other words, you can accomplish a great deal by understanding interpersonal and social factors without having to conduct abstract internal psychoanalysis. Plus, what you put "in there" (in your body) is an important factor too.

Chapter 79

Support serotonin naturally

Antidepressant drugs known as SSRIs (selective serotonin reuptake inhibitors) only work for about one in seven depressed patients. And that *one* patient out of seven probably only feels better because of a placebo effect.

Fortunately, you *do* have many natural treatment options if you suffer from depression. There are some encouraging findings about the role of omega-3 fatty acids (EPA and DHA) and vitamin D for improving the health of both the brain and the mind.

Unlike conventional medicine, in the world of natural medicine, there is no real distinction between brain and cognitive health versus emotion, mood and mental health. In other words, there is no artificial, imaginary barrier between "neurological" or "cognitive" disorders, thought of as brain conditions…and "psychiatric" disorders, thought of as mental conditions. Brain, mind and mood all function together naturally.

In a paper published in the *FASEB* journal (Federation of American Societies for Experimental Biology), researchers made four excellent points.

First, the researchers recognized the connection between "cognitive" and "psychiatric" disorders. And they theorized if a treatment works for "cognitive" disorders, it should also work for "psychiatric" disorders.

Second, they pointed to the wealth of previous research that shows omega-3 essential fatty acids (found in marine or fish oils) and vitamin D improve brain function.

Third, they theorized that omega-3s and vitamin D should then also work for "psychiatric" disorders like depression. The researchers even highlighted a "mechanism of action" that could help explain how and why omega-3s and vitamin D support mental health.

A mechanism of action explains *how* something works in the body. And this point is important because scientists in the 21st century can't just accept that a treatment works. They need to know *how* and *why* it works.

Fourth, the researchers brought up the very good point that the brain needs essential fatty acids and vitamin D to support normal production of serotonin. But drugs like SSRIs act by "blocking" the reuptake of serotonin back into brain cells.

As I've said before, drugs that chemically "block" normal metabolic processes are a bad bet. Whether it's a statin drug that "blocks" normal cholesterol. Or a bone density drug that "blocks" and kills normal bone cells. Or an SSRI that blocks the reuptake of serotonin. Using drugs that "block" normal functions don't follow a normal or natural path to good health. "Blockers" belong on a football team, but not in your body. I'm much more inclined to recommend nutrients that support normal functions so the body can preserve or restore normal health.

So back to the new research at hand…

First, let's take a look at vitamin D. As the researchers pointed out, vitamin D acts more like a hormone than a simple nutrient in the body. Also, it regulates the conversion of the essential amino acid tryptophan into serotonin.

Of course, serotonin isn't the only important neurotransmitter in the brain. But it *does* influence a wide range of cognitive functions and behavior. Including mood, decision-making, social behavior, impulsive behavior, and social decision-making.

Plus, research links many clinical conditions to disordered serotonin activity, including from autism (ASD), attention deficit hyperactivity disorder (ADHD), bipolar disorder, depression, and schizophrenia.

Next, let's look at essential fatty acids.

One type of fatty acid called eicosapentaenoic acid (EPA) facilitates serotonin release from brain cells into synapses between cells. EPA appears to act through its anti-inflammatory properties. It reduces inflammatory molecules in the brain called E2 prostaglandins. These inflammatory prostaglandins negatively impact serotonin in brain cells. They also block the release of serotonin into the synapses between cells.

Another type of fatty acid called docosahexaenoic (DHA) influences serotonin receptors. It makes the receptors more accessible by increasing cell membrane fluidity.

Now, how do vitamin D and essential fatty acids work *together*?

Your body converts vitamin D into a steroid hormone that regulates more than 1,000 different gene pathways, many in the brain. Then, the essential fatty acids interact with these pathways in the brain, including the serotonin pathway. These pathways are important for mood, cognition and decision-making.

The problem is, most people don't get enough fatty acids and vitamin D into their diets. Most people don't eat enough fish, which is the best source of omega-3 fatty acids such as EPA and DHA. Of course, your skin will produce plenty of vitamin D on its own if exposed to enough sunlight. But during fall and winter months, the sun isn't strong enough to activate vitamin D on the skin.

I suggest supplementation. Improving your intake of vitamin D, EPA and DHA with supplementation will naturally support serotonin activity in the brain. It will also help prevent and improve depression and other cognitive functions. The one thing it *won't* do is cause adverse side effects. The only "side effects" it will cause are other proven health benefits provided by these essential nutrients.

You can find EPA and DHA in high-quality fish oil supplements. But you want to make sure the manufacturer prepares the fish oil supplements according to specific procedures.

When it comes to vitamin D, I recommend everyone take 5,000 IU per day year-round. It's especially important during fall and winter months. You can find vitamin D in an easy-to-use liquid form, together with the carotenoid antioxidant powerhouse astaxanthin.

Chapter 80

Popular drugs help only 1 in 7 patients

Doctors dole out antidepressants far too easily. To far too many people. And for far too long. Plus, few antidepressants, if any, truly benefit their patients.

I've hounded this point many times before. And now, it seems I'm not the only doctor who is unafraid to speak the truth about these drugs. In the *British Medical Journal*, Des Spence, M.D., a general practitioner from Glasgow argued that antidepressants are far too overprescribed. He cites the Cochrane review that found only about one in seven depressed patients benefit from antidepressant drugs.

The newer antidepressant drugs like Zoloft and Wellbutrin are SSRIs. This stands for "synaptic serotonin re-uptake inhibitors." They artificially raise levels of serotonin in the brain by preventing their normal re-uptake into neurons or nerve cells. This artificially floods the brain with serotonin. Some argue this extra serotonin helps improve symptoms of depression.

But is that really true?

Through my work in forensic medicine, I see case after case of chronically depressed patients. They were "successfully" treated with SSRIs. But then they promptly committed suicide. The treatment was a success, but the patient died.

Here's part of the problem...

SSRIs treat only a symptom of depression. They do nothing about the *underlying* causes.

When people are depressed, they turn inward. They close themselves off. And they lack energy to carry out actions. Instead, they just endlessly think thoughts, many of them negative. But they take no action.

Now give that person Prozac. You haven't changed anything about the *cause* of the depression. But suddenly they have energy. Including the energy to carry out their suicidal thoughts. And that they do.

So, how do you start down this troubled road?

It begins with the very definition of clinical depression.

Let's look at both the old and the controversial, new editions of the *Diagnostic and Statistical Manual of Mental Disorders.* Both editions define clinical depression as two weeks of "low mood."

It doesn't take a doctorate to see that this definition is far too loose. Indeed, this very flawed definition of the disease may be the root of the problem. It led to the widespread "medicalization" of what should be just normal chapters in human life!

Is it any surprise that antidepressant prescriptions increased by almost 10 percent in 2011? This represents the largest increase in prescription medicines across the board! And this number is on track to continue to grow in coming decades.

And, some parties are in a good mood indeed about the overuse of antidepressants. In fact, three-quarters of those who write the definitions of "low mood" used in the psychiatric manual have links to drug companies!

Mental illness may be the perfect condition for the drug industry. And drug makers couldn't be happier with the growing numbers diagnosed with depression.

"Low mood" may be incurable—not surprising, considering the treatment with SSRIs. It's common—not surprising, given the definition. It's long-term—but why, if the treatment is in fact any good? And it involves multiple medications. Yes—I'd say it's *the* perfect disease for the drug industry!

Modern psychiatry's relationship with the drug industry has created a therapeutic drug mindset to treat mental illness. Now psychiatrists can simply write a prescription, just like…"real doctors!"

Have we completely abandoned the more time-intensive approaches involving psychoanalysis, talk therapies, and even spiritual dimensions?

I hope not.

Sometimes a "low mood" is an accurate and appropriate response to reality. You cannot simply medicate it away.

Studies show that mildly depressed people can more accurately assess circumstances. Plus, they're more effective at dealing with them. And they're better at predicting real outcomes.

Perhaps our "low mood" is our body's natural response to perceiving "all is not well." Perhaps it is part of the body's "fight-or-flight" defense system. But we lack the energy to fight. So we "stand down… conserve…and withdraw." All the while, we stay "on alert."

Perhaps these drugs take away some human wisdom that we all need to feel sometimes.

Guidelines from the National Institute for Health and Clinical Excellence do not support the use of antidepressants for mild depression. Or necessarily for moderate depression. Instead, it favors psychological talk-based therapies. And for mild to moderate depression, the use of herbal remedies such as St. John's can be effective.

Now, I'm not saying that depression isn't a real problem. It *is* debilitating for many millions of Americans. But I don't recommend trying to artificially manipulate your serotonin levels as a treatment for any disease.

There are several treatments you can try to help your body heal naturally and restore its own proper levels of serotonin, acetylcholine and other neurochemicals.

Chapter 81

A natural depression treatment
that works wonders

Seasonal Affective Disorder (SAD) is a type of depression that typically strikes during the winter, when days are shorter and there is less sunshine. Doctors often treat SAD with "light box" therapy. During light therapy sessions, you sit or work near a light box and the light enters your eyes indirectly.

Some researchers are finally "thinking outside the box" and have found light therapy also helps treat other types of depression not brought on by seasonal light deprivation.

In a recent study supported by the Canadian Institutes for Health Research, researchers randomly assigned 122 adults with major depression not related to SAD to one of four treatment groups.

The first group received 30 minutes of light treatment per day and a placebo pill. The second group used a "placebo" device that didn't provide actual light therapy and took Prozac. The third group used the placebo device and a placebo pill. And the fourth group received both actual light therapy and Prozac.

After eight weeks, researchers used a widely recognized depression scale to evaluate the participants' mental and emotional state.

Placebo outperforms antidepressant

First and foremost, Prozac showed no benefit over placebo.

No surprise there. Other studies consistently show the same thing (particularly when patients also receive a lot of attention from a health professional).

Among those who used a placebo device and took a placebo pill, about 30 percent of participants still showed improvement. Again, this finding demonstrates the benefits of a health professional paying any kind of attention to these patients.

By contrast, among those patients who used the placebo device and took Prozac, only 20 percent showed improvement.

So—the drug + placebo device performed worse than the placebo pill + placebo device. In other words, it appears the drug actually counteracted or negated any potential beneficial placebo effect!

And what about the group who got the real light therapy and the placebo pill? They fared even better yet—about 40 percent of them went into remission in just eight weeks.

Of course, the researchers still recommended giving Prozac together with light therapy because that combination saw a small bump in benefits. But antidepressants carry many harmful and dangerous side effects. In fact, a recent investigation shows that antidepressants cause 15 times as many suicides as the FDA reports.

From this study, I came away with two major impressions.

First, placebo continues to offer greater benefits than drugs for this major mental health condition. Secondly, light therapy performs even better than placebo alone.

Overall, patients tolerated the light treatment well. Researchers don't fully understand *why* it works. For seasonal affective disorder, it may help correct disturbances in the body's internal biological clock, or circadian rhythm. For non-SAD depression, it may work through the same "mechanism of action." But we just don't know at this point.

Isn't it enough — for now — to know it DOES work?

You can buy light boxes at drugstores and other retail outlets for less than $100. And some insurance even plans cover them. Treatment involves sitting in front of the light box for 30 minutes as soon as possible after waking. You can do it while eating breakfast or just working at your desk or on the computer.

Remember also that winter is the time of year when vitamin D levels decline, if you don't take regular vitamin D supplements. Research I reported from the U.K. a couple years ago demonstrated that those with low mood during winter had lower vitamin D levels, which explains a lot.

So make sure to take 10,000 IU daily of vitamin D. You can find it in liquid form, which may be easier to swallow with juice or water.

Chapter 82

Nature improves well-being in older adults

My daughter knows firsthand the power of spending time in Nature. She now works as a Maryland State Park Ranger. And under a wonderful governor, her state now funds a "Youth Park Ranger" program where urban children have an opportunity to get outside in Nature. I can't think of a simpler, healthier program for both mind and body.

My daughter's new Nature program is for children, but new research out of the University of Minnesota shows spending time in green and blue spaces (environments with running or still water) offers many health benefits to older people too.

As I often say, spending time in Nature every day improves your quality of life at any age. It measurably reduces stress. It also promotes physical, mental and spiritual healing. People can attain these health benefits by spending time outside to "get away from it all."

Fortunately, you don't have to embark on a Lewis & Clark expedition to gain the powerful benefits…

The new study shows exposure to small natural elements—such as a koi pond or a bench among flowers—benefitted older adults. In fact, these small green and blue spaces promoted feelings of renewal, restoration, and spiritual connection in adults ages 65 to 86.

They also provided places for social engagement and interaction, both planned and impromptu, with family and friends.

Researchers found access to blue and green spaces encouraged men and women to simply get out the door. It helped them maintain a structured daily schedule. Also, it helped offset the effects of chronic illness, disability and isolation. As a result, quality of life indicators showed decreases in boredom, isolation and loneliness. And improvements in their sense of accomplishment and purpose.

You can easily seek small connections to Nature. I always recommend spending time in and near water. I suppose it's only natural for me, since I spent a lot of time as a child on the coast of northern New England. And still do today, in New England and Florida.

Research shows movement in water is one of the best, healthiest, safest, and most restorative forms of physical activity. Also, simply spending time on the water or along the waterfront can help you relax and find a spiritual connection.

At the end of the fifth paragraph, in the very first chapter, of that great American novel *Moby Dick*, Herman Melville poetically writes, "Yes, as everyone knows, meditation and water are wedded forever."

I find many busy people think they don't have time or opportunities to connect with Nature or meditate on a daily basis.

But even in the middle of your busy life, you can find that "waterfront" for contemplation, spiritual connection and relaxation right in your own "mind's eye," anytime, every day.

You don't have to go away to a Buddhist Monastery, or even to the seashore, to get the benefits of practicing meditation.

Research shows practicing mindfulness as a young and middle-aged adult has many brain benefits. Imaging studies demonstrate that mindfulness meditation helps stave off dementia and can help you achieve healthy aging.

My advice for healthy aging is pretty simple:

1. Focus on overall wellbeing—mental and social health, as well as physical fitness.

2. Get out the door daily, even if it's just around the block or to the corner park.

3. Make contact with Nature an everyday priority. Sit in a park, listen to a water fountain, or sit among the plants in a garden.

Late summer and early fall is a special time of year, especially here along the New England coast. Here, the beaches are perfect for those contemplative and restorative walks along the water.

Chapter 83

Getting to the point of mood disorders

Today, modern psychiatrists like to talk about the semi-imaginary, chemical "imbalances" that cause mood disorders. They say they can correct the "imbalance" simply by adjusting the levels of certain chemicals in the brain, such as serotonin. Trouble is, they don't have any clue about the effects on all the <u>other</u> brain chemicals involved.

Plus, that approach assumes treating mood disorders is like doing an experiment with the Gibson chemistry set you used in middle school. Of course, according to all the latest research, this approach has been a disaster for mental health, public health, and even public safety.

The truth is—mental disorders are far more complex than most modern psychiatrists will admit.

Depressed men and women lived "normal lives" without drugs

In my view, we had a better understanding of the complexity of mental illness in the 19th century, when doctors considered the spiritual dimensions. And because they lacked modern drugs, doctors "prescribed" what they called "moral therapy" for patients with mental disorders such as depression.

Instead of locking away depressed patients—or numbing them with drugs—doctors allowed those struggling with mental disorders to live with others who were "normal." The mentally ill patients could then observe the ways other people reacted to and processed "reality." It helped the patients build a fund of positive experiences in their mental bank that they could draw from when they needed emotional reserves.

This approach isn't so different in principle from the 20th century's behavioral therapy and today's cognitive-behavioral therapies (CBI). Studies show these techniques are very effective, particularly in conjunction with other mind-body techniques like mindfulness meditation.

Spirit and consciousness are inherent to human existence…and certainly to our perception of it. But modern-day reductionists seem to think molecular models explain everything about our existence.

Fundamental physicists, who study the most basic aspects of reality itself, know better. They know life is far more complex than we currently comprehend.

In fact, astrophysicists made an observation that finally proved the final part of Einstein's General Theory of Relativity that he put forth a century ago. And many experts believe ancient Ayurveda and Chinese medicine probably understood some of these "cosmic" effects thousands of years before Einstein.

Chinese medicine offers deeper insights to depression

Practitioners of Chinese medicine have a deep understanding of the human existence as well. They too consider mood problems as spiritual problems. And they began using the acupuncture needle 2,000 years ago as a potent tool to tap into the essence or spirit, by bypassing the more material manifestations. In fact, an ancient description described acupuncture as the "spiritual pivot."

Now—let's go forward 2,000 years…

New research shows that acupuncture alleviates depression with insomnia. In Traditional Chinese Medicine, they call depression associated with insomnia "depressive insomnia." People with this condition have difficulty falling asleep. And they experience a disruption of sleep by dreams, generalized insomnia, and emotional volatility.

Western medical science is even beginning to understand the connection between these two disorders. In fact, in a recent study, researchers compared acupuncture to mirtazapine, an older antidepressant drug, in patients who suffer from depression with insomnia.

The researchers divided the participants into two groups. The first group received acupuncture. The second group received mirtazapine drug therapy. The drug caused drowsiness (not to be confused with healthful sleep), dizziness, and vision problems, as well weight gain associated with increased appetite and constipation. By comparison, acupuncture was effective in 90 percent of cases to improve duration and quality of sleep for patients with depression. And it caused no notable side effects.

The successful treatment protocol involved acupuncture sessions every other day. By comparison, the drug group took a pill daily.

Of course, some would argue taking daily pills is more "convenient." I suppose it is more convenient as long as you find going through the day in a drowsy stupor, with dizziness and visual disturbances to be convenient. And you can't mind gaining weight while struggling with increased appetite and constipation (enough to be depressed, right there).

In my view, anyone who still prescribes antidepressant drugs—when there are other safe and effective methods—simply misses the point.

PART 8

NATURAL ANSWERS FOR AN IRONCLAD IMMUNE SYSTEM

Chapter 84

Your immune system's most powerful ally

It seems every time I sit back down to my computer, another study pops up about the importance of vitamin D. It's no surprise really— Vitamin D appears to benefit virtually every part of your body. And it seems to help protect you against nearly every chronic disease. Now, three new studies even illustrate vitamin D's incredible effect on the immune system.

In the first study, researchers looked at vitamin D and its effect on colon cancer risk. They matched 318 people with colon cancer against a control group of 624 men and women without colon cancer. All the participants had given blood samples in the 1990s, before the appearance of any cancer.

The researchers measured the vitamin D levels in these samples and found the higher the participants' vitamin D blood levels at the outset, the less likely they were to develop colorectal tumors. Vitamin D, the authors suggest, interacts with the immune system to prevent the growth of this type of malignancy.

In a second study, researchers found that vitamin D prolongs survival time in people with metastasized colon cancer (cases in which the cancer has spread beyond the original site in the body).

For this study, researchers followed 1,430 people with metastatic colon cancer. The patients in the lowest fifth for vitamin D levels survived for an average of 25 months. By comparison, patients in the highest fifth for vitamin D levels survived for an average of 33 months. That's 33 percent longer. In addition, higher vitamin D delayed any progression of the cancer from 10 to 12 months.

These findings make perfect sense.

You see, malignant tumors contain other types of cells besides the actual cancer cells, including T-lymphocytes or T-cells. These immune cells influence how fast a tumor grows or spreads. They attack cancer cells, which they consider "foreign," and can limit tumor growth. And research has shown that vitamin D is necessary to activate these T-cells.

In yet another recent study, researchers linked low vitamin D with poorer recovery after major surgery. For this study, researchers at Massachusetts General Hospital and Harvard Medical School measured vitamin D levels of patients admitted to the hospital's surgical intensive care unit (ICU). They found that ICU patients with low vitamin D blood levels spent more time on artificial respiratory support. Evidence links mechanical ventilation itself with a number of negative health outcomes. So getting off those breathing machines is a critical goal in critical care—and vitamin D helps.

Of course, we already knew that low vitamin D aggravates asthma and Chronic Obstructive Pulmonary Disease (COPD). Conversely, we know that boosting vitamin D levels improves lung function.

So a lot may come back to vitamin D's role in supporting immune system function. It appears this critical nutrient inhibits inflammation in the lungs, while boosting the immune system to defend against respiratory bacteria and viruses. Indeed, a balanced immune system *decreases* unhealthy inflammation, while *increasing* healthy immune response against microbes.

No simple-minded, single-function drug can do anything like that. All they do is put the system out of balance. They either boost the immune system artificially, which increases inflammation. Or they deaden it, which reduces inflammation, but leaves you vulnerable to infection (as with steroids).

It's remarkable that vitamin D positively influences the body's reaction to so many diseases—from cancer to lung diseases. And that something as simple as keeping up your vitamin D levels (as with daily supplementation) can translate into measurable and meaningful benefits—well beyond the high-cost, high-tech, and invasive modern medicine that we throw at these devastating diseases.

Unfortunately, the government-industrial-medical guidelines for vitamin D are so pathetically constrained by their focus only on bone health, just following the RDA for vitamin D simply won't provide the benefits this nutrient is capable of conferring.

You really need to take 5,000 IU of vitamin D daily. Even better, combine it with the natural powerhouse astaxanthin. You can now take them together as an easy-to-use and easy-to-absorb liquid.

P.S. A quick reminder: If you come down with the flu, you can safely take up to 20,000 IU of vitamin D per day just for the duration of the illness. This course will help your immune system fight the infection more effectively. And it will undoubtedly be a whole lot more effective than relying on the pathetic flu vaccine or Tamiflu drug treatment.

Chapter 85

The simple, natural ingredient on your fruits and vegetables that can protect you from foodborne illness

You've probably been warned not to judge a book by its cover…and that beauty is only skin deep. But when it comes to food safety, it's all on the surface.

In an attempt to better understand what contributes to food contamination, researchers recently conducted an experiment on two dozen varieties of common salad greens and tomatoes.

What they found challenged the conventional wisdom that rougher surfaces (like a kale leaf) would hide viruses and bacteria and make them harder to wash away.

Instead, the researchers discovered that vegetables that have a waxy layer—which naturally protects the plant against diseases and dehydration—had fewer viruses on their surface after washing, compared to their non-waxy counterparts.

The cleanest greens you can eat

Specifically, the researchers found a *thousand-times fewer* viral particles left on vegetables with a wax layer after being washed, compared to vegetables without this type of layer.

The waxiest produce (and therefore least likely to harbor viruses) included:

- Collard greens (Top Bunch variety)
- Kale (Starbor and Red Russian
- Cabbage (Alcosa and Gonzales)
- Tomatoes (Indigo Rose, Rose, and Sungold)
- Romaine lettuce (Outredgeous)

Other lettuces, endive, spinach, radicchio, arugula, and mustard greens had the lowest amounts of wax.

The science behind food safety

So why did the researchers focus on produce used in salads? Well, fruits and vegetables are exposed to viruses and other microbial contaminants in a number of ways. Among the top offenders are contaminated irrigation water, animal waste on the plants, and handling by farm workers.

When produce is cooked, it typically kills microbial contaminants. But when it's eaten raw, like in a salad, food safety can be particularly problematic.

To conduct the experiment, the researchers swabbed 24 varieties of raw salad greens and tomatoes with a swine virus that mimics human rotavirus—a common pathogen responsible for gastrointestinal infections. (There is a vaccine for rotavirus, but safety and ethical questions have made it the subject of great controversy).

The researchers washed the contaminated greens and tomatoes twice in a standard salt solution.

Then, they evaluated the surfaces of the vegetables at different levels of magnification. Not only were they looking for viruses, but also the amount and composition of waxes on the produce.

While viruses typically adhere to waxes at the molecular level, the researchers found that when a wax completely covers the surface of a fruit or vegetable, it repels water and makes it harder for viruses to stick.

While the researchers did their best to make this sound chemically complicated (and relevant), it's basically the same reason it's simpler to keep floors clean when they are waxed. As we all know, waxed surfaces are easier to wash—whether they're floors or fruits.

Hidden sources of wax on your produce

While wax may help cut contamination on produce, it's important to note that not all wax on fruits and vegetables is natural.

Conventionally and even organically grown produce may be artificially waxed to prevent moisture loss and dehydration, protect it from bruising during shipping, and increase its shelf life.

That's why you'll often see wax on apples, cucumbers, eggplant, citrus fruits, peppers, and potatoes.

Some of this added wax is from natural sources like carnauba (from the carnauba palm tree), beeswax, and shellac (from the lac beetle). But some of it is petroleum-based.

To ensure you're not eating petroleum, buy organic fruits and vegetables, which, by law, can only use natural waxes. Or you can buy directly from the grower—just visit your local farmer's market or sign up for community-supported (CSA) deliveries.

Unfortunately, the only way to remove any type of added wax is to peel the fruit or vegetable. And that can remove the nutrients that lie right below the skin.

While you should carefully wash all produce before eating, your salad may be that much safer (and nutritious) if you load it up with kale, cabbage, collards, tomatoes, and red romaine.

Watch out for pesticides too

Of course, there are other contaminants on produce besides microbes that can cause health issues. Particularly pesticides.

According to the nonprofit Environmental Working Group, nearly three-quarters of conventional produce samples tested by the USDA in 2014 contained pesticide residues. And the really disturbing thing is that the pesticides remained on fruits and vegetables even after they were washed. And in some cases, even after they were peeled!

Every year, the EWG releases its "Dirty Dozen"—the 12 types of conventional fruits and vegetables that are most contaminated with pesticides.

The 2016 Dirty Dozen includes strawberries, apples, nectarines, peaches, celery, grapes, cherries, spinach, tomatoes, sweet bell peppers, cherry tomatoes, and cucumbers.

And the EWG notes that hot peppers, kale, and collard greens can be contaminated with insecticides and pesticides that are particularly toxic.

So how can you avoid these deadly chemicals? It's simple. Just eat organic produce—which, by law, can't be sprayed with pesticides, insecticides, or chemical fertilizers.

Chapter 86

"Wonder vitamin" reduces lung disease flare-ups by 40 percent

You've probably been subjected to those ridiculous commercials featuring an elephant sitting on top of breathless lung disease sufferers. Aside from the question of whether any animals (or humans) were harmed in the making of these commercials, do you want to know the real elephant in the room?

New drugs like the one featured in this ad really have little to offer (other than the long list of side effects rattled off at the end of those annoying commercials). But the benefits of vitamins are hiding in plain sight.

In fact, a new British study showed that simple vitamin D supplements reduced flare-ups of chronic obstructive pulmonary disease (COPD) by over *40 percent*.

COPD includes lung conditions like emphysema and chronic bronchitis, and affects more than 12 million people in the U.S. So it's no wonder drug companies have gravitated toward this disease like a herd of stampeding elephants.

But, once again, the real results—and relief for patients suffering from COPD—are coming from nature, not big pharma.

Less inflammation, easier breathing

The study included 240 people with COPD. Half were given vitamin D supplements, and the other half received a placebo.

The researchers found that everyone in the vitamin D group had less severe and shorter COPD flare-ups. And among people who started the study with low vitamin D levels, the results were even more dramatic.

Of course, people in darker, colder climates like the U.K. (and much of the U.S.) are generally deficient in vitamin D. In the study, 87 percent of participants had inadequate vitamin D status. The people who had D blood levels lower than 50 nmol/L had the most pronounced reduction in COPD flare-ups.

As you know, vitamin D has many effects in the body. In this case, the researchers believe it suppressed the inflammatory cells that trigger lung disease flare-ups.

How much is enough?

For optimum health, I recommend 5,000 IU of vitamin D3 daily to ensure there's a constant, adequate amount of the vitamin in the body at all times.

This dose is substantially more than the woefully inadequate 600 IU per day the government recommends for people under age 70 (if you're over age 70, you get a "whopping" 800 IU a day). But these outdated recommendations are based on old, inadequate vitamin D research and fearmongering about "excess" vitamin D.

Doctors often worry that fat-soluble vitamins, like D, can be dangerous because they are stored in the body. But lets look at it the other way around. In the COPD study, participants were given the equivalent of about 120,000 IU of vitamin D *all at once*, and then got another dose of the same size two months later.

Our ability to store high doses of vitamin D actually shows how much this vitamin is needed in the body at all times. Furthermore, it proves that large quantities can be and *are* safely stored in the body.

So a supposed "megadose" of vitamin D is simply safely stored away for later use. What's so dangerous about that, doc?

It's certainly far safer than the anti-inflammatory steroid drugs that many doctors prescribe for COPD. Steroids disrupt the body's metabolism and immune system about as much as vitamin D supports them.

But unfortunately, few people manage to leave a doctor's office without a drug prescription. And these days, vitamins are primarily used and tested in *addition to*, not *instead of,* drugs.

Imagine how healthy our lungs—and our entire bodies—might be in a properly nourished, drug-free world.

Chapter 87

Treat your cold or flu with echinacea and elderberry—not Tamiflu

As soon as you find yourself coming down with a cold or flu, there are effective, scientifically proven natural approaches you can take.

For decades, there has been growing research on the ability of the herb echinacea (the Native American purple cornflower) to prevent or limit the severity and duration of colds or flu.

And now, new research shows that echinacea combined with extract from elderberries is *just as effective* as the expensive and dangerous drug Tamiflu for reducing or ending flu symptoms.

Plus, people who take Tamiflu are over <u>twice </u>as likely to have their flu turn into pneumonia, bronchitis, or sinusitis than those who take echinacea and elderberry.

I wish I had known this when I was a young adult in medical training at the University of Pennsylvania—home to the nation's oldest hospital and medical school. There was not much that could keep me and my colleagues down. But we all dreaded getting the "chop rot" from the Children's Hospital of Philadelphia (CHoP). Mysterious viruses would emerge from children cooped up in this hospital. And they could "chop" down a healthy young adult in the prime of life—at least for a few days.

Fortunately for those kids and my colleagues, Tamiflu wasn't around then. As I have written in the past, this drug has serious side effects. Not only nausea, vomiting, and headaches—which are bad enough—but also kidney disorders and psychiatric syndromes.

But thanks to this new research, we now know an echinacea/elderberry combo is just as effective as Tamiflu, with none of the worrisome side effects.

How the flu flew away

Researchers in the Czech Republic recruited 473 people who previously had influenza symptoms for less than 48 hours. Each study participant was given either Tamiflu or a hot drink containing an echinacea extract supplemented with elderberry.

After one day, 2 percent of the echinacea group and 4 percent of the Tamiflu group had mild or no flu symptoms. After five days, 50 percent of the echinacea group and 49 percent of the Tamiflu group were symptom free. And after 10 days, 90 percent of the echinacea group and 85 percent of the Tamiflu group had recovered.

Echinacea and elderberry was particularly impressive when it came to preventing more serious health issues. Seven percent of the Tamiflu group ended up getting pneumonia, bronchitis, sinusitis, or gastrointestinal issues like nausea or vomiting. But only 3 percent of the echinacea group had these respiratory problems, and none of them suffered from the gastrointestinal issues.

While this study used a proprietary echinacea and elderberry blend from Europe, other studies indicate that a daily dose of echinacea tea spiked with elderberry extract is effective and makes a pleasant hot beverage. I don't think there is sufficient evidence to recommend doses. Like many herbal infusions, just brew a concoction that tastes good and drink it often. The key is to start this process within 48 hours after your first cold or flu symptoms.

And remember not to take echinacea unless you are coming down with a cold or flu. Otherwise, you run the risk of chronically overstimulating your immune system. Which, ironically, could increase your susceptibility to colds and flu.

Other ways to fight colds and flu

Of course, most basically healthy people eventually recover from colds and flu without any treatment. But why be miserable any longer than you have to?

Bolster your immune system throughout the year, and you'll make yourself much less susceptible to the viruses your family brings home from school or work.

A good approach is to take a good-quality B complex every day, along with 500 mg of vitamin C twice per day. And don't forget daily doses of 10,000 IU of vitamin D, 400 mg of vitamin E, 200 mcg of selenium, and 35 mg of zinc—which you want to be taking anyway for their many brain and body benefits.

There is a lot of talk about high-dose vitamin C, but your body can only effectively make use of 500 mg at a time.

You can, however, really stock up on vitamin D. Some of my natural physician colleagues say from their personal and clinical experience, it's best to take 20,000 IU of D per day when you feel you are coming down with a cold or flu. I'm not aware of any studies on that higher dose, however.

Finally, if you're reading this on a touch screen, make sure you frequently wash your hands or use alcohol-based hand sanitizers. That's a good idea in any circumstance, but particularly for touch screens, which are a great invention—for viruses and other diseases that are passed along by touching.

Chapter 88

The hidden, ugly truth about vaccines

Since the start of the measles outbreak in California, we've heard plenty about vaccines from the usual "experts" in the media and the talking heads in the academic-industrial-government medical complex. The U.S. Surgeon General finally weighed in on the topic with nothing more than a deafening echo of what the lame stream media reports were already spouting.

Of course, vaccination is a complex issue. And we could really use a non-politicized Surgeon General who's actually an expert on infectious diseases to guide us through these complex times. For example, when I worked with former Surgeon General C. Everett Koop during the Reagan administration, he always led the charge on important public health issues. But the Obama administration chose the current Surgeon General because he's an expert on gun control and partisan, political fundraising.

Politics aside, it's very distressing that we never hear about so many of the scientific facts concerning vaccines. Perhaps they think we can't handle the truth. Because the truth is not pretty.

You see, the measles outbreak in California involved many vaccinated people who nonetheless contracted the disease. Similarly, there was an outbreak of mumps among healthy, young professional hockey players, many of whom had been vaccinated.

You may wonder why and how all these people contract these infectious diseases when they've already been vaccinated.

The truth is, getting vaccinated doesn't guarantee you won't get the disease.

In fact, in an interview, Gabe Mirkin, M.D., explained the situation perfectly. He said, "It's not that vaccines don't work at all, it's that we were led to believe they offer lifelong immunity when they don't. How on Earth do 20-year-old men on the Pittsburgh Penguins hockey team all come down with mumps if they were vaccinated as kids?"

Gabe is actually an old friend and colleague from back in the days when we lived in Maryland. Now, he lives here in Florida like me. During the 1990s, he was one of two regular physicians in the D.C. area (the other was Michael Emmer, M.D.) who I ever visited as a patient. And I recommended them both to my family and friends. Gabe actually practiced science-based medicine, instead of just handing out pills as prescribed by big pharma.

And Gabe nailed the hidden, ugly truth about vaccines: They aren't guarantees.

In fact, the only way to *guarantee* you'll get full immunity is to get the disease itself. This also confers natural immunity to members of the population.

When I was a child, everyone came down with chicken pox, German measles, measles, and mumps. Mostly, we were sick for a few days from school and that was all. Then we had lifelong immunity.

Anyone who missed getting these largely self-limiting infections naturally as a child ran the risk of coming down with them as an adult—when the infections could be far more dangerous. Nobody worried about exposing children in school because parents *wanted* their children to get, and get over, these common infections quickly while they were young.

In addition, when children are breastfed, they continue to receive "passive immunity" from the mother during the most vulnerable period of infancy. Then, well-nourished and healthy children who spend time outdoors generally develop stronger immune systems that can withstand the common childhood infections.

On the other side of the coin, some vaccines can and *do* have deadly and debilitating consequences. For example, the HPV vaccine—given to innocent young girls and boys—is a national scandal. In some cases, patients develop devastating neurological diseases as a direct consequence of vaccination.

Unlike our gun control expert Surgeon General, Senator Rand Paul, a physician, is one of the few "talking heads" in Washington, D.C., actually qualified to give a medical opinion. As he quickly pointed out, no one seems to talk about the millions of reports citing the negative consequences of vaccines. We only hear the parroting of the party line about the "indisputable" evidence supporting vaccines.

But even well-established vaccines have their problems. In fact, there is a pending lawsuit against the MMR (mumps, measles, rubella) vaccine, which states the U.S. government purchased an estimated four million doses of mislabeled and misbranded vaccine for over a decade or more.

Plus, vaccines contain many dangerous ingredients. According to the Centers for Disease Control (CDC) itself, common additives include: aluminum, antibiotics, albumin, formaldehyde, monosodium glutamate (MSG), and thimerosal (containing mercury).

Many people have deadly allergic reactions to antibiotics, albumin or MSG. Mercury is toxic to brain and nervous tissue. Experts suspect aluminum has the same side effects. And, of course, formaldehyde is a metabolic poison used to embalm dead tissue.

Amazingly, the Environmental Protection Agency, California, and other states have banned dumping several of these chemicals into the environment. Yet the CDC encourages doctors to dump them into the bodies of our children!

So—what's the result of all this vaccination in our children?

American children are the most highly vaccinated people on the planet. These poor little pin cushions receive some 49 doses of 14 different vaccines before the age of six. But they're also among the most chronically ill children in Western nations.

A final note that nobody else seems to be catching on to...

Doctors often give Tylenol (acetaminophen) before, during, and/or after administering a vaccine. This practice conveniently but inappropriately prevents the presence of a fever from stopping administration of a "scheduled" vaccine. But a child with a fever should never receive a vaccine because it's a sign the immune system is already over-stimulated.

Furthermore, Tylenol is a metabolic poison. In fact, one researcher recently uncovered a link between children who received Tylenol at the time of vaccination and the development of autism.

The vaccine industry is a risk-free proposition for big pharma. In fact, federal law prevents anyone from suing the manufacturer of a vaccine for the harm it does. Nor is it a risk for the academic-government-industrial medical complex. The public bears *all* the risk. And there's no recourse for the citizens who ultimately pay for it all.

Chapter 89

Which vaccines do you really need?

I've talk about the pressure we're all under to get an annual flu vaccine. But you and I both know your healthcare providers aren't likely to be content with just one vaccination. They want to inoculate you against a whole host of health conditions.

Pneumonia. Shingles. Tetanus. Even childhood diseases like mumps and measles.

But do you really need all—or *any*—of these vaccines?

Confusing immunization "facts" can spread as quickly as…a virus. So it's no wonder you may be concerned about vaccinations. Especially as you age, and are bombarded with propaganda about more "essential" vaccines you "must" have.

At the same time, there are increasing concerns that the more vaccines you get, the more imbalanced your immune system becomes. And an imbalanced immune system can make you more susceptible to chronic diseases. Not to mention the public health consequences of eliminating natural immunity in the population.

Then there's the shocking lack of science (*and* lack of effectiveness) of the government's influenza vaccine. It's certainly enough to make you wonder whether it's worth getting jabbed with *any* vaccination needle.

Based on my concerns about the flu vaccine, you may think I'm against vaccines in general.

But let me be clear. I am not anti-vaccine. I am pro-science.

Throughout my career, I have witnessed important developments in the history and science of vaccines. And I've found that some of the more recent vaccines are ones we would actually be better off *not* getting.

So let's take a look at the science behind common vaccines. And whether that science suggests you should—or <u>shouldn't</u>—get a particular vaccine.

But first, it's helpful to know the dramatic history of vaccines. And how that has led to where we are today. An environment where healthcare workers feel increasing pressure to inoculate everybody for everything.

Immunization goes back over 200 years

Some of the greatest advancements in modern medicine resulted from the ability to vaccinate people against deadly infections.

For instance, Dr. Edward Jenner's experiments with cowpox in England led to average village doctors throughout the Western world being able to provide smallpox immunity to their patients by the late 1700s. Centuries before, Eastern doctors accomplished the same thing for some residents of the vast Chinese empire.

Of course, neither East nor West knew then about viruses or the germ theory of disease. They just based their findings on trial and error and observation.

When the germ theory did become widely understood and accepted, it led to the development of more vaccines during the late 19th and early 20th centuries. Some were developed by doctors who worked in the same job I held myself, almost 100 years later, at Walter Reed Army Medical Center (including Dr. Walter Reed himself.)

One of the most notable vaccines to emerge in the mid-20th century was the injectable polio vaccine, created by Dr. Jonas Salk, whom I once had the privilege of meeting later in his career.

The debate over polio vaccines

Interestingly, Salk's vaccine kills the polio virus once it enters the bloodstream from the gastrointestinal tract. This is important because if polio gets into the bloodstream, it can then migrate into the central nervous system (CNS)—causing the dreaded "infantile paralysis." But the vast majority of younger children who are exposed to the polio virus just end up with a GI infection. The virus never gets into the CNS. And children who get this GI polio infection develop lifelong immunity to the disease—without being vaccinated.

Dr. Albert Sabin later developed the oral polio vaccine. But there is a problem with the oral polio vaccine—it prevents natural GI infections caused by the virus, which means that children can't develop the natural immunity I mentioned above.

Without natural immunity, doctors have to make sure to vaccinate each and every child. Otherwise, there would be pockets where there was no immunity at all—and every child would be susceptible to polio when it periodically came through the population. And potentially at older ages, when contracting the virus is more likely to cause paralysis (as in the case of Franklin D. Roosevelt, who got polio as a young adult).

Scientific debate between oral and injectable polio vaccines continues to this day. I had my own "debatable" encounter with polio when I was doing fieldwork in Southeast Asia in 1977.

There was an outbreak of polio in a jungle village, and the local government health officials refused to investigate it. Fortunately, Catholic priests from the nearby Columbian Mission were happy to guide me and help map the outbreak—which we traced to a contaminated common water source.

I turned in the maps and data to the local health authorities, who refused to do anything. Instead, they castigated me as a foreigner for interfering and "insulting" what must have been their very fragile egos. They even lodged incendiary complaints against me with my sponsoring organization back in the U.S. It was a shocking and dispiriting introduction to government public health for me.

The eradication of smallpox

Like the polio vaccine, smallpox vaccination was another great global achievement. It was so successful that during the late 1970s, medical teams working for the World Health Organization were able to isolate the last remaining pockets of smallpox in the horn of Africa.

As a new medical anthropologist, I was asked by a senior health professional at the CDC (which was good at doing its job back then because it still focused on its mission against infectious diseases) to speak at an annual American Anthropological Association meeting in the 1980s. You see, these infectious disease doctors realized they needed anthropologists to figure out the cultural and social factors that were keeping people from getting vaccinated. So the CDC wanted me to help generate awareness about completing the eradication of smallpox and other infections.

Unfortunately, I learned the ivory-tower anthropologists were not really interested in anything as relevant as helping to eradicate an infectious disease that had been a scourge of human populations since earliest recorded history. Although many did make politically correct careers writing about how smallpox and other diseases introduced by Europeans had decimated Native American and other populations hundreds of years ago.

But in terms of contemporary medical practice, these academic anthropologists were more interested in studying how indigenous concepts of belly buttons related to beliefs about causes of illness (or maybe it was their own belly buttons they were interested in studying—I never quite got that straight).

Thankfully, my faculty advisor for my MD/PhD in anthropology, Nobel laureate Baruch Blumberg, wasn't one of those ivory-tower investigators. He did early research with Dr. Irving Millman to develop a hepatitis B vaccine before Merck took over the research. (Blumberg was awarded the Nobel Prize in 1976 for discovery of the virus.)

How the "golden age" is turning into a bureaucratic rage

The idea of being inoculated against every conceivable virus may sound appealing in terms of disease prevention. But as with pharmaceutical drugs, it seems the last generation of vaccines has really stuck us with some problems.

Part of this is due to the emergence of a sub-specialized field of "virology" that includes many scientists and physicians. These careerists see every health issue as a nail that needs to be pounded. So they focus on developing the technology to "hammer" viruses with vaccines.

Take the human papillomavirus (HPV) vaccine, for instance. This vaccine is very controversial, as I have often reported. In fact, some doctors and whistleblowers have described it as the greatest medical scandal of the century.

Why? First of all, in terms of the actual infection, HPV is not any more dangerous than viruses that cause the common cold. And there is no data showing the vaccine actually prevents cervical cancer. Finally, the vaccine works against only a few of the HPV strains—and the latest concern is that vaccinated women may be more likely to get infected with higher-risk strains of the virus.

Plus, there are already excellent, safe screening techniques that effectively help prevent cervical cancer (which is already relatively rare and becoming more rare) without any vaccination.

Sadly, the push to give every girl the HPV vaccine is less about public health and more about profits. Which is ironic because previous generations of vaccine developers, including Dr. Jonas Salk, gave away their creations for the benefit of humankind.

But that all changed when today's big pharma entered the vaccine industry. Drug companies started complaining they couldn't make enough money from vaccines. So our "public servants" in Congress got into the act of vaccination.

These bureaucrats were convinced to pass legislation making drug companies "immune" from malpractice lawsuits for all of the harm done by their vaccines. Instead, there is a vaccine injury compensation fund (which the taxpayers are stuck with). But according to many consumers, trying to get compensation for vaccine injuries is like trying to pass the proverbial camel through the eye of a needle.

So where are we today? Certainly, there are too many useless and dangerous vaccines. But that doesn't mean all of the current vaccines are worthless.

Vaccines you should consider

Pneumonia. Dr. Robert Austrian, my former professor at the University of Pennsylvania and colleague at the College of Physicians of Philadelphia, spent his career developing an effective vaccine for pneumonia.

Pneumonia is the eighth leading cause of death in Americans. And people over age 65 are particularly at risk. The good news is that the vaccine prevents pneumonia in 60 to 80 percent of people over age 65. That's why I think older people—and younger people with chronic diseases or immunological problems—may want to consider getting this vaccine. One vaccination will usually last your entire lifetime.

Chickenpox/shingles. Painful (and now distastefully well-publicized) shingles outbreaks are triggered by the same virus that causes chickenpox during childhood. If you had chickenpox or were vaccinated against it, the virus may be reactivated in later life as shingles.

One clinical trial of 38,000 people age 60 or older found that the shingles vaccine reduced the chance of suffering an outbreak by 51 percent. You've got better odds if you're under age 70—the vaccine was effective for 64 percent of that age group. But for those age 70 or older, the vaccine only reduced the risk of shingles by 34 percent.

So consider those odds when deciding whether to have a shingles vaccine.

Another factor to take into account is that shingles appears to have become much more common since universal childhood vaccination for chickenpox started. So that suggests you may have more protection from shingles if you actually had chickenpox as a child—rather than receiving the vaccine.

If you've never had chickenpox or been vaccinated against it, I recommend getting the vaccine. It can be very dangerous to get chickenpox as an adult. You may end up with serious complications like encephalitis, myocarditis (inflammation of the heart), or pancreatitis.

Vaccines that probably aren't worth it

Measles, mumps, rubella (MMR). Healthcare workers may try to tell you that even if you had this trifecta of diseases as a child, you still need a vaccination as an adult. But there is no reason for older adults to get this vaccine.

Even the vaccine-pushing CDC admits that if you were born before 1957, you're "generally considered immune" to measles and mumps.[3] You don't need any so-called "booster shot."

But today's children must have the MMR vaccine to be allowed to go to school (and of course, children have to go to school—typically without choice of public schools). So that means natural measles, mumps, and rubella immunity will soon be gone from the general population, requiring all children in every new generation to get the vaccine. Forever. What a gold mine in those steel needles.

Meningitis. The only time this vaccine is really useful is for young people who live in close quarters like college dorms, boarding schools, and camps where the disease has been known to spread. It seems that today the typical college student is more interested in having multiple "close contacts" than, say, hitting the books, so it might make sense for them.

But for older adults, the risk of getting meningitis is very low, making the vaccine unnecessary.

Tetanus. This vaccine doesn't protect against a virus, but rather against a toxic chemical made by anaerobic bacteria that hide deep in the soil. This bacteria can burrow deep into your injured tissues and cause infection.

Many doctors say they have never seen a single case of tetanus (lockjaw) in their entire medical careers. And the vaccine requires a booster every 10 years—which may unbalance the immune system. Taking all of that into account, tetanus vaccines may simply not be worth it—at any age.

Don't succumb to the politics of vaccinations

The big questions when it comes to all vaccines are really a matter of elementary logic. If vaccines work so well and provide immunity to those who get them, why are so many parents, teachers, physicians, and government bureaucrats so insistent about taking away all choice and forcing *everyone* to get potentially dangerous vaccines—because somehow the unvaccinated are a threat to others?

If you get a vaccine and become immune, then you are protected from that infection. Regardless of whether someone, or anyone, else is vaccinated and protected. So why bully, hector, and strong-arm everyone around you to get a vaccine for your own protection?

This issue came up in a recent Republican presidential debate. Three of the candidates, including two who are licensed physicians, raised serious questions about mandatory vaccination.

No matter where you come down on the subject, one thing is true. Without universal vaccination, there is still the opportunity for natural immunity to develop in the population (as it can with polio). But universal vaccination requires that everyone—everywhere, forever—get vaccines.

Bottom line: eliminating all natural immunity in the population may have long-term, unforeseen consequences for the human immune system and health.

So be aware and be informed the next time you hear you "must have" a certain vaccine. I always say the least medicine that works is the best medicine. Likewise, the fewer vaccines needed to sensibly protect your health, the better.

Chapter 90

7 natural ways to stay cold and flu free—
without vaccines

As you know, I and many others are troubled by the flu vaccine side effects that are reported in other countries (but that only some people, including my readers, ever seem to hear about in the U.S.). Serious side effects like convulsions, narcolepsy, and compromised immune systems.

And then there's the lack of evidence that this vaccine really works.

There is no evidence it really helps older people. There is no evidence it works in children. And last year's vaccine did not appear to work at all in anybody, anywhere.

So here's what I recommend. Every time a doctor, nurse, or pharmacist asks you to get a vaccine, ask them how much research they have done on the safety and effectiveness of the vaccine.

I estimate that I perform about 20 hours of research per month on the latest findings worldwide on vaccines, including the flu vaccine. That's 240 hours per year. Does your doctor, nurse, or pharmacist do that much research on what he or she recommends?

If you really want to stump your healthcare providers, ask them why they're pushing flu vaccines when there are 7 simple steps everyone can do to protect themselves from cold and flu viruses *better* than a flu vaccine can.

And then hand them the following list.

My top cold and flu fighters

1.) Don't automatically shake hands. Did you know that Donald Trump may be the first politician not to shake hands? This is because "The Donald" practices germ avoidance. Maybe it is because the one thing he cannot afford is to be sick. After all, cold and flu viruses are spread by contact, and who knows where someone's hands have been?

2.) Regularly wipe down your keypads and phones. Hilary Clinton is another politician who is good at "wiping" things clean (or maybe not so good, according to the FBI)—like personal computer servers that hold government classified documents. But I digress. Wiping down surfaces can be a very healthy practice.

Phones and keypads can be germ-breeding grounds. And they come into close contact with mouths, eyes, ears, and hands—all of which are disease transfer and entry points. So wipe down these devices regularly with alcohol, an alcohol-based hand sanitizer, or slightly soapy water (do not soak!) regularly.

3.) Stay sanitary in public restrooms. You already know to wash your hands after using the bathroom. But public restroom sanitation goes beyond that. As I reported in the past, public restroom door handles, toilets, faucets, soap dispensers, and hand driers are all loaded with bacteria and viruses.

After you wash your hands with soap and water, avoid the hand dryer. Research shows it just blows bacteria and viruses throughout the restroom. Instead, dry your hands with a paper towel and then use that towel to open the door when you exit the bathroom. Doorknobs are *teeming* with bacteria and viruses—especially in public restrooms.

In your own bathroom, close the lid before you flush to cut down on airborne germs.

4.) Carry hand sanitizer in your car. Now that we have to pump our own gasoline (except on the New Jersey Turnpike), gas pumps have become some of the most contaminated surfaces anywhere.

Visit the restroom and wash up after pumping gas, or clean your hands with sanitizer. In fact, you should always keep alcohol-based hand sanitizer (that doesn't contain the toxic chemical triclosan) in your car. Spritz your steering wheel and stick shift (or run your hands over them while they're still wet after applying gel sanitizer) whenever you get in the car—especially after pumping gas.

5.) Give your purse, briefcase, or bag a boost. Think of how many germs your satchels literally sit on when you put them on the floor in public places. And then how those germs can transfer to your hands when you pick up your bag.

Hang the strap or handle of your briefcase or purse over the back of a chair or other hook, or simply put your bag on a chair or bench—not on the dirty floor.

6.) Hold your breath. If someone in a public place is sneezing or coughing, just turn away and hold your breath for a few seconds. This will help keep you from inhaling the germs released into the air. Then, avoid touching surfaces—and don't touch your face—until you can get to a less contaminated area.

This precaution reminds me of school sports physicals. To check for a hernia, the doctor says, "Turn your head and cough." The cough increases the pressure inside the abdomen, which can cause any hernia to appear. I used to wonder about the complex pressure dynamics involved in coughing while turning the head. When I got to medical school and asked about it, the professor laughed and said the school doctor was just avoiding getting repeatedly coughed in his face.

7.) Don't ever underestimate the importance of sleep. There's plenty of evidence showing that lack of sleep increases your risk of getting a cold, flu, or other illness.

And now a new study quantifies that risk. Researchers found that people who sleep less than six hours a night are over *four times* more likely to get a cold than those who get more shuteye. (The study was done in Pittsburgh rather than New York because, you know…it's the "city that never sleeps.")

The researchers sequestered 164 volunteers in a hotel. Each study participant was given a cold virus via nasal drops, and then monitored for a week. The researchers discovered that the people who slept fewer than six hours per night were 4.2 times more likely to come down with a cold compared to people who slept seven or more hours per night. And people who spent less than five hours sleeping were 4.5 times more likely to get a cold.

In other words, just one extra hour in bed each night can help you avoid having to spend days in bed with a severe cold.

In fact, lack of sleep was the biggest risk factor for coming down with a cold in this study—more than age, stress levels, alcohol intake, ethnicity, education, or income. Even the great villain of government public health, smoking, was less likely to cause a cold than lack of sleep.

So if you're wondering why it seems so many people these days always seem to have a cold, it may simply be because of lack of sleep. Something the CDC has identified as yet another public health "epidemic."

Along with illnesses, the CDC says insufficient sleep is linked to motor vehicle accidents, industrial disasters, and medical errors. (When I was in medical training, we were told that young physicians don't need sleep, but apparently, sleep-deprived doctors finally "woke up" to the fact that doctors are human too).

The National Sleep Foundation did a survey in 2013 that found one out of five Americans get less than six hours of sleep on work nights, and more than half get less than seven hours' sleep. The U.S. ranked lowest in total sleep hours among the six countries surveyed.

Another new study sheds light on how the relationship between sleep and immunity works.

It has to do with how your body has a built-in 24-hour "clock" that regulates hormonal functions, physiology, and behavior. This clock is called the circadian cycle. And this cycle is found in every animal and plant that has a lifespan longer than 24 hours, including single-celled organisms. It's another factor that shows how closely we are tied to nature, or should be.

The researchers who conducted this study noted that disruption of the circadian cycle affects almost everyone in modern society, due to factors like artificial lighting, working at night and shift work, jet lag, and even the light emitted at night by cell phones and tablets.

In the study, the researchers disrupted the normal 24-hour clock of mice by putting them on 20-hour clock out of synch with the day-and-night, light-and-dark cycle.

The researchers found that even though the mice still got enough sleep, their immune response wasn't normal. Which made them more vulnerable to illness. That suggests that for good health and immunity, not just the *amount* of sleep but the *quality* and *timing* of that sleep are important.

In other words, if you want to fight flu, colds, and other viruses, get enough sleep *and* go to bed and wake up around the same time each day. (This gives new meaning to the old Italian-American saying about "going to the mattresses.")

And of course, help keep your immune system strong with a healthy diet and a supplement regimen that includes a high-quality B vitamin complex every day, 250 mg of vitamin C twice a day, and 10,000 IU of vitamin D per day.

Chapter 91

A cure for the common cold
(hiding in plain sight)

My late father-in-law, Jack O'Leary, used to ask me long ago why, with all their billions in tax-payer provided research money, the NIH wasn't working on a cure for the common cold (instead of all the arcane pursuits I would tell him about). As a journalist and advertising executive, he knew that kind of cure would provide the story—and the sale—of the century. Not to mention save millions of days of lost work and discomfort for Americans.

I had to break it to him that addressing such a "common" concern just wouldn't be in keeping with the "elevated pursuits" and self-opinions of the Mandarins of Medicine at the NIH. Which made him wonder, as a lifelong hard-working man and taxpayer, what exactly <u>we</u> (who pay the bills) are really getting out of all this research at NIH?

I only wish he were still here to see the results of a new study on what may very well be the elusive cure he asked about. Granted, this research didn't, and wouldn't, come from the NIH. But it should finally give many, many people some much needed relief.

As it turns out, the well-known herbal product *Echinacea* can reduce the symptoms and duration of a cold once you catch one.

Of course, Echinacea is well-known these days. It's been a common-sense folk remedy for centuries. And research on it has also been around for a long time. In fact, we published a study showing Echinacea's benefits for colds back in 1994—in the very first issue of the first medical research journal on CAM, which I had founded. And, even then, the results were "nothing to sneeze at."

But this new research should silence the critics and the skeptics once and for all. It's the largest clinical trial on Echinacea ever conducted. The study took place at the Common Cold Center in Cardiff, Wales, and involved 755 people over a period of four months. Those taking Echinacea had fewer colds, of shorter duration, with fewer recurrences of symptoms. The Echinacea treated group also used fewer over-the-counter remedies. And it was effective against influenza viruses as well. And this study is just in time to provide some hope for the flu since both the flu vaccine and the flu treatment, Tamiflu, have now been shown to be victims of more bad science in favor of drug profits.

In addition to being the largest study on Echinacea to-date, it is also the first to track its effectiveness against specific viruses of different varieties. And the fact that it fared so well makes sense, because Echinacea acts by stimulating the immune system to do its job—and get a jump on viruses before they multiply.

We rely on the immune system for combatting all germs—whether they're viral or bacterial. So immune-stimulators like Echinacea are a much better way to tackle infections of any type. Instead of just endlessly searching for antibiotics that are effective against only certain bacteria. Plus, antibiotics don't work at all for the viruses that cause colds and flus.

But Echinacea does. And now the research has become incontrovertible.

The dose used in this study to effectively prevent colds was 2,400 mg per day of a standardized, liquid Echinacea extract. The dose was increased to 4,000 mg per day if a participant came down with cold symptoms. Both doses were effective for their intended purposes. But one helpful hint to keep in mind is if you decide to use Echinacea this winter...

Participants in this study were asked to hold the liquid in their mouths for 10 seconds to ensure it would make direct local contact with any potential viruses in the upper throat.

Chapter 92

Defend against superbugs
with 5 simple steps

Antibiotics can certainly save lives. But their overuse allowed untreatable, antibiotic-resistant superbugs to develop.

One of the deadliest superbugs—called Clostridium difficile (C. difficile)—causes about 250,000 infections and leads to nearly 14,000 deaths each year, according to the Centers for Disease Control (CDC). It also costs the health care system at least $1 billion each year. In a moment, I'll tell you about five steps you can take to defend against C. difficile.

The term C. difficile comes from the Latin word meaning "difficult." And that word certainly applies here. The main symptom with C. difficile is deadly, dehydrating diarrhea (like cholera).

People who take antibiotic drugs are most at risk of getting a C. difficile infection because the drugs wipe out the good bacteria of the normal, healthy microbiome. These good bacteria influence digestion, nutrition, and inflammation, and probably other health factors, in addition to protecting against infectious diarrhea.

Age is also a factor. In fact, according to a new CDC study, one in every three C. difficile infections occurs in people ages 65 years and older. Plus, more than 100,000 cases occur in U.S. nursing homes, spreading from the hands and medical equipment of health professionals. Hospital surfaces are also rife with dangerous bacteria.

Unfortunately, the problem is only getting worse.

In fact, between 2000 and 2010, C. difficile-related hospitalizations doubled. And the rate is still climbing. The CDC attributes part of the dramatic increase to a dangerous new strain of C. difficile called NAP1.

Experts say antibiotics are clearly driving the whole problem. Yet poor detection and diagnostic methods also play a part. For example, in one recent case, a healthy 56-year-old woman developed sudden, painful diarrhea one morning. After a phone consultation, her doctor prescribed the wrong treatment. She went to the emergency room and died less than 36 hours later.

So until the CDC figures out how to turn the tide (don't hold your breath), I suggest you focus on prevention.

Here are some common sense, preventative steps you can take to protect yourself from antibiotic-resistant bacteria. Your choices will also help stem this growing public health problem:

1. **Practice good hygiene.** The simplest step you can take is to wash hands well with regular soap (*not antibacterial agents!*) and water. If you can't get to a wash basin, use alcohol-based hand sanitizers.

2. **Don't take antibiotics** unless you have a bacterial infection that requires treatment with an antibiotic. The best way to determine whether you really need an antibiotic—and which one(s)—is for your doctor to take a sample of the infected area. For example, take a swab of your sore throat and then submit it to the lab to (a) detect the presence of bacteria, (b) determine which bacteria and (c) test to see which antibiotics will work against it. Without taking these steps, it's guesswork.

3. If your doctor determines you *do* have an infection and need an antibiotic, **take the full dose for the full course of treatment**. Up to one-third of the time, patients don't take prescriptions correctly. And inappropriate practices double the use of antibiotics without any clinical benefit whatsoever.

4. **Only choose "organic" meat and dairy** that comes from animals raised without antibiotics.

5. **Keep your immune system in good working order**. This step is probably the single most important thing you can do for your health. Unfortunately, it's also probably the single most overlooked step in fighting deadly "superbugs."

You can keep your immune system healthy by taking a high-quality daily B vitamin complex, 500 mg of vitamin C twice per day, and 10,000 IU of vitamin D daily. Also, get selenium and zinc in your diet from healthy meats and seafood.

You can also boost your immune system when coming down with a cold or flu by taking the herb Echinacea purpurea (purple coneflower).

So while the CDC continues to wring its hands about C. difficile, keep washing yours. And follow my simple, sensible advice for good health and immunity. After all, the best offense we have against deadly superbugs is still a good defense.

PART 9

NATURAL WAYS TO NURTURE YOUR HEALTH

Chapter 93

10 signs you may have low vitamin D

I recommend having your vitamin D levels checked every 12 months through a routine blood test. Your doctor will order the test during your annual check-up. But between visits, and especially at the end of a long, dark winter, you should keep an eye out for 10 signs you may have a vitamin D deficiency. I'll tell you all about those important signs in a moment. But first, let's back up...

As you know, vitamin D is a critical nutrient used by every cell in your body. But an alert *Daily Dispatch* reader informed me that the U.S. Preventive Services Task Force (USPSTF) released a taxpayer-supported report claiming they did not find any evidence supporting the health benefits of supplemental vitamin D.

This report shows exactly what's wrong with healthcare in America. Not only do I *not* trust their findings. I don't trust the bureaucrats who fabricated the report.

These bureaucrats rely on government grants to keep studying the same old questions, using the same old failed approaches. No wonder they never find any solutions. Of course, they don't really want to find any new solutions—because that could put them out of a job or out of a cushy government committee assignment.

The problems start with the flawed and outdated Recommended Daily Allowances (RDAs).

The quasi-government committees that make up the RDAs still focus on preventing 19th century nutritional deficiency diseases. They steadfastly ignore the mounds of scientific evidence published by independent scientists. These well-designed, independent studies support the idea that higher, optimal doses of nutrients can prevent, treat and even cure common diseases.

But the government continues to spend your tax money on regular, ritualistic reviews that use incredibly small doses of vitamins. Then, when the study shows no benefit for the vitamin, they say, *see–that independent study was wrong*.

Today's academic-government-industrial-medical complex will never admit to knowing what the leading natural scientists and philosophers have known for ages—that nutrition is critical for all health and it's involved in all disease.

Though, if they *did* admit this truth, they would find themselves in the company of every genius from Hippocrates to Thomas Sydenham and Thomas Jefferson to Thomas Alva Edison.

But somehow, the bureaucrats believe they know better.

So nothing ever changes—officially.

But, as I said earlier, an incredible amount of scientific evidence supports the need for higher levels of many nutrients for optimal health, including vitamin D.

Actually, the case with vitamin D is even a little different.

You see, with vitamin D, we are not just talking about how higher levels can prevent many common cancers, increase survival time, and improve quality of life in cancer patients. We're not just talking about how higher levels can help prevent heart disease, kidney disease, neurological diseases like multiple sclerosis, and other common problems.

There is, in fact, an actual worldwide deficiency of vitamin D. And evidence links many medical problems with this deficiency.

But government health experts wear blinders when it comes to vitamin D. They still only focus its role in bone health, which is based on discoveries made in the 1920s.

But in the last century, science proved that vitamin D is critical to every cell, tissue and organ in the body—not just the bones.

Medically speaking, there are 10 clear warning signs that you may have a vitamin D deficiency. Doctors see these signs every single day.

1. Bone pain

If you suffer from ongoing bone pain not explained by a "pathologic" diagnosis, you may have low vitamin D.

2. Muscle weakness

Muscles have vitamin D receptors and must have a constant supply to function.

3. Chronic infections and respiratory illnesses

Scientific studies show that vitamin D helps defend against infections and respiratory illnesses, especially in children. In fact, chronic respiratory infections in children are a strong indicator of a vitamin D deficiency. Instead of addressing this issue, the Centers for Disease Control wants all children to get the flu vaccine, which does not prevent the flu and appears to cause a six-fold increase in the risk of respiratory illness.

Thankfully, some doctors are getting the message. In fact, doctors with the prestigious Mayo Clinic advise that you need vitamin D to help your body fight infections. And if you're troubled by frequent infections, they advise getting a vitamin D blood measurement at your doctor's office.

4. Low mood

We know vitamin D helps produce adequate levels of serotonin, a critical neurotransmitter in the brain that produces feelings of well-being. And many solid, independent studies link low vitamin D levels with depression.

Of course, the popular "antidepressant" drugs on the market artificially raise serotonin levels through the roundabout way of preventing its re-uptake from the synapses.

Unfortunately, these selective serotonin reuptake inhibitors (SSRIs) only work in one out seven patients. And new research suggests the one patient who *does* feel better after taking the SSRI probably *only* does so because of a placebo effect. Not because the drug actually works.

Plus, SSRIs cause a wide range of harmful side effects.

Evidence links low vitamin D with increased anxiety, which frequently accompanies depression. Aside from clinical conditions like anxiety or depression, vitamin D's effect on serotonin can impact mood in anybody. So if your mood is off, it may be a sign of vitamin D deficiency.

5. Abnormal sweating

Abnormal sweating can be a sign of vitamin D deficiency. In fact, years ago, doctors commonly asked pregnant mothers if they experienced heavy sweating, since nutritional deficiency can occur under the strenuous demands of a growing baby.

6. Congestive heart failure

Maintaining sufficient vitamin D is a long-term, lifetime proposition. And if you don't maintain adequate levels over your lifetime, it even affects your heart muscle. In fact, the National Institutes of Health now recognizes scientific studies that show vitamin D deficiency can lead to congestive heart failure.

7. High blood pressure

Researchers link high blood pressure, a major cause of heart disease, with low vitamin D. In fact, a prospective study on women conducted by Harvard University over many years found that women with low vitamin D had 66 percent higher risk of high blood pressure compared to women with the highest levels of D.

8. Chronic pain

Studies show low vitamin D levels increase the risk of suffering from chronic pain. In fact, general malaise or fatigue may also be associated with lack of vitamin D. In athletes, lack of endurance may be a sign of low vitamin D levels.

9. Skin conditions

Your skin improves with moderate sun exposure. And studies show you can improve a variety of common skin conditions—such as dermatitis and eczema—by supplementing with vitamin D. In fact, many forward-thinking doctors now use vitamin D therapy to treat psoriasis patients. Plus, according to the Mayo Clinic, no matter what treatment is used, psoriasis is harder to manage unless vitamin D levels are adequate.

10. Kidney problems

Vitamin D is also important for the kidneys, which help make the active form of vitamin D in the body. So if you have kidney disease caused by cardiovascular disease or diabetes, low vitamin D contributes to this vicious cycle. Simply getting older can make it harder for you to get enough vitamin D. The body just doesn't activate as much of it as you age. Of course, most the medical conditions I mentioned above also become more common with age. So while vitamin D is important throughout your life, it's especially important as you get older. Which is why it's critical to stay vigilant. Be on the lookout for any of the telltale symptoms listed above. And again, have your levels checked annually. The ideal vitamin D level for optimal health is 30 ng/ml or more.

To reach and maintain this optimal level, make sure to supplement with 5,000 IU of vitamin D daily. If you don't like taking pills, you can get vitamin D in a liquid form, which is now available together with astaxanthin, which you can take straight on the tongue or add to a small glass of natural fruit juice or milk in the morning.

Chapter 94

Avoid antibiotics, fight gum disease, and more with the all-natural little blue wonder

We already know blueberries are helpful for memory and cognition, and research shows they also help protect against cardiovascular disease, diabetes, and obesity. Research has even uncovered the beneficial effects of blueberries on dental health and reducing the use of antibiotics.

It's quite an extensive array of benefits, considering this berry has only recently come under scientific scrutiny.

Wild blueberries are three times better for you than farm-grown fruit

There are two major types of blueberries that grow in the U.S. The low-bush blueberry, which is the wild variety (*Vaccinium angustifolium*) and a high-bush variety. High bush blueberries have been cultivated to grow at a higher elevation than wild blueberries would typically grow in their rocky native soil.

Blueberries are rich sources of phenolic acids, which have both antioxidant and anti-inflammatory properties.

Of course, the reason that plants produce bioactive phenols and other constituents is to protect them under the strenuous conditions of the wild. Cultivated plants have it "easy" by comparison and need to produce far fewer phenolic and other bioactive compounds for their growth and protection.

Research shows that total phenolic content is over three times higher in the wild compared to the cultivated varieties. Which means wild blueberries are three times better for your health.

Beyond phenols, there are many other constituents in blueberries that contribute to their total antioxidant capacity.

For instance, blueberries also have abundant anthocyanins, which give them their characteristic dark blue color. Like phenols, anthocyanins have anti-inflammatory properties and act as natural antioxidants.

Heart benefits that rival pharmaceutical drugs

One study looked at the benefits of blueberry anthocyanins at protecting the linings of blood vessels from damage.

Blueberries have also been studied for their ability to prevent atherosclerosis, or hardening of the arteries.

One study looked at the effects of wild blueberry powder on **fat accumulation in white blood cells** — which is one of the culprits in atherosclerosis.

The researchers found that even low concentrations of blueberry anthocyanins reduced fat accumulation. And two other blueberry components—syringic and gallic acid—were also found to be effective at lowering fat accumulation in white blood cells.

Best of all, the concentrations of blueberry anthocyanins found to be effective in these studies are readily achievable in your everyday diet with proper supplementation.

Another clinical trial showed that daily blueberry consumption improved **blood pressure** and **arterial stiffness** in postmenopausal women suffering from early-stage high blood pressure.

The study involved 48 participants who received either 22 grams of freeze-dried blueberry powder or 22 grams of a placebo powder daily. After eight weeks, the blueberry group's blood pressure was significantly lower. Systolic pressure dropped from 138 to 131 mmHg, and diastolic pressure dropped from 80 to 75 mmHg.

An effect that significant may very well allow older individuals to opt for blueberry supplements instead of blood pressure drugs to treat hypertension.

Biochemical measurements were also done on the study participants. The women who ate blueberries had increased production of nitrous oxide, a very powerful relaxant of blood vessels. Basically, nitrous oxide widens the vessels and reduces blood pressure, while supplying good blood circulation to the brain and other tissues.

To recap, in terms of cardiovascular benefits, research shows that blueberries do it all—reducing the oxidation and inflammation that damage blood vessels, curtailing the accumulation of fats that causes atherosclerosis in damaged arteries, and lowering blood pressure and arterial stiffness—which are both major factors for heart disease.

But the benefits of blueberries don't stop with the heart.

The new "brain food"

Other research shows that whole, fresh, high-bush blueberries (*Vaccinium corymbosum*) help reduce the **oxidative stress** that can lead to **age-related brain damage**.

In one study, lab animals that ate blueberries were protected from oxidation and destruction of brain cells. And their brain tissue was actually able to repair damage due to age-related changes.

Biochemical measurements also demonstrated that blueberries supported antioxidant activity in a number of the animals' cellular functions. In addition, key neurotransmitter activity was increased in the animals' brain and nervous tissues.

Tiny berries offer big immune benefits

For the immune system, one study showed that six weeks of daily ingestion of blueberry powder **increased natural killer cells** (T cell counts) in sedentary men and women. These white blood cells are key to protecting the body from infections, cancer, and other diseases. My colleague Dr. Jerry Thornthwaite discovered natural killer cells back in the 1970s, and their importance continues to be uncovered.

Blueberries may also be an unexpected weapon in the war against obesity and diabetes.

Based on the research I reported above about reducing fat accumulation, you might be wondering if blueberries have a role in preventing obesity. Indeed, scientific research shows blueberry anthocyanins can help **prevent weight gain, support weight loss, and help prevent the metabolic complications of obesity like diabetes.**

When certain white blood cells (macrophages) infiltrate fat tissue, they contribute to complications like type 2 diabetes. But anthocyanin-rich fractions from blueberries were found to reduce inflammation and fat tissue formation in one study.

These compounds also restored insulin and glucose uptake of fat tissue.

Wild blueberry consumption also showed benefits regarding glucose metabolism in a lab animal model of metabolic syndrome and diabetes.

The important advice your dentist won't give you

Latest research demonstrates how blueberries can help fight **gum disease** (periodontitis) and also **reduce the use of antibiotics**.

Gum disease can result when dental bacteria build up plaque on teeth, causing the gums to become inflamed. Researchers found that wild blueberry extract (remember, wild blueberry is about three times more potent than domestic) helps prevent dental plaque formation, providing a new natural therapy for periodontitis and reducing the need for antibiotics.

Blueberry polyphenols have already been shown to work against foodborne disease-causing bacteria, so the scientists tested whether they also fight a microbe called Fusobacterium, which is one of the main culprits in periodontitis.

In the lab, they tested extracts from the wild, low-bush blueberry and found they inhibit growth of this bacteria and its ability to form plaque. The blueberry extracts also blocked a molecular pathway involved in causing inflammation.

The researchers believe the best approach would be to develop a special oral device to slowly release blueberry extract into the mouth and onto the teeth after deep dental cleaning. But you don't necessarily have to wait for development and FDA approval of expensive treatments with new device, or a trip to the dentist for an unpleasant deep cleaning.

Blueberry extract is available in a water-soluble, powdered form that can be added to any beverage. It's designed to be swallowed so it can be absorbed in the blood and tissues. But you can also hold the beverage in your mouth for a while to savor the flavor before swallowing—and do some good for your teeth and gums too.

Look for a dietary supplement or water-soluble powder containing 400 mg of blueberry extract.

Chapter 95

African "tree of life" yields a nutritional gold mine—proving this is one superfood worthy of the title

Every other week it seems something new is being touted as the next "superfood." So it's hard to take the claims seriously. But when it comes to baobab, there's plenty of truth behind the hype. Making it a true "superfood" worthy of your attention.

The fruit, leaves, and seeds of this massive tree have more vitamin C than oranges. More calcium than milk. More antioxidants than strawberries.

Plus, baobab fruit is packed with minerals like magnesium—which is essential for everything from heart to bone health.

If you've never heard of baobab (pronounced bay-oh-bab), that's because it's virtually impossible to find the fruit in the U.S. But the good news is that you can now get the benefits of this healthful fruit without having to travel all the way to Africa.

How one massive tree provides such an abundance of sustenance?

In Africa, baobab is known as the "tree of life." Fitting, since some of these massive trees are thought to be up to 6,000 years old.

Baobab grows throughout the woodlands, grasslands, and savannahs of sub-Saharan Africa. It can reach heights of 75 feet, and its roots can spread even further.

African communities rely on the whole tree for their daily existence. The cork-like bark is used to make cloth and rope. The trunk stores water during times of drought. The leaves are used in traditional medicines. And the coconut-sized fruit is both tasty and nutritious.

And here's the impressive amount of nutrients in this "tree of life."

Calcium. Research shows that baobab leaves are very rich in calcium—between 1,500 to 2,250 mg in every 100 grams. Only amaranth, okra, onion leaves, and sorrel provide better plant-based sources of calcium. And the same amount of whole milk only has 113 mg of this essential mineral.

Vitamin C. Baobab fruit pulp has between 150 to 500 mg of this disease-fighting vitamin per 100 grams. How does that stack up to other food sources of C? Well, oranges only have 53 mg, kiwis have 93 mg, and yellow bell peppers have 184 mg.

Magnesium. Baobab pulp has an average of 195 mg of magnesium per 100 grams. In contrast, magnesium-rich foods like dark leafy greens have 79 mg. Mackerel has 97 mg. Only squash and pumpkin seeds have more magnesium than baobab.

Antioxidants. Baobab's antioxidant levels are (almost) off the charts. One gram of baobab fruit pulp has an integral antioxidant capacity (IAC) reading of 11, and the leaves have an IAC of 9. Check out how that compares to the IACs of popular high-antioxidant fruits: strawberries (1), kiwi (0.3), apple (0.2), and orange (0.1).

Polyphenols. Baobab is loaded with these disease-fighting compounds. In fact, one study showed that baobab extract mixed into water helped people digest dietary starch better—and reduced their blood glucose levels. Which suggests that baobab may be effective at helping fight diabetes. Other studies have revealed that the fruit has potent anti-inflammatory effects.

And the above list is just the beginning… research also shows baobab is a good source of manganese, phosphorus, potassium, and zinc. It also has A and B vitamins and lutein—which is essential for eye health.

So how can you benefit from this tree of life?

As I mentioned earlier, you're not likely to find the actual baobab fruit in your produce section. Unfortunately it just doesn't travel well. So most Americans can't sit down to a menu of dishes made from baobab leaves or fruit.

However, baobab is now more readily available as a powdered ingredient. And can be found as a dietary supplement. A combination of dried baobab powder with other supplement ingredients can provide a potent addition to your daily regimen.

I recommend 500-1,000 mg per day.

Since the optimal quantities of baobab don't really fit into a pill or capsule, the best form is a water-soluble powder. Mix the powder with water, tea, or juice, and you'll get a health boost you'll never achieve with sports drinks, so-called "hydration" drinks, or energy drinks.

Chapter 96

The single most important thing you can do to prevent premature death

As the U.S. government science bureaucrats continue dithering over recommendations about vitamin D intake, some real scientists in Germany (and yes, even some right here at home) are making it perfectly clear: Vitamin D prevents premature death. Plus, it reduces death rates from all causes.

So why is the U.S. hemming and hawing—and confusing patients and doctors alike?

Blind leading the blind

Over the past three decades, many scientists who study chronic diseases have stumbled into studying diet and nutrition. They often lack any understanding of nutrition as a fundamental part of human biology and behavior. And despite their ignorance on matters of nutrition, they publish their findings. And the government science bureaucrats jump on the research—and the politically correct bandwagon.

But one source has always been an exception to the rule. *The American Journal of Clinical Nutrition* (AJCN) doesn't report spurious statistical findings like those that can be found in other journals.

And across the Atlantic, German scientists tend to put out reliable information on nutrition. That's because they know how to conduct scientific investigations on human biology. They have consistently been way ahead of the United States in investigating natural and nutritional approaches to health and medicine.

Research you can trust

The trustworthy team at AJCN published a report in their April 2013 issue that takes a close look at vitamin D.

In it, a team of scientists measured vitamin D levels in nearly 10,000 people ages 50 to 74 years. Another 5,500 participants were measured at 5 year-follow-up. All deaths were recorded during an average follow-up period of 9.5 years. During the follow-up period about 10 percent of study participants died: 43.3 percent from cancer, 35.0 percent from heart disease, and 5.5 percent of respiratory diseases.

People with the lowest vitamin D levels were more likely to have died of any cause, and of cancer, heart disease, and respiratory disease specifically.

They also found a dose-response relationship between low vitamin D levels and death—that is, the lower the vitamin D, the higher the mortality rate.

This is the best kind of epidemiological study, with the strongest kind of results that can be performed on human populations. It makes it perfectly clear: Higher vitamin D levels protect against premature death—as well as all the leading causes of death.

It's never too late to up your D

Plenty of studies prove the dangerous effects of lack of vitamin D in childhood, but these highlight the fact that even in adults—and older adults at that—low levels of D have bad health effects.

On the flip side, that means that even later in life, you can improve your health and longevity by increasing your vitamin D intake.

And here's some more good news: Vitamin D can be free. All you need to do is expose your skin to the sun and your body will activate its own vitamin D.

During the Fall and Winter months you can build up healthy vitamin D levels with appropriate high-quality supplements. If you have any reason to believe you are not getting enough vitamin D, ask your doctor to measure your levels the next time you have a routine blood sample taken for testing. If you're below 75 nmol/L—and especially below 30 nmol/L—it's time to add a high-quality supplement.

Chapter 97

Today's TRUE nutrient deficiencies

Fourteen years ago, two landmark studies were published in the *Journal of the American Medical Association (JAMA)*. They revealed that the dietary standards set by the U.S. government are grossly inadequate.

These two studies should have changed the way doctors viewed the role of optimal nutrition in preventing and treating chronic diseases.

Yet, here we are—over a decade later. And the government recommended dietary allowances (RDAs) are still the only benchmark conventional doctors acknowledge and recommend.

The information on nutrition and health that the public is given (and not given) by the government sometimes reminds me of the book *Catch-22* by Joseph Heller. Really one scene in particular that depicts an aviator being hit by anti-aircraft flak. The protagonist, Yossarian (Alan Arkin in the movie), labors carefully to bandage the relatively superficial wounds on the injured flyer's arms and legs. Yet, when he finishes, he opens the flyer's heavy flight jacket only to find his intestines spilling out through a fatal abdominal wound.

Bloody and graphic, yes. But not that far off from how the government handles its RDAs. Follow them, and we're all like poor, well-intentioned Yossarian. Applying Band-Aids to potentially fatal health problems.

The government guidelines on nutrient intakes are hopelessly outdated.

They were designed to prevent frank vitamin and nutritional deficiencies. And diseases like beri-beri, kwashiorkor, pellagra, rickets, and scurvy.

So yes, the government is keeping us safe from some deadly scourges— *of the 19th century*. But what about what's killing us in the 21st century?

Will they ever move on to the true nutritional medicine proposed 10 years ago in those landmark *JAMA* articles?

Government RDAs don't even come close

In those old *JAMA* articles, the researchers gathered more than 150 studies. And after carefully examining all the data, they determined just how much of several common vitamins most people need each day to help prevent today's chronic diseases. Including heart disease, cancer, diabetes and osteoporosis, as well as infectious diseases.

But, in many cases, what they found was vastly different from even the most current government RDAs.

Take a look at the chart at the end of this chapter, which shows the current RDA of several specific nutrients, compared to the optimal amounts determined by the *JAMA* articles back in 2002.

Obviously, the government is still hopelessly out of touch with what the human body really needs for optimal health.

One step forward, two steps back

Today the government does (finally) recognize that vitamin D deficiency is a serious problem—even by their standards. Current estimates show that up to 30 percent of the population isn't getting the RDA. But the true dimensions of the worldwide vitamin D deficiency epidemic are likely a lot higher from the standpoint of optimal nutrition. Meanwhile, at the same time, they tell everyone to avoid sun exposure, which is critical for achieving and maintaining even the RDA vitamin D levels. (For the record, you should aim for 15-20 minutes of direct sun exposure—on the arms and legs—per day, at least three times per week. *Without* sunscreen.)

The government also continues to dwell on nutritional "problems" that don't really exist. For example, they still focus on iron deficiency as a "major" public health issue. (Despite the fact that it occurs only in 11 to 16 percent of *some* subgroups of children and child-bearing women.) Granted, they now recognize that their old iron measurement techniques leave a lot to be desired. Of course, they haven't done anything about their standards.

And one troubling new development that no one is currently talking about is the prevalence of iodine deficiency—especially in young women. We thought we had that problem ended by adding iodine to our salt supply. But with the CDC constantly telling people to lower their salt intake (to potentially dangerously low levels at that), it's really no wonder this problem has emerged.

The best way to get everything you need for optimal health

Those landmark *JAMA* articles also pointed out, as I have for 30 years, that the stand-alone nutrients recognized by the RDAs actually fall short in yet another way when it comes to helping you get the optimal nutrition you need...

You see, on their own, these vitamins don't include the other critical nutritional components in healthy foods and vegetables (like lycopene and lutein, for instance).

It stands to reason that plants, which thrive outdoors, must have some built-in protection from the elements. Indeed, they've developed antioxidants to protect them from oxidation and "free radicals" that are inevitable parts of constant exposure to oxygen in the atmosphere and to regular climatic events.

So eating a nutritious, balanced diet is truly the only way to get all the biologically-active and beneficial compounds you need for optimal health, whether the RDAs recognize them or not.

Of course, I don't mean to diminish the importance of those RDA nutrients. It's just that you'll get even more benefits if you opt for whole foods that contain them. Because these food sources also offer other benefits that still aren't even on the government's RDA radar screen yet.

The following is a chart comparing the current government RDA and the optimal amount of nutrients you truly need.

Nutrient	Current government RDA	Optimal amount (via 2002 JAMA articles)
Folate	400 micrograms	800 micrograms
Vitamin A	3,000 IU for men 2,333 IU for women	15,000 IU
Vitamin B6	1.3 milligrams for adults up to 50 1.7 milligrams for men over 50 1.5 milligrams for women over 50	3 milligrams
Vitamin B12	2.4 micrograms	9 micrograms
Vitamin C	90 milligrams for men 75 milligrams for women	2,000 milligrams
Vitamin D	600 IU	2,000 IU (but safe in doses up to 30,000 IU)
Vitamin E	15 milligrams	70 milligrams

Here are the best food sources for the RDA nutrients listed in the chart above.

Folate: dark green, leafy vegetables (like broccoli, Brussels sprouts, cabbage, kale, spinach); asparagus; avocados; bananas; beans; oranges; yeast

Vitamin A: organ meats, fish, shellfish, egg yolks, fruits and vegetables (some carotenoids in fruits and vegetables are converted to vitamin A in the body)

Vitamin B6: poultry, fish, shellfish, soybeans, bananas, nuts, peas

Vitamin B12: poultry, fish, meat, eggs

Vitamin C: broccoli, citrus fruits, melons, peppers, strawberries, tomatoes

Vitamin D: saltwater fish, fish liver oil, liver, fortified milk (and while it's not a food, don't forget about a critical source of vitamin D: sunshine)

Vitamin E: nuts, vegetable oils, wheat germ

One quick note for vegetarians and vegans. Take another look above at vitamins A, B6, B12, and D. Most of these key nutrients come from animal sources. Unfortunately, the average human just can't get optimal nutrition from a diet that doesn't include meat. So vegetarians and vegans should always take high-quality supplements to achieve optimal levels.

Getting to the "guts" of the problem

Unfortunately, the government is no closer today to giving people truly sound nutritional advice than they were a decade ago. Like poor, misguided Yossarian from *Catch-22*, the "experts" can't seem to get at the real "guts" of the problem.

I remember exchanging communications a few years ago with one of the leading Ph.D. nutritional experts at Johns Hopkins in Baltimore. He's a very influential figure in the American Society for Clinical Nutrition and plays a big role in helping determine the RDAs. I asked him flat out why he still didn't accept that optimal nutrient intakes need to be higher than the established RDAs. He responded simply, "There is no evidence."

By what standard?

Maybe he and his colleagues haven't been reading the *Journal of the American Medical Association* for the past 10+ years.

But if we wait for all the evidence sought by some of these non-medical, Ph.D., career scientists we'll all be dead. Probably from some preventable disease.

The evidence is here—and has been for over a decade. So do yourself, and your health, a favor and forget about the "bare minimum" RDAs. Instead, strive for optimal nutrition.

Focus your diet on the foods listed above, and fill in any gaps with good, high-quality nutritional supplements.

Chapter 98

The dangerous delusion of "detox" drinks

Here we go again…A tried and true tenet of natural healing is being potentially misunderstood by mainstream medicine and meanwhile exploited by the quick-fix (and quick-buck) "health" marketeers.

This time it's with the delusion of so-called "detox" products and drinks. But unfortunately, the detox-in-a-blender fad bears no resemblance to any authentic detox regimen.

What is detox, anyway?

Some of the new drink marketeers may not know it, but it actually stands for detoxification. And that can mean two very different things from a health perspective:

1. To the medical establishment, it's about appropriate treatment for drug or alcohol intoxication or addiction.

2. In natural medicine, it's a way of restoring the body, mind, and spirit to their most cleansed, balanced and healthful state.

The characters running around promoting "detox" drinks (who seem hyped up on their own adrenaline) could use a good detox themselves. They need to slow down, and take time (and even lie down) for an authentic, natural detox treatment…as I'll demonstrate in just a moment.

Heavy metals and other "toxins"

A really unfortunate thing about the wildly incorrect messages about detox is that real detoxification is an important cornerstone of good health. It's something we should all do periodically to get rid of toxic accumulations that slow down our bodies and cloud our minds.

The human body accumulates toxins, like heavy metals, that the liver can't effectively metabolize and the kidney can't adequately excrete. Metals like **lead** or excess **iron** can accumulate and poison virtually any and all tissues of the body. Fortunately, there is a real medical treatment for effectively eliminating lead that I will tell you about shortly. Other toxins, including chemicals from pesticides, for example, accumulate in body fat.

Note to dieters: One of many reasons I recommend slow, steady weight loss is that accumulated toxic chemicals trapped in fat tissues are released into the blood and body when fat is metabolized due to caloric restriction. A sudden release of toxins into the bloodstream can temporarily poison other tissues in the body, causing symptoms that may convince you that your weight loss is doing more harm than good, at least temporarily.

But back to the medical treatment I mentioned for eliminating excess lead from the body. Chelation therapy using infusion with a substance called EDTA has been approved for use by the FDA for lead poisoning. The EDTA chemically traps the heavy metal so it can be eliminated in the urine. After many years of study, research recently established that chelation therapy with EDTA, together with vitamin C, is effective for treating and reversing cardiovascular disease.

Mainstream medical "experts" were quick to claim it was the vitamin C—not the chelation therapy itself—that was responsible for the positive effect. (Yes, these are indeed the same "experts who are usually quick to claim that vitamins have no effect on heart disease, or anything else, for that matter!)

Is your body poisoning itself?

"Alternative" or natural medicine holds that everyday food consumption results in toxic buildup. The idea is that when we break down the food's constituents and our gut bacteria carry out their own metabolism, the result is that we produce chemical products that are "foreign" to the body—termed "auto-intoxication."

This is a 19th century concept that we now realize is more complex in terms of the microbiome and the role of probiotics and fiber.

Modern research validates genuine detoxification

Some of my own research in the late 20th century actually validated some of the 19th century ideas about auto-intoxication. Based on a theory from Dr. Nicholas Petrakis at University of California, San Francisco, I performed an analysis with colleagues at the National Cancer Institute (NCI) on the US National Health and Nutrition Examination Survey.

We found that less frequent bowel movements (constipation) in women is related to higher rates of breast cancer.

Dr. Petrakis thought that constipation allowed toxic, carcinogenic breakdown products to accumulate in the intestines, which would then be absorbed back into the blood and could cause cancer in tissues. We found such results for the most common cancer in women. But we were quietly told by our political bosses at NCI not to pursue this research because nobody really believed in those old ideas anymore… despite the evidence we had just found.

Change your body and your life with true detoxification

So far I've covered two types of detoxification: alcohol/drug detox and removal of heavy metals and chemicals from the body. But it's the cleansing of this "auto-intoxification" that applies to the vast majority of us.

What I hope you take away from this is that the true detoxification, or cleansing, that I'm about to describe, can change your body and your life. All those ways in which you feel sluggish, "stuck," or foggy—this type of detoxification can reverse them.

But here's the thing: You'll have to slow down and take your time to reap the rewards (in fact, the slowing down is a reward in itself). *This detox does not come in a bottle*. Rest and relaxation, good air, pure water, and "energy" form the foundation of any authentic detox.

This approach is bound to be good for whatever ails you.

Ancient detoxification rituals get new life

The idea of accumulated toxins actually goes back before the 19th century—*way before*.

Ayurveda, the 5,000-year-old healing system of India, recognizes toxic buildup, and that's why purification plays such a crucial role in Ayurvedic medicine. The difference is that while Western natural medicine is concerned with *products of digestion*, Ayurveda places emphasis on the toxic effects of poorly or *undigested food* (or thoughts, or experiences—all known as *ama*).

Did you notice I referred to "purification," and not "detoxification"? Rather than thinking of the process as "de-" anything, Ayurveda takes a more positive approach. The mainstay of Ayurvedic purification is an intensive treatment regimen that's custom tailored to each individual based on constitution, season, medical or emotional conditions, and other factors.

Panchakarma (PK), or "five actions," is not a just a quick "do-it-yourself" detox in a bottle. It requires the help of an Ayurvedic practitioner, who will design a program just for you. The program entails a customized, combination herbal remedy, modified diet of easily digestible foods, a schedule that honors nature's daily cycles, and daily treatments performed by highly trained therapists. PK can last anywhere from a few days to more than a month. Some facilities offer outpatient services, but many people choose to stay at the treatment center so they can focus without distraction on the intense purification they're undergoing.

And the treatments? While they're not quite like what you'll experience at a typical spa, they are incredibly relaxing and balancing. Well—most of them anyway.

Some of the actions of PK are not practiced in the west because they're somewhat extreme and unpleasant. One, the *basti*, or enema, is frequently included as a substitute, but may not constitute what you might consider a typical day at the spa. But together with the PK's heat-based massages, aromatherapy, and stimulating treatments, it creates a purification experience like no other.

While PK is based on age-old understanding of toxic buildup, it may address the more modern variety as well. Preliminary research has shown that its treatments can mobilize and remove toxic, fat-soluble pesticides and agrochemicals from the body.

So as you can see, an authentic detox is nothing like downing an energy drink (which the FDA is now warning are actually toxic themselves). A major benefit to following any of the authentic, natural approaches is that they make you slow down and take time to focus, relax, and rejuvenate. No one has figured out how to put that in a bottle just yet.

As former Surgeon General Dr. C. Everett Koop used to tell me, sometimes the "tincture of time" is the best medicine of all.

If you need help finding an Ayurvedic practitioner near you, try the National Ayurvedic Medical Association at www.ayurvedanama.org. Their website has a directory of practitioners.

Chapter 99

7 sneaky foods that pretend to be healthy

Every day, people choose foods that seem healthy but really aren't. Here's a look at seven of these sneaky "health" foods.

#1: Banana chips. These snacks are made from a fruit that is naturally high in potassium—and fruits and vegetables are generally healthy foods. But just like their unhealthy potato chip cousins, banana chips are deep fried in high-calorie oil.

Just half a cup of banana chips can have around 200 calories and 10 grams of saturated fat.

Meanwhile, a large, fresh banana is virtually fat free and contains only about 120 calories. Plus, it has more vitamins and minerals than banana chips, because frying can destroy vital nutrients. If you like bananas, you're much better off sticking with the whole, uncooked fruit.

#2: Energy bars. You can find energy bars sneaked into the grocery aisle with healthy foods, or even in the weight-loss section. But beware. Many of these crazed concoctions average 200 to 250 calories each. And since most energy bars tend to be small, it's not unusual to down a couple a day as a supposedly nutritious "snack."

But then you find that you've eaten as many calories as you'd get in a healthy, large lunch or moderate dinner. In that sense, energy bars are meal "replacements," with all of the calories (and more) but few of the nutrients—and none of the enjoyment, satisfaction, or benefits of eating a real meal.

The sugar content can also be quite high, accounting for many of energy bars' empty calories, and making some of them no better than candy bars. And they're not even as tasty.

If you need a portable, "on-the-go" snack, try a hard-boiled egg or a fresh banana.

#3: Muesli. This is a health food store staple and hard to pronounce, so it must be good for you, right?

Muesli is marketed as a healthy alternative to sugary breakfast cereals. And while there are some brands that have fewer than 200 calories per serving, there are others that have a whopping 600 calories per cup—with high fat content and ridiculous amounts of added sugar, to boot.

If you like having some sort of cereal in the morning, you can make your own healthy version. Buy bulk oats, sunflower seeds, dried fruits (cut into small bits), and some nuts, mix them together, and add milk. Alternately, eggs are a great, nutritious way to start the day.

#4: Prepared salads. There is nothing healthier than a fresh, green salad. But when you order a salad at a restaurant, watch out for the extra calories, fat, and sugar often used to dress it up so it tastes better.

If you trust the basic ingredients, ask for the dressing on the side. Or ask for olive oil and vinegar (or lemon) and dress your own salad at the table. And of course, you can also make these dressings at home. Don't ever buy or use prepared salad dressings. To keep your olive oil fresh, only buy as much as you will use in a three-month period.

#5: Sushi. This trendy food is bound to be good for you, right? After all, what could be healthier than raw fish (even if you're not a seal)?

While the nutrient content of sushi is indeed healthy, any uncooked food can pose a risk of infection or infestation with parasites. Although the high standards of real sushi restaurants present a minimal risk, watch out for the proliferation of "sushi-on-the-side" eateries where chefs aren't well versed in proper sushi preparation.

You also need to be careful of mercury contamination. Mercury is common in fish, and because many of the fish used in sushi are large predators at the top of the marine food chain, they can have high concentrations of mercury.

Tuna is particularly problematic. Some experts say adults should avoid eating more than 6 ounces of tuna sushi per week to make sure they don't consume too much mercury. And pregnant women and children should eat even less.

#6: Low-fat yogurt. I have often warned that many of the processed foods labeled as "low-fat" contain extra sugar to make them taste better. And studies are showing this added sugar—*not* naturally occurring fat—is the real culprit behind many chronic diseases.

You are better off with a real, full-fat yogurt. Real yogurt is made from milk, which we all know is a good source of calcium and vitamins A and D. It also contains beneficial bacteria (probiotics) that digest the sugar found in milk and thus naturally lower yogurt's sugar content.

#7: Trail mix. We have now reached the end of the unhealthy food trail. Which seems appropriate because trail mix, while supposedly nutritious, may be the sneakiest snack of all.

A basic trail mix made solely of dried fruits and nuts is a good, healthy snack. Nuts and fruits eaten in moderation are natural, high-nutrient foods. In fact, they form a basis of the "Bear Diet," which I recommend for healthy weight loss and weight maintenance.

But prepackaged trail mixes typically contain lots of "tasty" ingredients like milk chocolate candies, sugar-coated nuts, yogurt-covered raisins, corn syrup, and fried banana chips. These ingredients are packed with refined sugars, and can boost the calorie content of a trail mix to a whopping 44 calories *per tablespoon.* That's more than 700 calories per cup!

This caloric load can also include a hefty amount of trans-fats, which should be completely banned from any diet (and are finally being banned by the FDA over the next couple of years).

The alternative is to make your own trail mix with nuts and dried berries from your health food store. Not only will you save a lot of money and calories, but you'll also have a very nutritious snack that you can eat anywhere, whether you're waiting in traffic or scaling the Sierra Nevada Mountains.

Why nuts and berries? Nuts are high in vitamins and minerals and are associated with a lower risk of heart disease, high blood pressure, diabetes, metabolic syndrome, cancer, gallstones, and obesity. Berries have been linked to a lower risk of cancer, cardiovascular disease, and urinary tract infections. They also boost immune function.

And if that weren't impressive enough, nuts and berries together are an antioxidant and immune-system powerhouse. The combo also shows benefits for brain and nerve function. A growing number of clinical studies demonstrate that moderate consumption of berries and nuts improves cognitive performance. The dynamic duo may also delay, or even reverse, the effects of age-related dementia.

The truth is, eating healthy doesn't have to be a guessing game.

A little common sense goes a long way. And when in doubt, you can't go wrong by always opting for whole, natural foods over processed, prepackaged products—no matter how sneakily nutritious they may seem.

Chapter 100

7 simple food-safety tips to keep you and your family healthy

We hear a lot of horror stories about outbreaks of foodborne illnesses. And that can make you wonder whether any fruit, vegetable, meat, or dairy you buy is really safe—even if it's organic.

But while the media make it seem like foodborne illnesses are on the rise, the CDC reports that actually isn't the case. In 1999, the CDC estimated there were about 76 million cases of foodborne illnesses each year in the U.S., resulting in 325,000 hospitalizations and 5,000 deaths. In 2011, those numbers dropped to 48 million cases, with 128,000 hospitalizations and 3,000 deaths.

That's still a shocking number of food safety incidents, but the good news is that the vast majority of cases are mild.

Still, the crony-capitalist government never wants to let a good crisis go to waste, and lobbyists have influenced new "food safety" legislation to actually hide provisions that favor big food and agriculture—and take away control from small farmers and consumers.

But you can still avoid some of these big-government intrusions in the name of "food safety." Just buy locally grown foods. Foods sold within 50 miles of their points of origin are not subject to some of the most restrictive and ridiculous regulations of the FDA and USDA. Most grocery stores of all sizes and descriptions now have sections for locally grown foods. Ask your grocer.

Knowing where and how your food is grown goes a long way toward helping protect you and your family from foodborne illnesses. But there are also other steps you can take. Here are my top recommendations to keep you and your family safe from E. coli, salmonella, listeria, and other bacteria linked to foodborne illnesses.

Don't automatically assume meat is the culprit

Often when we hear about E. coli and salmonella outbreaks, it may actually be due to contaminated produce—not meat (although big government sometimes confuses the facts).

Case in point: the recent E. coli outbreaks at Chipotle restaurants.

There's a theory that big food and agriculture corporations were threatened by this large food chain's popularity and commitment to using clean, organic ingredients. But despite talk that the meat used in Chipotle's menu items was responsible for the outbreaks, it may have really been the lettuce. And the theory is that the lettuce may have been purposefully infected with E. coli by Chipotle's rivals.

Whether or not this this is true, the bottom line is that the Chipotle outbreak was most likely not caused by meat. Indeed, despite the fact that the politically correct love to jump onto the anti-meat bandwagon whenever possible, themajority of foodborne illness outbreaks are not from meat.

Like the case of Chipotle, they're actually caused by contaminated produce. Which leads me to my next point…

Wash produce—even (and especially) if it's bagged

You need to wash all produce before you eat it, even if you think it's been washed before. And don't be fooled by bagged produce claiming to be "triple washed."

Some of the largest salmonella outbreaks have been due to bagged lettuce. And in January, there were listeria outbreaks throughout the U.S. due to bagged lettuce produced at a Dole facility.

That's why the simplest way to protect yourself from deadly bacteria is to neverbuy bagged produce.

Why? Well, bagged produce claims to be "ready to eat," but that doesn't mean it's safe. Much of this produce is washed but not sanitized. And conventional bagged produce may be "washed" with dangerous chemicals.

You won't run into that with organic produce, but I still don't recommend eating any type of packaged vegetables or fruits. Not only because of the potential microbial contamination, but because I think it's a good idea to avoid all packaged foods.

After all, why package a healthy food like greens? It's wasteful and unnatural. Not to mention that there have been reports that some lettuce can be two weeks old before it's even stuck in a bag.

That's why I always recommend buying your produce in bulk from the grocery store or farmer's market, where you can inspect it without the camouflage of a plastic bag. And you can wash it yourself.

The CDC recommends washing all produce under running water at room temperature (using a soft brush to remove any stubborn dirt). If the water is too hot or cold, it can open up pores in fruits and vegetables that could trap bacteria and other contaminants.

Cook meat at the right temperature to kill bacteria

While you're busy washing your produce, you might be wondering if you should also wash your meat and poultry before cooking it.

Don't!

Salmonella bacteria are frequently present on chicken, but rinsing poultry simply contaminates your sink. And that can spread salmonella to other foods…or even your family.

The right way to kill dangerous bacteria on poultry and all other meat is to cook it to a proper internal temperature.

All types of cooked poultry should have an internal temperature of 165 degrees, regardless of whether you use an oven, skillet, or outdoor grill. This cooks the meat all the way through, especially around any bones that may be harboring bacteria.

You can check the temperature by using an oven thermometer—but do notleave the thermometer in the meat while cooking.

Metal thermometers conduct heat and make the area around the thermometer cook faster—throwing off the temperature measurement for the entire piece of meat. (And it will also ruin your thermometer!) Instead, use a thermometer only to sample the temperature when you think the meat is done.

Combination meat dishes, such as lasagna, casseroles, and reheated leftovers, should also reach 165 degrees for at least 15 seconds. Ground meats should hit 155 degrees. And eggs (fried, poached, or scrambled), pork, lamb, seafood, and steaks should cook to 145 degrees.

And the good news for rare-meat lovers is that this temperature still allows for plenty of pink in a juicy steak.

Give yourself a (clean) hand

Of course, you should always wash your hands when preparing food. In fact, improper food handling causes most cases of foodborne illness. Fortunately, there are simple steps you can take to protect you and your family.

Before you start preparing a meal, make sure to remove all accessories, including bracelets, rings, and wristwatches. (This is one case where you don'twant to take a licking and keep on ticking). And avoid artificial fingernails (which are unhealthy for nails anyway, especially in people with metabolic and pituitary conditions, as well as diabetes).

All of these accessories can harbor germs, which can contaminate food you touch. (Not that the analogy is appetizing, but as a pathologist who handled human tissue, I never wore jewelry because I got tired of taking it on and off and potentially misplacing or losing it).

Make sure to wash your hands properly and frequently while handling food, and especially after touching raw produce, meat, poultry, or seafood. You need to rub soap on your hands for at least 15 seconds to kill germs.

And avoid antibacterial soaps, which can lead to development and survival of dangerous, resistant strains of bacteria. My daughter's middle school science project demonstrated that simple concept 20 years ago—not to mention all the science that has come out since. But many food safety "experts" still miss this fundamental point.

"Cleaning" kitchen tools isn't the same as sanitizing them

Another thing to watch out for when preparing foods is cross-contamination.

For instance, cutting boards are great for preparing, presenting, and serving foods. But be careful not to use a cutting board to slice raw meat...and then chop vegetables. Even if you wash the board in between, that still may not eliminate all germs left over from the meat.

That's because there is a difference between cleaning and sanitizing. Cleaning removes the visible debris, but sanitizing removes or kills germs at the microscopic level.

To sanitize a cutting board, use hot soap and water, and then wipe with a little bleach solution in water. Or better yet, keep separate cutting boards for meats and for vegetables.

It also matters what type of cutting board you choose. Studies show that wood cutting boards are safer than plastic ones. That's because bacteria can be caught in knife grooves in plastic, and are impossible to clean out. On the other hand, the natural pores in wood are thought to trap and immobilize the bacteria, which eventually and naturally kills it.

When you are done preparing your food, put any ceramic, metal, or plastic utensils in the dishwasher to sanitize them. You can also run sponges through the dishwasher as long as you use a high-heat setting.

Of course, you'll damage wood cutting boards, bowls, or utensils in the dishwasher, so hand wash and sanitize them as I recommended above. And wooden bowls that contain only vegetables or fruit can be wiped clean and "seasoned" with some salt and olive oil to keep them safe.

Store your food properly

Just as heating certain foods is important to kill bacteria, so is keeping them cool.

The FDA recommends you keep your refrigerator at or below 40 degrees Fahrenheit. Most average refrigerator settings are between 35 and 40 degrees, so you should be fine. But if you're concerned, test the temperature with a thermometer. And while you're at it, test the freezer to make sure it's at zero degrees Fahrenheit.

Here's another handy thermostat tip: If you don't keep a fully stocked refrigerator or freezer, or are going to be away for a while, fill the empty spaces with plastic jugs of water. The higher specific heat of water will help your fridge or freezer stay at a constant cold temperature—without using extra energy.

If you want to save leftovers, put them in the refrigerator or freezer within three to four hours after cooking. But don't just place hot food directly in the fridge. Not only does that waste energy, but it may play havoc with the thermostat.

Instead, any cooked food should be allowed to cool to room temperature (this takes about two hours), and then placed in the refrigerator or freezer.

Can't wait for your leftovers to cool? Place the cooking pot in a sink of cold or ice water until the contents get to room temperature.

If you want to freeze your leftovers, put them in smaller, sealable containers labeled with the contents and date. That's important because frozen foods are best consumed within six months.

When it comes time to thaw your food, transfer it from the freezer to the refrigerator a day in advance. But if you are in a hurry, place the frozen food under running warm water, or in a bath of hot water in the sink. Once thawed, eat the food within three days.

Trust your nose and your eyes

Finally, remember to always use a healthy dose of common sense, which eliminates most of the cases of foodborne illness in the home.

That includes using common sense when it comes to "use by" dates stamped on dairy, bread, or other foods you need to buy in packages.

Of course, you should select the packages with the later dates at the store. But don't automatically throw out these foods as soon as they hit the "use-by" date, especially if the package has never been opened. Instead, use your eyes and nose to detect any spoilage.

After all, we have millions of years of biologic adaptation to back us up. If it looks and smells good, it is likely still good to eat.

Know the warning signs of foodborne illness

If you experience the following symptoms, you may have eaten contaminated food. Check with a doctor immediately—especially if you're over age 65 or have a compromised immune system. Both factors can make you more susceptible to developing life-threatening complications from a foodborne illness.

- E. coli infection. Common symptoms include diarrhea, which can range from mild to severe; abdominal cramping; nausea; and vomiting. In severe cases, kidney failure may develop. Most symptoms show up within four days of eating contaminated meat, dairy, or produce.

- Salmonella infection. Often, there are no symptoms. But some people develop diarrhea, abdominal cramps, and fever within eight to 72 hours after eating contaminated food. In rare cases, salmonella can cause acute dehydration or serious diseases like meningitis or infections of the heart (endocarditis) or bones (osteomyelitis).

- Listeriosis. The main symptoms are fever, chills, and severe headaches. Advanced cases may lead to life-threatening septic shock, meningitis, or encephalitis. And beware—although most symptoms appear within a couple days of eating contaminated vegetables or fruits, you can develop listeriosis as long as two months later.

SOURCES

Part 1: Cancer Answers from a True Insider

http://www.angio.org

Cavallo T, Sade R, Folkman J, Cotran RS (1972) Tumor angiogenesis: Rapid induction of endothelial mitoses demonstrated by autoradiography. J Cell Biol 54:408–420

Folkman J, Klagsbrun M (1987) Angiogenic factors. Science 235:442–447

Ausprunk DH, Falterman K, Folkman J (1978) The sequence of events in the regression of corneal capillaries. Lab Invest 38:284–294

Nature (impact factor: 36.28). 01/2006; 438(7070):932-6. DOI:10.1038/nature04478

http://www.angio.org/understanding/fact.php

http://www.scienceofcancers.org/brain-cancer-clinical-trials.php

"Vitamin C and Cancer," in Nutrition and Cancer Prevention: Investigating the Role of Micronutrients. New York: Marcel Dekker, 1989

"How Vitamin C Stops Cancer." ScienceDaily, 9/10/07. (Retrieved 5/29/12, from http://www.sciencedaily.com/releases/2007/09/070910132848.htm)

"Effect of vitamin C on prostate cancer cells in vitro: Effect on cell number, viability, and DNA synthesis," The Prostate 1997; 32(3): 188-195

Cancer Epidemiol Biomarkers Prev 1992; 1: 119

"Can dietary beta-carotene materially reduce human cancer?" Nature 1981; 290: 201-208

"Carotenoid analyses of foods associated with a lower risk for cancer," Journal of the National Cancer Institute 1990; 82: 285-292.

Omenn, G. S. (1998). "Chemoprevention of lung cancer: The rise and demise of beta-carotene," Annual Review of Public Health 1998; 19: 73–99

"Vitamins for Chronic Disease Prevention: Scientific Review and Clinical Applications." Journal of the American Medical Association 2002; 287(23): 3,116-3,129.

"Phase I clinical trial to evaluate the safety, tolerability, and pharmacokinetics of high-dose intravenous ascorbic acid in patients with advanced cancer." Cancer Chemother Pharmacol. 2013; 72(1): 139-146

"Phase I Evaluation of Intravenous Ascorbic Acid in Combination with Gemcitabine and Erlotinib in Patients with Metastatic Pancreatic Cancer," PloS One 2012; 7(1): e29794

"Anti-angiogenic effect of high doses of ascorbic acid," J Transl Med. 2008; 6: 50

Complementary and Integrative Medicine in Cancer Care and Prevention. New York: Springer, 2007, pg. 188-193

www.californiaavocado.com

Aggarwal BB, Bhardwaj A, Aggarwal RS, Seeram NP, Shishodia S, Takada Y. Role of resveratrol in prevention and therapy of cancer: preclinical and clinical studies. Anticancer Res. 2004 Sep-Oct;24(5A):2783-840. http://www.ncbi.nlm.nih.gov/pubmed/15517885?dopt=Abstract

E. Brakenhielm, R. Cao, Y. Cao. FASEB J., 15, 1798–1800 (2001).

K. Igura, T. Ohta, Y. Kuroda, K. Kaji. Cancer Lett., 171, 11–16 (2001).

In Vivo. 2007 Mar-Apr;21(2):365-70

Journal of Experimental & Clinical Cancer Research 2009; 28:124

Drug News Perspect 2009; 22(5): 247-254

Molecular Cancer 2011, 10:12

Bhat TA, Nambiar D, Pal A, Agarwal R, Singh RP. Fisetin inhibits various attributes of angiogenesis in vitro and in vivo—implications for angioprevention. Carcinogenesis. 2012 Feb;33(2):385-93. doi: 10.1093/carcin/bgr282. Epub 2011 Dec 1

"Piperine inhibits PMA-induced cyclooxygenase-2 expression through downregulating NF-kB, C/EBP and AP-1 signaling pathways in murine macrophages," Food Chem Toxicol 2012; 50(7): 2,342-2,348

"Piperine inhibits cytokine production by human peripheral blood mononuclear cells," Genet Mol Res. 2012; 11(1): 617-627

"Piperine suppresses tumor growth and metastasis in vitro and in vivo in a 4T1 murine breast cancer model," Acta Pharmacol Sin 2012; 33(4): 523-530

Crowley 1994:92; Lebot, Merlin and Lindstrom 1992:51-3

Henderson B.E., Kolonel L.N., Dworshy R., Kerford D., Mori E., Sing K and Thevenot H. Cancer incidence in the islands of the Pacific. Nat. Cancer Inst. Monogr. 1985;69:3-81.

Le Marchand L., Hankin J., Bach F., Kolonel L., Wilkens L., Stacewicz- Sapuntzakis M., Bowen P., Beecher G., Laudon F., Baque P., Daniel R., Seruvatu L., Henderson B. An ecological study of diet and lung cancer in the South Pacific. Int. J. Cancer 1995;63:18-23.

Thevenot H., Germain R., Chaubet M. Cancer occurrences in developing countries. IARC Scientific Publication No. 75, Lyon, International Agency for Research on Cancer, 1986;323-329.

http://www.steinerlabs.com/publications/alpha-pyrone-research-on-cancer-incidence/

Castleman, Michael. "Kava Safety Update." Mother Earth Living; January, 2008

http://news.uci.edu/features/can-kava-cure-cancer

Mol Cancer. 2013; 12: 55. Published online 2013 Jun 10.

Nutrition and cancer 06/2012; 64(6):838-46. DOI PubMed

Kava Blocks 4-(Methylnitrosamino)-1-(3-pyridyl)-1-Butanone–Induced Lung Tumorigenesis in Association with Reducing O6-methylguanine DNA Adduct in A/J Mice. Cancer Prevention Research; January, 2014

"Chemotherapy-induced neurotoxicity: the value of neuroprotective strategies." Neth J Med. 2012; 70(1): 18-25

"Metabolic approach to the enhancement of antitumor effect of chemotherapy: a key role of acetyl-L-carnitine," Clin Cancer Res 2010; 16(15): 3,944-3,953

"Induction of ER Stress-Mediated Apoptosis by a-Lipoic Acid in A549 Cell Lines," Korean J Thorac Cardiovasc Surg 2012; 45(1): 1-10

"Lipoic acid - biological activity and therapeutic potential," Pharmacol Rep 2011; 63(4): 849-858

"Coenzyme Q10 for Prevention of Anthracycline-Induced Cardiotoxicity," Integr Cancer Ther 2005; 4(2): 110-130

"Improved survival in patients with end-stage cancer treated with coenzyme Q(10) and other antioxidants: a pilot study," J Int Med Res 2009; 37(6): 1,961-1,971

"Vitamin C and Cancer," in Nutrition and Cancer Prevention: Investigating the Role of Micronutrients. New York: Marcel Dekker, 1989

Complementary and Integrative Medicine in Cancer Care and Prevention. New York: Springer, 2007, pg. 178-186

"Ascorbic acid and cancer: A review," Cancer Research 1979; 39: 663

"A Prospective Study on Folate, B12, and Pyridoxal 5'-Phosphate (B6) and Breast Cancer,"Cancer Epidemiology Biomarkers & Prevention 1999; 8(3): 209–217

"Multivitamin Use, Folate, and Colon Cancer in Women in the Nurses' Health Study,"Annals of Internal Medicine 1998; 129(7): 517-524

Complementary and Integrative Medicine in Cancer Care and Prevention. New York: Springer, 2007, pg. 187-188

"Calcium Supplements for the Prevention of Colorectal Adenomas," New England Journal of Medicine 1999; 340: 101–107

Complementary and Integrative Medicine in Cancer Care and Prevention. New York: Springer, 2007, pg. 269-270

Mian L, et al. Review: The Impacts of Circulating 25-Hydroxyvitamin D Levels on Cancer Patient Outcomes: A Systematic Review and Meta-Analysis. DOI: http://dx.doi.org/10.1210/jc.2013-4320

"Curcumin and its analogues: Potential anticancer agents," Medicinal Research Reviews 2009; 30(5): 818-860

"Curcumin inhibits the migration and invasion of human A549 lung cancer cells through the inhibition of matrix metalloproteinase-2 and-9 and Vascular Endothelial Growth Factor (VEGF)," Cancer Letters 2009; 285(2): 127-133

"Effects of curcumin on bladder cancer cells and development of urothelial tumors in a rat bladder carcinogenesis model," Cancer Lett 2008; 264(2): 299-308

"Effect of curcumin on lung resistance-related protein (LRP) in retinoblastoma cells," Curr Eye Res 2009; 34(10): 845-851

"Allicin inhibits cell growth and induces apoptosis in U87MG human glioblastoma cells through an ERK-dependent pathway," Oncol Rep. 2012; 28(1): 41-48

"Allium vegetables and risk of prostate cancer: a population-based study," J Natl Cancer Inst 2002; 94(21): 1,648-1,651

"Inhibition of the Growth of Human Pancreatic Cancer Cells by the Arginine Antimetabolite L-Canavanine," Cancer Res 1994; 54(23); 6,045-6,048

"GABA's control of stem and cancer cell proliferation in adult neural and peripheral niches," Physiology 2009; 24: 171-185

"African herbal medicines in the treatment of HIV: Hypoxis and Sutherlandia. An overview of evidence and pharmacology," Nutrition Journal 2005; 4: 19

"Medicinal plant 'fights' AIDS," BBC News, 11/30/01. (Retrieved 6/1/12, from http://news.bbc.co.uk/2/hi/africa/1683259.stm)

"Anthropological study of health beliefs, behaviors and outcomes. Traditional folk medicine and ethnopharmacology." Human Organization 1983; 42(4): 351-353

"Chrysanthemum indicum L. Extract Induces Apoptosis through Suppression of Constitutive STAT3 Activation in Human Prostate Cancer DU145 Cells," Phytother Res. 2012 (published online Mar 22)

"Anti-inflammatory effects of the Nigella sativa seed extract, thymoquinone, in pancreatic cancer cells," HPB 2009; 11(5): 373-381

Vitamin D deficiency and mortality risk in the general population: a meta-analysis of prospective cohort studies. Am J Clin Nutr. 2013(97):782-793

American Cancer Society. What are the key statistics about cervical cancer? http://www.cancer.org/cancer/cervicalcancer/detailedguide/cervical-cancer-key-statistics. Updated April 11, 2013. Accessed October 16, 2013

JAMA Intern Med. 2013;():1-9. doi:10.1001/jamainternmed.2013.2912

Doyle, K. (2013, February 27). Screnning might avert many lung cancer deaths: Study. Retrieved 2013, from http://www.reuters.com/article/2013/02/27/us-lung-cancer-idUSBRE91Q16F20130227

Rosenthal, Elisabeth. "Let's (not) get physicals," The New York Times, Sunday Review, June 2, 2012.

"Treating you better for less," The New York Times, Sunday Review, June 3, 2012, pg. 12.

"Quantifying the Benefits and Harms of Screening Mammography," JAMA Intern Med (http://archinte.jamanetwork.com/article.aspx?articleid=1792915), December 30, 2013

"Rethinking Screening for Breast Cancer and Prostate Cancer," JAMA 2009;302(15):1685-1692

Institute of Medicine (US) and National Research Council (US) Committee on New Approaches to Early Detection and Diagnosis of Breast Cancer; Joy JE, Penhoet EE, Petitti DB, editors. Saving Women's Lives: Strategies for Improving Breast Cancer Detection and Diagnosis. Washington (DC): National Academies Press (US); 2005.8. "Saving Women's Lives: Strategies for Improving Breast Cancer Detection and Diagnosis," National Institutes of Health (www.ncbi.nlm.nih.gov) 2005

"Cancer? Not!" Medscape (www.medscape.com); Aug 29, 2013

"The $2.7 trillion medical bill: Colonoscopies explain why the U.S. leads the world in health expenditures," The New York Times (www.nytimes.com), 6/1/13

"Can colorectal cancer be prevented?" The American Cancer Society (www.cancer.org), accessed 8/2/13

"Comparative Effectiveness and Cost-effectiveness of Screening Colonoscopy vs. Sigmoidoscopy and Alternative Strategies," Am J Gastroent 2013 108(1):120-132 (http://www.medscape.com/viewarticle/779647_4)

"Less is More: Not 'Going the Distance' and Why," JNCI 2011; 103(23): 1,726-1,728 (http://jnci.oxfordjournals.org/content/early/2011/11/09/jnci.djr446.full)

"The $2.7 trillion medical bill: Colonoscopies explain why the U.S. leads the world in health expenditures," The New York Times (www.nytimes.com), 6/1/13

"Study: Colonoscopies often come with costly, unnecessary sedation," CBS News (www.cbsnews.com), 3/20/12

Utilization of Anesthesia Services During Outpatient Endoscopies and Colonoscopies and Associated Spending in 2003-2009," JAMA 2012; 307(11): 1,178-1,184 (http://jama.jamanetwork.com/article.aspx?articleid=1105089)

"Reducing Mortality from Colorectal Cancer by Screening for Fecal Occult Blood," NEJM 1993; 328:1365-1371

"Colorectal-Cancer Incidence and Mortality with Screening Flexible Sigmoidoscopy," NEJM 2012; 366:2345-2357

"Once-only flexible sigmoidoscopy screening in prevention of colorectal cancer: a multicentre randomised controlled trial." Lancet 2010;375:1624-1633

"Once-Only Sigmoidoscopy in Colorectal Cancer Screening: Follow-up Findings of the Italian Randomized Controlled Trial—SCORE," JNCI 2011; 103(17):1310-1322

What are the key statistics about breast cancer? (2014, September 9). Retrieved 2014, from http://www.cancer.org/cancer/breastcancer/detailedguide/breast-cancer-key-statistics

"Rethinking the Standard for Ductal Carcinoma In Situ Treatment." JAMA Oncol. 2015;1(7):881-883.

"Specific serum carotenoids are inversely associated with breast cancer risk among Chinese women: a case–control study." Br J Nutr. 2015 Oct 20:1-9.

"Meta-analysis of vitamin D sufficiency for improving survival of patients with breast cancer." Anticancer Res. 2014 Mar;34(3):1163-6.

"Effects of selenium supplements on cancer prevention: meta-analysis of randomized controlled trials." Nutr Cancer. 2011 Nov;63(8):1185-95.

Lung Cancer Facts. (n.d.). Retrieved 2014, from https://www.lungcancerfoundation.org/about-us/lung-cancer-facts/

"Vitamin D and lung cancer risk: a comprehensive review and meta-analysis."Cell Physiol Biochem. 2015;36(1):299-305.

"Cloud cover-adjusted ultraviolet B irradiance and pancreatic cancer incidence in 172 countries." J Steroid Biochem Mol Biol. 2015 Apr 9.

"Vitamin D status and surgical outcomes: a systematic review." Patient Safety in Surgery 2015, 9:14.

"Changing Incidence of Serum 25-Hydroxyvitamin D Values Above 50 ng/mL: A 10-Year Population-Based Study." Mayo Clin Proc. 2015 May;90(5):577-86.

Henderson BE, et al. Cancer incidence in the islands of the Pacific. Nat. Cancer Inst. Monogr. 1985;69:3-81.

Leitzman, P, et al. Kava blocks 4-(methylnitrosamino)-1-(3-pyridyl)-1-butanone-induced lung tumorigenesis in association with reducing O6-methylguanine DNA adduct in A/J mice. Cancer Prev Res (Phila). 2014 Jan;7(1):86-96.

Abu N, et al. In vivo antitumor and antimetastatic effects of flavokawain B in 4T1 breast cancer cell-challenged mice. Drug Des Devel Ther. 2015 Mar 6;9:1401-17.

Liu Z, et al. Kava chalcone, flavokawain A, inhibits urothelial tumorigenesis in the UPII-SV40T transgenic mouse model. Cancer Prev Res (Phila). 2013 Dec;6(12):1365-75.

Ji T, et al. Mol Cancer. Flavokawain B, a kava chalcone, inhibits growth of human osteosarcoma cells through G2/M cell cycle arrest and apoptosis. Mol Cancer. 2013 Jun 10;12:55.

Triolet J, et al. Reduction in colon cancer risk by consumption of kava or kava fractions in carcinogen-treated rats. Nutr Cancer. 2012 Aug;64(6):838-46.

Eskander RN, et al. Flavokawain B, a novel, naturally occurring chalcone, exhibits robust apoptotic effects and induces G2/M arrest of a uterine leiomyosarcoma cell line. J Obstet Gynaecol Res. 2012 Aug;38(8):1086-94.

Li X, et al. Kava components down-regulate expression of AR and AR splice variants and reduce growth in patient-derived prostate cancer xenografts in mice. PLoS One. 2012;7(2):e31213.

The Coca-Cola Company. Product Nutrition. http://productnutrition.thecoca-colacompany.com. Accessed April 17, 2015.

"The Effect of Curcumin on Breast Cancer Cells," J Breast Cancer. 2013 Jun; 16(2): 133–137

"Serum lycopene reduces the risk of stroke in men," Neurology 2012; 79(15): 1,540-1,547

"Are organic foods safer or healthier than conventional alternatives?: a systematic review." Ann Intern Med 2012; 157(5): 348-366

"The Impact of Organic Farming on Quality of Tomatoes Is Associated to Increased Oxidative Stress during Fruit Development," PlosONE 2013; 8(2): e56354

"Lycopene Content Among Organically Produced Tomatoes," Journal of Vegetable Science 2006; 12(4): 93-106

Part 2: Healing Pain Instead of Treating Pain

Goadsby, P.J., MD, D Sc, & Silberstein, S.D., MD. (2013, January 23). Migraine triggers: Harnessing the messages of clinical practice. Neurology, 80(5), 424-425

"Perceived triggers may not actually provoke migraine." Medscape. Jan. 24, 2013.

Holland, S., Silberstein, S., Freitag, F., Dodick, D., Argoff, C., & Ashman, E. (2012, April 24). Evidence-based guidelines update: NSAIDs and other complementary treatments for episodic migraine prevention in adults: Report of the Quality Standards Subcommittee of the American Academy of Neurology and the American Headache Society. Retrieved 2012, from http://www.ncbi.nlm.nih.gov/pubmed/22529203

Diener, H., Rahifs, VW., & Danesch, U. (2004). The First Placebo-controlled Trial of a Special Butterbur Root Extract for the Prevention of Migraine: Reanalysis of Efficacy Criteria. European Neurology Eur Neurol, 51(2), 89-97. Doi: 10. 1159/000076535

The Lancet. "Paracetamol no better than placebo for lower back pain." ScienceDaily. ScienceDaily, 24 July 2014. <www.sciencedaily.com/releases/2014/07/140724094025.htm>

"Food and Drug Administration. Assessment of Safety of Aspirin and Other Nonsteroidal Anti-Inflammatory Drugs (NSAIDs)." Available at: http://www.fda.gov/ohrms/dockets/ac/02/briefing/3882b2_02_mcneil-nsaid.htm. Accessed February 18, 2014

Rabago D, et al. Dextrose Prolotherapy for Knee Osteoarthritis: A Randomized Controlled Trial. Ann Fam Med May/June 2013 vol. 11 no. 3 229-237.

"Drug Resistance and Pseudoresistance: An Unintended Consequence of Enteric Coating Aspirin" Circulation. 2012;CIRCULATIONAHA.112.117283 published online before print December 4 2012, doi:10.1161/CIRCULATIONAHA.112.117283

"Could tarantula venom help fight pain?" Medical News Today (www.medicalnewstoday.com) 2/29/2016

Astone, N.M., Martin, S., & Aron, L.Y. (2015, March 5). Death Rates for US Women Ages 15 to 54. Retrieved 2015, from http://www.urban.org/research/publication/death-rates-us-women-ages-15-54

Rising morbidity and mortality in midlife among white non-Hispanic Americans in the 21st century." Proc Natl Acad Sci U S A. 2015 Dec 8;112(49):15078-83.

"Acceptability of a Guided Imagery Intervention for Persons Undergoing a Total Knee Replacement." Orthop Nurs. 2015 Nov-Dec;34(6):356-64.

"Effectiveness of mindfulness meditation on pain and quality of life of patients with chronic low back pain." Int J Yoga. 2015 Jul-Dec;8(2):128-33.

"Observing the Effects of Mindfulness-Based Meditation on Anxiety and Depression in Chronic Pain Patients." Psychiatr Danub. 2015 Sep;27 Suppl 1:S209-11.

"Management of osteoarthritis (OA) with the pharma-standard supplement FlexiQule (Boswellia): a 12-week registry." Minerva Gastroenterol Dietol. 2015 Oct 22.

"Curcumin loaded solid lipid nanoparticles ameliorate adjuvant-induced arthritis in rats." Eur J Pain. 2015 Aug;19(7):940-52.

"A new curcuma extract (flexofytol®) in osteoarthritis: results from a belgian real-life experience." Open Rheumatol J. 2014 Oct 17;8:77-81.

"Co-analgesic therapy for arthroscopic supraspinatus tendon repair pain using a dietary supplement containing Boswellia serrata and Curcuma longa: a prospective randomized placebo-controlled study." Musculoskelet Surg. 2015 Sep;99 Suppl 1:S43-52.

"Efficacy and Safety of Fish Oil in Treatment of Knee Osteoarthritis." J Med Assoc Thai. 2015 Apr;98 Suppl 3:S110-4.

"Fish oil in knee osteoarthritis: a randomised clinical trial of low dose versus high dose." Ann Rheum Dis. 2016 Jan;75(1):23-9.

"An aerobic walking programme versus muscle strengthening programme for chronic low back pain: a randomized controlled trial," Clinical Rehabilitation 2013; 27(3): 207-214

"Repetitive Transcranial Magnetic Stimulation Once a Week Induces Sustainable Long-Term Relief of Central Poststroke Pain," Neuromodulation: Technology at the Neural Interface June 2015; 18(4): 249–254

Part 3: Brain-Healers from Behind the Curtain

"Higher normal fasting plasma glucose is associated with hippocampal atrophy: The PATH Study,"Neurology 2012; 79:1,019-1,026

"Impaired insulin and insulin-like growth factor expression and signaling mechanisms in Alzheimer's disease—is this type 3 diabetes?" J Alzheimers Dis 2005; 7(1): 63–80

"Berberine: A potential multipotent natural product to combat Alzheimer's Disease," Molecules 2011; 16: 6,732-6,740

"Oren-gedoku-to and its Constituents with Therapeutic Potential in Alzheimer's Disease Inhibit Indoleamine 2, 3-Dioxygenase Activity In Vitro," J Alzheimers Dis 2010; 22(1):257-66

Molecular Basis of Inhibitory Activities of Berberine against Pathogenic Enzymes in Alzheimer's Disease," The Scientific World Journal vol. 2012, Article ID 823201 (doi:10.1100/2012/823201)

Effect of Vitamin E and Memantine on Functional Decline in Alzheimer Disease – The TEAM-AD VA Cooperative Randomized Trial," JAMA. 2014; 311(1): 33-34

"Current evidence for the use of coffee and caffeine to prevent age-related cognitive decline and Alzheimer's disease," Journal of Nutrition, Health & Aging 2014: 18(4): 383-392

"Self-Reported Increased Confusion or Memory Loss and Associated Functional Difficulties Among Adults Aged ≥60 Years — 21 States, 2011," Centers for Disease Control (www.cdc.com) 5/10/2013

Desideri G, et al. Benefits in cognitive function, blood pressure, and insulin resistance through cocoa flavanol consumption in elderly subjects with mild cognitive impairment: the Cocoa, Cognition, and Aging (CoCoA) study. Hypertension. 2012 Sep;60(3):794-801. doi: 10.1161/HYPERTENSIONAHA.112.193060. Epub 2012 Aug 14.

Brickman AM, et al. Enhancing dentate gyrus function with dietary flavanols improves cognition in older adults. Nat Neurosci. 2014 Dec;17(12):1798-803. doi: 10.1038/nn.3850. Epub 2014 Oct 26.

Harwood ML, et al. Tolerance for high flavanol cocoa powder in semisweet chocolate. Nutrients. 2013;5(6):2258-2267.

Fox, M, Knapp, LA, Andrews, PW, Fincher, CL, Hygeine and the world distribution of Alzheimer's disease, Evolution, Medicine and Public Health, 2013, DOI: 10.1093/emph/eot015.

Ratner, E and Atkinson, D, J Am Geriatr Soc 2015: 63(12): 2612-2614

"Meta-analysis of modifiable risk factors for Alzheimer's disease," J Neurol Neurosurg Psychiatry (www.jnnp.bmj.com) 8/20/2015

"Neurological diseases remain neglected and ignored." Lancet 2012; 379: 287

"The road to 25×25: how can the five-target strategy reach its destination?"Lancet Global Health 2014; 2:e126.

"Forecasting the global burden of Alzheimer's disease." Alzheimers Demen2007; 3: 186–91.

"Neurodegenerative diseases: an overview of environmental risk factors."Environ Health Perspect 2005; 113: 1250–6.

"The role of environmental exposures in neurodegeneration and neurodegenerative diseases." Toxicol Sci 2011; 124: 225–50.

"Mitochondrial dysfunction in Parkinson's disease: molecular mechanisms and pathophysiological consequences." EMBO J. 2012; 31(14): 3038-62.

"Occupational and environmental risk factors for Parkinson's disease."Parkinsonism Relat Disord 2002; 8: 297–309.

"What we truly know about occupation as a risk factor for ALS: a critical and systematic review." Amyotroph Lateral Scler 2009; 10: 295–U70.

"Severely increased risk of amyotrophic lateral sclerosis among Italian professional football players." Brain 2005; 128: 472–6.

"Preventing Alzheimer's disease-related gray matter atrophy by B-vitamin treatment." PNAS 2013; 110(23): 9523–9528

"Vitamin D and the risk of dementia and Alzheimer disease." Neurology2014; 83(10):920-8

"New Studies Focus on Vitamin D and MS." National MS Society (www.nationalmssociety.org). Accessed 9/16/14.

"Effect of Vitamin E and Memantine on Functional Decline in Alzheimer Disease – The TEAM-AD VA Cooperative Randomized Trial," JAMA 2014; 311(1): 33-34.

"Nicotine from edible Solanaceae and risk of Parkinson disease." Annals of Neurology 2013; 74(3): 472–477.

"Age at obesity and association with subsequent dementia: record linkage study." Postgrad Med J 2014; 90(1,068): 547-51

"The effects of an 8-week hatha yoga intervention on executive function in older adults." J Gerontol A Biol Sci Med Sci. 2014; 69(9): 1109-16.

Part 4: Master Your Heart Health

"Blood tests for heart disease." http://www.mayoclinic.org/diseases-conditions/heart-disease/in-depth/heart-disease/art-20049357. Accessed March 24, 2014.

"Moderate elevation of body iron level and increased risk of cancer occurrence and death." Int J Cancer. 1994 Feb 1;56(3):364-9.

Muller H, et al. The Serum LDL/HDL Cholesterol Ratio Is Influenced More Favorably by Exchanging Saturated with Unsaturated Fat Than by Reducing Saturated Fat in the Diet of Women. J. Nutr. January 1, 2003 vol. 133 no. 1 78-83.

Nichols AB, et al. Daily nutritional intake and serum lipid levels. The Tecumseh study.Am J Clin Nutr. 1976 Dec;29(12):1384-92.

Dreon DM, et al. Change in dietary saturated fat intake is correlated with change in mass of large low-density-lipoprotein particles in men. Am J Clin Nutr. May 1998 vol. 67 no. 5 828-836.

Siri-Tarino, PW. Meta-analysis of prospective cohort studies evaluating the association of saturated fat with cardiovascular disease. Am J Clin Nutr. January 2010 ajcn.27725

Lemos da Luz P, et al. High Ratio of Triglycerides to HDL-Cholesterol Predicts Extensive Coronary Disease. Clinics. Aug 2008; 63(4): 427–432

Sachdeva A, et al. Lipid levels in patients hospitalized with coronary artery disease: an analysis of 136,905 hospitalizations in Get With The Guidelines

Weverling-Rijnsburger AWE, et al. Total cholesterol and risk of mortality in the oldest old. The Lancet. Volume 350, Issue 9085, 18 October 1997, Pages 1119–1123

Neaton JD, et al. Serum Cholesterol Level and Mortality Findings for Men Screened in the Multiple Risk Factor Intervention Trial. Arch Intern Med.1992;152(7):1490-1500. doi:10.1001/archinte.1992.00400190110021

Lack of Vitamin D Linked to CVD Biomarkers, Inflammation," Medscape (www.medscape.com) 2/27/2014

"Vitamin D deficiency is associated with inflammation in older Irish adults," J Clin Endocrinol Metab 2014

"Demographic Differences and Trends of Vitamin D Insufficiency in the US Population, 1988-2004" Arch Intern Med. 2009;169(6):626-632

"Total Joint Arthroplasty and the Risk of Myocardial Infarction: A General Population, Propensity Score-Matched Cohort Study." Arthritis Rheumatol. 2015 Oct;67(10):2771-9.

"Plasma total homocysteine, B vitamins, and risk of coronary atherosclerosis."Arterioscler Thromb Vasc Biol. 1997 May;17(5):989-95.

"The kidney and homocysteine metabolism." J Am Soc Nephrol. 2001 Oct;12(10):2181-9.

"Metformin activates an atypical PKC-CBP pathway to promote neurogenesis and enhance spatial memory formation." Cell Stem Cell, volume 11, issue 1, 23-25, 6 July 2012.

The New York Times. Declining Lethality.http://www.nytimes.com/interactive/2014/01/05/sunday-review/declining-lethality.html?_r=0. Accessed January 24, 2015.

Ingenbleek Y, McCully KS. Vegetarianism produces subclinical malnutrition, hyperhomocysteinemia and atherogenesis. Nutrition. 2012 Feb;28(2):148-53. doi: 10.1016/j.nut.2011.04.009. Epub 2011 Aug 27.

Selhub J, et al. Vitamin status and intake as primary determinants of homocysteinemia in an elderly population. JAMA 1993;270:2693–8.

Saposnik G, et al. Homocysteine-lowering therapy and stroke risk, severity, and disability: additional findings from the HOPE 2 trial. Stroke. 2009 Apr;40(4):1365-72. doi: 10.1161/STROKEAHA.108.529503. Epub 2009 Feb 19.

Spence JD, et al. Vitamin Intervention For Stroke Prevention trial: an efficacy analysis. Stroke. 2005 Nov;36(11):2404-9. Epub 2005 Oct 20.

"Factors associated with no apparent coronary artery disease in patients with type 2 diabetes mellitus for more than 10 years of duration: a case control study," Cardiovasc Diabetol 2015; 14(146)

Henry, J.P. and Micozzi, M.S. (1977) Influence of psychosocial stimulation and early experience on blood pressure in infancy and childhood, Medical College Pennsylvania, Ciba Symposium on Hypertension in Children, Adolescents and Young Adults, Philadelphia, Pennsylvania.

Micozzi, M.S. (1980) Childhood hypertension and academic standing in the Philippines, American Journal of Public Health 70: 530-532.

James PA, et al. 2014 Evidence-Based Guideline for the Management of High Blood Pressure in Adults. Report From the Panel Members Appointed to the Eighth Joint National Committee (JNC 8). JAMA. 2014;311(5):507-520. doi: 10.1001/jama. 2013.284427.

Rodriguez C, et al. Waste and Harm in the Treatment of Hypertension. Journal of the American Medical Association Internal Medicine June 10, 2013; 173(11): 956-957.

Sim JJ, et al. Impact of Achieved Blood Pressures on Mortality Risk and End-Stage Renal Disease Among a Large, Diverse Hypertension Population. J Am Coll Cardiol 2014; 64(6), 588-597.

Risky Drugs: Why the FDA Cannot be Trusted. http://www.bibliotecapleyades.net/ciencia/ciencia_industryweapons295.htm. Accessed August 21, 2014.

Alzheimer's Association International Conference (AAIC) 2014. Abstract P2-083. Presented July 14, 2014.

Gottesman RF, et al. Midlife Hypertension and 20-Year Cognitive Change: The Atherosclerosis Risk in Communities Neurocognitive Study. JAMA Neurol. 2014 Aug 4. doi: 10.1001/jamaneurol.2014.1646.

"Conjugated linoleic acid in adipose tissue and risk of myocardial infarction," Am. J Clin Nutr 2010 Jul;92(1):34-40

"Cellular and molecular mechanisms of statins: an update on pleiotropic effects." Clin Sci (Lond). 2015 Jul 1;129(2):93-105.

Howard BV, et al. Low-fat dietary pattern and weight change over 7 years: the Women's Health Initiative Dietary Modification Trial. JAMA. 2006; 295:39-49.

Brinton EA, et al. A low-fat diet decreases high density lipoprotein (HDL) cholesterol levels by decreasing HDL apolipoprotein transport rates. J Clin Invest. Jan 1990; 85(1): 144–151.

Dreon DM, et al. Reduced LDL particle size in children consuming a very-low-fat diet is related to parental LDL-subclass patterns. Am J Clin Nutr. June 2000 vol. 71 no. 6 1611-1616.

"Processed foods: contributions to nutrition," Am J Clin Nutr 2014; Apr 23 (epub ahead of print)

Muller H, et al. The Serum LDL/HDL Cholesterol Ratio Is Influenced More Favorably by Exchanging Saturated with Unsaturated Fat Than by Reducing Saturated Fat in the Diet of Women. J. Nutr. January 1, 2003 vol. 133 no. 1 78-83.

Nichols AB, et al. Daily nutritional intake and serum lipid levels. The Tecumseh study.Am J Clin Nutr. 1976 Dec;29(12):1384-92.

Dreon DM, et al. Change in dietary saturated fat intake is correlated with change in mass of large low-density-lipoprotein particles in men.Am J Clin Nutr. May 1998 vol. 67 no. 5 828-836.

Siri-Tarino, PW. Meta-analysis of prospective cohort studies evaluating the association of saturated fat with cardiovascular disease. Am J Clin Nutr. January 2010 ajcn.27725.

American Heart Association. Trans Fats.http://www.heart.org/HEARTORG/GettingHealthy/FatsAndOils/Fats101/Trans-Fats_UCM_301120_Article.jsp. Accessed April 16, 2014.

Lemos da Luz P, et al. High Ratio of Triglycerides to HDL-Cholesterol Predicts Extensive Coronary Disease. Clinics. Aug 2008; 63(4): 427–432.

Sachdeva A, et al. Lipid levels in patients hospitalized with coronary artery disease: an analysis of 136,905 hospitalizations in Get With The Guidelines.

Am Heart J. 2009 Jan;157(1):111-117.e2. doi: 10.1016/j.ahj.2008.08.010.

Weverling-Rijnsburger AWE, et al. Total cholesterol and risk of mortality in the oldest old. The Lancet. Volume 350, Issue 9085, 18 October 1997, Pages 1119–1123.

Neaton JD, et al. Serum Cholesterol Level and Mortality Findings for Men Screened in the Multiple Risk Factor Intervention Trial. Arch Intern Med.1992;152(7):1490-1500. doi:10.1001/archinte.1992.00400190110021.

Gillman MW, et al. Margarine intake and subsequent coronary heart disease in men. Epidemiology. 1997 Mar;8(2):144-9.

Ramsden CE, et al. Use of dietary linoleic acid for secondary prevention of coronary heart disease and death: evaluation of recovered data from the Sydney Diet Heart Study and updated meta-analysis BMJ 2013;346:e8707

USDA. Adoption of Genetically Engineered Crops in the U.S. http://www.ers.usda.gov/data-products/adoption-of-genetically-engineered-crops-in-the-us/recent-trends-in-ge-adoption.aspx#.U07t4sbjPgl. Accessed April 16, 2014.

Russo, GL. Dietary n-6 and n-3 polyunsaturated fatty acids: from biochemistry to clinical implications in cardiovascular prevention. Biochem Pharmacol. 2009 Mar 15;77(6):937-46. doi: 10.1016/j.bcp.2008.10.020. Epub 2008 Oct 28.

O'Keefe, S, et al. Levels of trans geometrical isomers of essential fatty acids in some unhydrogenated U.S. vegetable oils. Journal of Food Lipids.Volume 1, Issue 3, pages 165–176, September 1994.

"Potent anti-obese principle from Rosa canina: structural requirements and mode of action of trans-tiliroside." Bioorg Med Chem Lett. 2007;17:3059–3064.

"Rosehip extract inhibits lipid accumulation in white adipose tissue by suppressing the expression of peroxisome proliferator-activated receptor gamma." Prev Nutr Food Sci. 2013;18:85–91.

"Effects of rose hip intake on risk markers of type 2 diabetes and cardiovascular disease: a randomized, double-blind, cross-over investigation in obese persons." Eur J Clin Nutr. 2012;66:585–590.

"Daily intake of rosehip extract decreases abdominal visceral fat in preobese subjects: a randomized, double-blind, placebo-controlled clinical trial." Diabetes Metab Syndr Obes. 2015; 8: 147–156.

"Is Organic Agriculture 'Affluent Narcissism'?" Forbes (www.forbes.com) 11/7/2012

"Distinguishable Epidemics of Multidrug Resistant Salmonella Typhimurium DT104 In Different Hosts," Science 9/27/2013; 341(6153):1514-1517

"Organic foods vs. supermarket foods: Element levels," Journal of Applied Nutrition 1993; 45:35-39

"New Evidence Settles a Lingering Question – Is Organic Food More Nutritious?," Organic Consumers Association (www.organicconsumers.org) 3/19/2008

"Natural Sunscreen Agents: A Review," Sch. Acad. J. Pharm., 2013; 2(6):458-463

"Comparison of antioxidant potency of commonly consumed polyphenol-rich beverages in the United States." J Agric Food Chem. 2008 Feb 27;56(4):1415-22.

Daley, C. A., Abbott, A., Doyle, P.S., Nader, G. A., & Larson, S. (2010). A review of fatty acid profiles and antioxidant content in grass-fed and grain-fed beef. Nutrition Journal Nutr J, 9(1). doi:10.1186/1475-2891-9-10

EWG's Shopper's Guide to Pesticides in Produce. (n.d). Retrieved 9/1/2015, from http://www.ewg.org/foodnews/dirty_dozen_list.php

EWG's Shopper's Guide to Pesticides in Produce. (n.d). Retrieved 9/1/2015, from https://www.ewg.org/foodnews/clean_fifeteen_list.php

Food Storage Chart for Cupboard/Pantry, Refrigerator and Freezer. (n.d). Retrieved 9/1/2015, from http://food.unl.edu/food-storage-chart-cupboardpantry-refridgerator-and-freezer

Food Waste: The Facts. (n.d.). Retrieved 9/1/15, from http://www.worldfooddayusa.ord/food_waste_the_facts

Pendick, D. (2015, March 05). Peanuts linked to same heart, longevity benefits as more pricey nuts – Harvard Health Blog. Retrieved 9/1/2016, from http://www.health.harvard.edu/blog/peanuts-linked-to-heart-longevity-benefits-pricey-nuts-201503057777

Part 5: Conquering Everyday Health

"Vitamin D and gastrointestinal diseases: inflammatory bowel disease and colorectal cancer," Therap Adv Gastroenterol. 2011 January; 4(1): 49–62

"Plasma 25-hydroxyvitamin D and colorectal cancer risk according to tumour immunity status," Gut; published online 1/15/2015

Vitamin D status and survival of metastatic colorectal cancer patients: Results from CALGB/SWOG 80405," J Clin Oncol 2015; 33

"The phytoestrogen prunetin affects body composition and improves fitness and lifespan in male Drosophila melanogaster." The FASEB Journal 2016; 30(2): 948-958

"Individual variability in human blood metabolites identifies age-related differences." Proceedings of the National Academy of Sciences, 2016; 113(16):4252-9

"Effects of blueberry supplementation on measures of functional mobility in older adults." Appl Physiol Nutr Metab. 2015 Jun;40(6):543-9.

"Effects of Lifestyle Modification on Telomerase Gene Expression in Hypertensive Patients: A Pilot Trial of Stress Reduction and Health Education Programs in African Americans." PLoS One. 2015 Nov 16;10(11):e0142689.

"Metformin promotes lifespan through mitohormesis via the peroxiredoxin PRDX-2." Proc Natl Acad Sci U S A. 2014 Jun 17;111(24):E2501-9.

"Metformin improves health span and lifespan in mice." Nat Commun.2013;4:2192.

Life Extension. (2015, December 16). Anti-aging human study on metformin wins FDA approval. Retrieved 2015, frim http://www.prnewswire.com/news-releases/anti-aging-human-study-on-metformin-wins-fda-approval-300193724.html

"A nutrigenomics approach for the study of anti-aging interventions: olive oil phenols and the modulation of gene and microRNA expression profiles in mouse brain." Eur J Nutr. 2015 Dec 22.

"Brain atrophy in cognitively impaired elderly: the importance of long-chain ω-3 fatty acids and B vitamin status in a randomized controlled trial." Am J Clin Nutr July 2015 vol. 102 no. 1 215-221.

Hearing Loss Association of America. Basic Facts About Hearing Loss.http://www.hearingloss.org/content/basic-facts-about-hearing-loss. Accessed January 26, 2015.

Bush AL, et al. Peripheral Hearing and Cognition: Evidence From the Staying Keen in Later Life (SKILL) Study. Ear Hear. 2015 Jan 13.

Chen DS, et al. Association of Hearing Impairment with Declines in Physical Functioning and the Risk of Disability in Older Adults. J Gerontol A Biol Sci Med Sci. 2014 Dec 3. pii: glu207.

Choi YH, et al. Antioxidant vitamins and magnesium and the risk of hearing loss in the US general population. Am J Clin Nutr. 2014 Jan;99(1):148-55. doi: 10.3945/ajcn.113.068437.

Brown KD, et al. Activation of SIRT3 by the NAD+ Precursor Nicotinamide Riboside Protects from Noise-Induced Hearing Loss. Cell Metabolism, Volume 20, Issue 6, p1059–1068, 2 December 2014.

Kyle ME, et al. Impact of Nonaspirin Nonsteroidal Anti-inflammatory Agents and Acetaminophen on Sensorineural Hearing Loss: A Systematic Review.

Otolaryngol Head Neck Surg. 2015 Jan 5. pii: 0194599814564533.

"Impact of Statins on Biological Characteristics of Stem Cells Provides a Novel Explanation for Their Pleotropic Beneficial and Adverse Clinical Effects," American Journal of Physiology – Cell Physiology; 7/29/2015

"Vitamin C Is Associated with Reduced Risk of Cataract in a Mediterranean Population," J. Nutr. June 1, 2002; 132(6): 1299-1306

"Prospective Study of Dietary Fat and Risk of Cataract Extraction among US Women," American Journal of Epidemiology December 14, 2004; 161(10): 1-12

"Black and Green Teas Equally Inhibit Diabetic Cataracts in a Streptozotocin-Induced Rat Model of Diabetes," J. Agric. Food Chem., 2005, 53 (9): 3710–3713

"Dietary carbohydrate in relation to cortical and nuclear lens opacities in the melbourne visual impairment project," Invest Ophthalmol Vis Sci. 2010 Jun;51(6): 2897-905

"Green Tea Catechins and Their Oxidative Protection in the Rat Eye," J. Agric. Food Chem., 2010, 58 (3): 1523–1534

Part 6: 9 Secrets to Stop Aging in its Tracks

"The phytoestrogen prunetin affects body composition and improves fitness and lifespan in male *Drosophila melanogaster.*" *The FASEB Journal* 2016; 30(2): 948-958

"Individual variability in human blood metabolites identifies age-related differences." Proceedings of the National Academy of Sciences, 2016; 113(16):4252-9

"Effects of blueberry supplementation on measures of functional mobility in older adults." Appl Physiol Nutr Metab. 2015 Jun;40(6):543-9.

"Effects of Lifestyle Modification on Telomerase Gene Expression in Hypertensive Patients: A Pilot Trial of Stress Reduction and Health Education Programs in African Americans." PLoS One. 2015 Nov 16;10(11):e0142689.

"Metformin promotes lifespan through mitohormesis via the peroxiredoxin PRDX-2." Proc Natl Acad Sci U S A. 2014 Jun 17;111(24):E2501-9.

"Metformin improves healthspan and lifespan in mice." Nat Commun.2013;4:2192.

Life Extension. (2015, December 16). Anti-aging human study on metformin wins FDA approval. Retrieved 2015, from http://www.prnewswire.com/news-releases/anti-aging-human-study-on-metformin-wins-fda-approval-300193724.html

"A nutrigenomics approach for the study of anti-aging interventions: olive oil phenols and the modulation of gene and microRNA expression profiles in mouse brain." Eur J Nutr. 2015 Dec 22.

"Brain atrophy in cognitively impaired elderly: the importance of long-chain ω-3 fatty acids and B vitamin status in a randomized controlled trial." Am J Clin Nutr July 2015 vol. 102 no. 1 215-221.

Hearing Loss Association of America. Basic Facts About Hearing 11Loss.http://www.hearingloss.org/content/basic-facts-about-hearing-loss. Accessed January 26, 2015.

Bush AL, et al. Peripheral Hearing and Cognition: Evidence From the Staying Keen in Later Life (SKILL) Study. Ear Hear. 2015 Jan 13.

Chen DS, et al. Association of Hearing Impairment with Declines in Physical Functioning and the Risk of Disability in Older Adults. J Gerontol A Biol Sci Med Sci. 2014 Dec 3. pii: glu207.

Choi YH, et al. Antioxidant vitamins and magnesium and the risk of hearing loss in the US general population. Am J Clin Nutr. 2014 Jan;99(1):148-55. doi: 10.3945/ajcn.113.068437.

Brown KD, et al. Activation of SIRT3 by the NAD+ Precursor Nicotinamide Riboside Protects from Noise-Induced Hearing Loss. Cell Metabolism, Volume 20, Issue 6, p1059–1068, 2 December 2014.

Kyle ME, et al. Impact of Nonaspirin Nonsteroidal Anti-inflammatory Agents and Acetaminophen on Sensorineural Hearing Loss: A Systematic Review. Otolaryngol Head Neck Surg. 2015 Jan 5. pii: 0194599814564533.

"Impact of Statins on Biological Characteristics of Stem Cells Provides a Novel Explanation for Their Pleotropic Beneficial and Adverse Clinical Effects," American Journal of Physiology – Cell Physiology; 7/29/2015

"Vitamin C Is Associated with Reduced Risk of Cataract in a Mediterranean Population," J. Nutr. June 1, 2002; 132(6): 1299-1306

"Prospective Study of Dietary Fat and Risk of Cataract Extraction among US Women," American Journal of Epidemiology December 14, 2004; 161(10): 1-12

"Black and Green Teas Equally Inhibit Diabetic Cataracts in a Streptozotocin-Induced Rat Model of Diabetes," J. Agric. Food Chem., 2005, 53 (9): 3710–3713

"Dietary carbohydrate in relation to cortical and nuclear lens opacities in the melbourne visual impairment project," Invest Ophthalmol Vis Sci. 2010 Jun;51(6): 2897-905

"Green Tea Catechins and Their Oxidative Protection in the Rat Eye," J. Agric. Food Chem., 2010, 58 (3): 1523–1534

Part 7: A Drug-Free Guide to Defeating Your Depression

"The impact of whole-of-diet interventions on depression and anxiety: a systematic review of randomised controlled trials," Public Health Nutr. 2014 Dec 3:1-2

Food and the brain. Program and abstracts of the American Psychiatric Association 168th Annual Meeting; May 16-20, 2015; Toronto, Ontario, Canada. Workshop

Mollusks, oyster, eastern, wild, raw Nutrition Facts & Calories. (2014). Retrieved 2014, http://nutritiondata.self.com/facts/finfish-and-shellfish-products/4189/2

"Mediterranean dietary pattern and depression: the PREDIMED randomized trial," BMC Medicine 2013;11: 208

"Discrepancy between the Atwater factor predicted and empirically measured energy values of almonds in human diets." Am J Clin Nutr. 2012 Aug; 96(2): 296-301.

"Vegetarian diet and mental disorders: results from a representative community survey." Int J Behav Nutr Phys Act. 2012 Jun 7; 9: 67.

"Prevalence of celiac disease and gluten sensitivity in the United States clinical antipsychotic trials of intervention effectiveness study population." Schizophr Bull. 2011 Jan; 37(1): 94-100.

"A randomized controlled trial to test the effect of multispecies probiotics on cognitive reactivity to sad mood." Brain Behav Immun. 2015 Aug; 48:258-64.

"Research update: healthy aging and prevention of late-life mood and cognitive disorders." American Association for Geriatric Psychiatry 2015 Annual Meeting, session 303.

Cosgrove, L., Bursztajn, H. J., Erlich, D. R., Wheeler, E. E. and Shaughnessy, A. F. (2012), Conflicts of interest and the quality of recommendations in clinical guidelines. *Journal of Evaluation in Clinical Practice*. doi: 10.1111/jep.12016

Presented at the American Academy of Neurology's 65th Annual Meeting in San Diego, March 16 to 23, 2013

"Vitamin D and the omega-3 fatty acids control serotonin synthesis and action, part 2: relevance for ADHD, bipolar, schizophrenia, and impulsive behavior," FASEB journal (Federation of American Societies for Experimental Biology), Published online before print February 24, 2015

"Efficacy of Bright Light Treatment, Fluoxetine, and the Combination in Patients With Nonseasonal Major Depressive Disorder," JAMA Psychiatry 2016;73(1):56-63

"Therapeutic Observation of Acupuncture for Depressive Insomnia," Shanghai Journal of Acupuncture and Moxibustion 2014; 6: 539-541

"Acupuncture Rivals Antidepressants For Insomnia And Depression," Health CMI (www.healthcmi.com) 2/13/2016

Part 8: Natural Answers for an Ironclad Immune System

"Influence of Epicuticular Physicochemical Properties on Porcine Rotavirus Adsorption to 24 Leafy Green Vegetables and Tomatoes." PLoS One. 2015 Jul 16;10(7):e0132841.

http://pdf.usaid.gov/pdf_docs/Pnacy849.pdf

http://nwhort.org/wp-content/uploads/2015/07/FreshFruitLabelingManual-rev-070115.pdf

https://www.ewg.org/foodnews/summary.php

Martineau AR, et al. Vitamin D3 supplementation in patients with chronic obstructive pulmonary disease (ViDiCO): a multicentre, double-blind, randomised controlled trial. *The Lancet Respiratory Medicine*, 2014; DOI:10.1016/S2213-2600(14)70255-3.

American Lung Association. Chronic Obstructive Pulmonary Disease (COPD) Fact Sheet. http://www.lung.org/lung-disease/copd/resources/facts-figures/COPD-Fact-Sheet.html. Accessed December 17, 2014.

"The relationship between cold temperature and risk of ischemic stroke in patients with atrial fibrillation." Eur Heart J (2015) 36 (suppl 1).

"How cold is too cold: the effect of seasonal temperature variation on risk of STEMI." Eur Heart J (2015) 36 (suppl 1).

"The relationship between the environmental factors and severity of clinical status and short-term prognosis for the patients with non-ST elevation acute coronary syndromes." Eur Heart J (2015) 36 (suppl 1).

"Echinaforce Hotdrink versus Oseltamivir in Influenza: A randomized, double-blind, double dummy, multicenter, non-inferiority clinical trial."http://dx.doi.org/10.1016/j.curtheres.2015.04.001.

The American Heart Association. Learn About Influenza. (n.d.). Retrieved 2015, from http://www.lung.org/lung-disease/influenza/in-depth-resources/pneumonia-fact-sheet.html

http://www.cdc.gov/vaccines/vpd-vac/shingles/hcp-vaccination.htm

http://www.cdc.gov/vaccines/schedules/hcp/imz/adult.html

"Behaviorally Assessed Sleep and Susceptibility to the Common Cold." Sleep.2015 Jan 17. pii: sp-00619-

https://sleepfoundation.org/sleep-polls-data/other-polls/2013-international-bedroom-poll

"Environmental disruption of the circadian clock leads to altered sleep and immune responses in mouse." *Brain Behav Immun*. 2015 Jul;47:14-23.

"Safety and efficacy profile of *Echinacea purpurea* to prevent common cold episodes: a randomized, double-blind, placebo-controlled trial." *Evid Based Complement Alternat Med.* 2012:841315. Epub 2012 Sep 16

"Antibiotic resistance," Centers for Disease Control (www.cdc.gov) 9/16/2013

"Clostridium difficile Infection," N Engl J Med 2015; 372:1539-1548

Part 9: Natural ways to Nurture Your Health

"Plasma 25-Hydroxyvitamin D Levels and Risk of Incident Hypertension Among Young Women," Hypertension Nov 2008;52(5):828-32

"Phenolic acids of the two major blueberry species in the US Market and their antioxidant and anti-inflammatory activities." Plant Foods Hum Nutr. 2015 Mar;70(1):56-62.

"Anti-inflammatory effect of the blueberry anthocyanins malvidin-3-glucoside and malvidin-3-galactoside in endothelial cells." Molecules. 2014 Aug 21;19(8):12827-41.

"Anthocyanins and phenolic acids from a wild blueberry (Vaccinium angustifolium) powder counteract lipid accumulation in THP-1-derived macrophages." Eur J Nutr. 2015 Jan 17.

"Daily blueberry consumption improves blood pressure and arterial stiffness in postmenopausal women with pre- and stage 1-hypertension: a randomized, double-blind, placebo-controlled clinical trial." J Acad Nutr Diet. 2015 Mar;115(3):369-77.

"Blueberry treatment decreased D-galactose-induced oxidative stress and brain damage in rats." Metab Brain Dis. 2015 Jun;30(3):793-802.

"Six weeks daily ingestion of whole blueberry powder increases natural killer cell counts and reduces arterial stiffness in sedentary males and females." Nutr Res. 2014 Jul;34(7):577-84.

"Anthocyanins from fermented berry beverages inhibit inflammation-related adiposity response in vitro." J Med Food. 2015 Apr;18(4):489-96.

"The Effects of Wild Blueberry Consumption on Plasma Markers and Gene Expression Related to Glucose Metabolism in the Obese Zucker Rat." J Med Food. 2014 Nov 10. [Epub ahead of print].

"Wild Blueberry (Vaccinium angustifolium Ait.) Polyphenols Target Fusobacterium nucleatum and the Host Inflammatory Response: Potential Innovative Molecules for Treating Periodontal Diseases." Journal of Agricultural and Food Chemistry, 2015; 63 (31): 6999.

"Baobab food products: a review on their composition and nutritional value."Crit Rev Food Sci Nutr. 2009 Mar;49(3):254-74.

USDA National Nutrient Database for Standard Reference Release 27http://ndb.nal.usda.gov/ndb/search/list.

"The use of photochemiluminescence for the measurement of the integral antioxidant capacity of baobab products." Food Chemistry Volume 102, Issue 4, 2007, Pages 1352–1356.

"The polyphenol-rich baobab fruit (Adansonia digitata L.) reduces starch digestion and glycemic response in humans." Nutr Res. 2013 Nov;33(11):888-96.

"Vitamin D deficiency and mortality risk in the general population: a meta-analysis of prospective cohort studies," Am J Clin Nutr 2013 97: 782-793

"Vitamins for Chronic Disease Prevention in Adults: : Scientific Review," JAMA2002; 287(23): 3,116-3,126
2 "Vitamins for Chronic Disease Prevention in Adults: : Clinical Applications," JAMA 2002; 287(23): 3,127-3,129

"Alternative therapy produces intriguing results in some heart patients but many questions remain." American Heart Association Late-Breaking Clinical Trial Report. November 4, 2012.

Micozzi, MS, Fundamentals of Complementary & Altenative Medicine, 2010, Elsevier Health Sciences

CalorieKing. Calories in Banana Chips. http://www.calorieking.com/foods/search.php?keywords=banana+chips&go=Go. Accessed June 16, 2014.

CalorieKing. Calories in Energy Bars. http://www.calorieking.com/calories-in-energy+bars.html. Accessed June 16, 2014.

CalorieKing. Hodgson Mill Apple & More Muesli Cereal, dry.http://www.calorieking.com/foods/calories-in-breakfast-cereals-to-be-cooked-apple-more-muesli-dry_f-ZmlkPTE4MzAyMA.html. Accessed June 16, 2014.

National Resources Defense Council. Guide to Mercury in Sushi.http://www.nrdc.org/health/effects/mercury/sushi.asp. Accessed June 16, 2014.

Lowenstein, JH, et al. DNA barcodes reveal species-specific mercury levels in tuna sushi that pose a health risk to consumers. 21 April 2010 doi: 10.1098/rsbl.2010.0156 Biol. Lett.

CalorieKing. Calories in Trail Mix. Average All Brands, Trail Mix: Regular, with Chocolate Chips, Unsalted Nuts & Seeds.http://www.calorieking.com/foods/calories-in-trail-mix-regular-with-chocolate-chips-unsalted-nuts-seeds_f-ZmlkPTYxNDg5.html. Accessed June 16, 2014.

About the Author

Marc S. Micozzi, M.D., Ph.D.

In his 35-year career, physician, medical anthropologist and epidemiologist Marc S. Micozzi M.D., Ph.D., has accomplished something no other physician has been able to achieve.

He thrust the STAGGERING PROOF of complementary alternative therapies in the faces of mainstream medicine AND DEMANDED THEY LISTEN. In fact, some of the world's most recognized natural research—on things like lycopene, lutein, brassica vegetables, and excess iron—would not even exist without his courage to stand up for true science.

His medical career is all but unrivaled—especially given his vast and unique mixture of experience within mainstream medicine and complementary and alternative medicine (CAM).

Dr. Micozzi was the founding editor-in-chief of the first U.S. journal in Complementary and Alternative Medicine and organized and edited the first U.S. textbook in the field, *Fundamentals of Complementary & Integrative Medicine* in 1996, continuously in print for 20 years, now it its 5th edition. He has published nearly 300 articles in medical literature and is the author or editor of over 40 books.

As the Senior Investigator for cancer prevention at the National Cancer Institute, Dr. Micozzi published the original research on diet, nutrition, and chronic disease. He continued this line of research as the Associate Director of the Armed Forces Institute of Pathology and Director of the National Museum of Health and Medicine.

He has served as the Executive Director of the College of Physicians of Philadelphia (the same city where he completed medical and graduate training at the University of Pennsylvania).

In recent years, Dr. Micozzi has served as the Founding Director of the Policy Institute for Integrative Medicine, working to educate policy makers, the health professions, and the general public about the opportunities for integrative medicine and the need for clean, clear science within our modern medical establishment.

As Editor of his monthly newsletter *Insiders' Cures*, Dr. Micozzi's message of taking what's rightfully yours is already changing the lives of people just like you…

Dr. Micozzi has written or edited over 40 books, including (with

Michael Jawer), *The Spiritual Anatomy of Emotion* and *Your Emotional Type: Key to the Therapies That Will Work for You*. He was the founding editor-in-chief of the first U.S. journal on the subject of CAM (in 1994), and he organized and edited the first U.S. textbook, *Fundamentals of Complementary & Alternative Medicine*, now going into it's fifth edition.

"*The Spiritual Anatomy* of Emotion presents a unique and arresting view of such topics as mind, body, memory, illness, perception, and emotion. The authors show us an altogether novel way of understanding who we are and what we're about. There's more to being human than we ever imagine, and this book is an excellent road map for anyone who wants to take that journey."

ERIC LESKOWITZ, M.D.,
Department of Psychiatry, Harvard Medical School

"*Your Emotional Type*, may be the Rosetta Stone we've been waiting for—a code for matching a particular therapy to a particular patient. Micozzi and Jawer... have found gold."

LARRY DOSSEY, M.D.
Author of *Healing Words: The Power and Prayer and the Practice of Medicine* and *The Power of Premonitions*

"By helping patients understand the connection between their personality type, their symptoms, and treatment choices, Jawer and Micozzi help patients become more informed consumers of alternative health care."

ILENE A. SERLIN,
Psychologist and Dance Movement Therapist

You can read more about all of Dr. Micozzi's titles and purchase them online at www.drmicozzi.com.